Healing Cultures

Healing Cultures:

The Sri Lankan Experience

By

Nirekha De Silva

Cambridge
Scholars
Publishing

Healing Cultures: The Sri Lankan Experience

By Nirekha De Silva

This book first published 2023

Cambridge Scholars Publishing

Lady Stephenson Library, Newcastle upon Tyne, NE6 2PA, UK

British Library Cataloguing in Publication Data
A catalogue record for this book is available from the British Library

ISBN (10): 1-5275-3162-7
ISBN (13): 978-1-5275-3162-8

This book is dedicated to,
My Son, Anuk Randev De Silva
My Parents Nirmalee and Mohan De Silva
My Supervisors and Mentors, Prof. Jay Sanderson,
Prof. Fiona Kumari Campbell, Prof. Afshin Akhtarkhavari
and Prof. Kieran Tranter, Dr. Sinharaja Tammita-Delgoda
and Dr. Sanjay Garg
All the Healers in Sri Lanka

CONTENTS

Summary xii

Acknowledgements xiv

Chapter 1 1
Living Practices in Health and Wellbeing in Sri Lanka
Part 1 Background 1
1.1 Reflection 1: Spirit Healer Ghana Manio 1
1.2 Reflection 2: Spiritual Healer Venerable Wellawatthe Seelagawesi Thero 8
1.3 Reflection 3: Inter-generational Healing Practice of Horiwila Kadum Bidum 10
1.4 Reflection 4: Traditional Siddha Doctor 14
Part 2: Living Practices in Health and Wellbeing in Sri Lanka 15
Part 3: Why Sri Lanka matters 19
Part 4: Research Question 27
Part 5: Key Terms and Concepts 28
Part 6: Methodology 33
Part 7: Overview of the Book 64

Chapter 2 68
Recognising and Regulating Traditional Practices related to Health and Wellbeing
Introduction 68
Part 1: International schemes dealing with traditional practices related to health and wellbeing 73
1.1 Indigenous Peoples, Self-determination 74
1.2 Access and benefit sharing 78
1.3 Intellectual Property 83
Part 2: How Traditional Practices Related to Health and Wellbeing are Regulated in Sri Lanka 85
2.1 Sri Lanka's Role in Application of International Laws Related to Traditional Practices in Health and Wellbeing 86
2.2 Sri Lanka's Domestic Laws and Mechanisms Related to Traditional Practices in Health and Wellbeing 88

2.3 Changes in traditional legal systems 93
2.4 Changes in Health and Wellbeing 94
Part 4: Revitalisation Efforts of Traditional Knowledge and its Impact on Traditional Healing and Wellbeing Practices of Sri Lanka 96
4.1 Religious revival 96
4.2 Educational revival 98
4.3 Revival of language 99
4.4 Health care revival 99
Conclusion 100

Chapter 3 103
The Diversity of Healing Practices in Sri Lanka
Introduction 103
Part 1: Government Recognised Traditional Healing Practices in Sri Lanka 104
1.1 Ayurveda 105
1.2 Siddha (South Indian traditional medicine) 114
1.3 Unani (medicine of Unan origin) 117
1.4 Homeopathy 120
1.5 Acupuncture 123
1.6 Deshiya Chikithsa 125
Part 2: Diversity of Healing Practices in Sri Lanka 127
2.1 Inter-Generational Healing 128
2.2 Cosmic Healing 130
2.3 Adopted Traditional Healing 133
2.4 Biomedical Healing 134
2.5 Integrated Healing 135
Part 3: Dynamics and Complexities of Diverse Healing Practices ... 142
Conclusion 147

Chapter 4 149
The Role of Sri Lankan Government in Recognising, Supporting and Regulating 'Traditional' Healing Practices and the Impact on Culture
Introduction 149
Part 1: Public Demand and the Establishment of a Government Controlled Traditional Medicine System in Sri Lanka 151
Part 2: Administration of Traditional Health Care 156
2.1 The Ministry of Indigenous Medicine 156
2.1 Department of Ayurveda 158
2.3 Provincial Administration of Indigenous Medicine 160
2.4 Sri Lanka Ayurveda Medical Council 161

Part 3: Education 164
3.1 Ayurveda Education and Hospital Board 164
3.2 National Institute of Traditional Medicine 166
3.3 Institute of Indigenous Medicine, University of Colombo ... 169
3.4 Gampaha Wickramarachchi Ayurveda Institute 173
3.5 Diploma in Ayurveda 178
Part 4: Hospitals and Curative Services 184
4.1 Borella Ayurveda Teaching Hospital 186
4.2 Kaitady Siddha Teaching Hospital 187
4.3 Gampaha Wickramarachchi Ayurveda Teaching Hospital ... 188
4.4 Government Homeopathy Hospital 189
Part 5: Medicines and Drugs 189
5.1 Ayurveda Formulary Committee 190
5.2 Sri Lanka Ayurvedic Drugs Corporation 190
Part 6: Research and Herb Gardens 192
6.1 The Ayurveda Research Committee 193
6.2 Bandaranaike Memorial Ayurveda Research Institute 193
6.3 Herbal Gardens 195
6.4 Herbal farmer village project of the Ministry of Indigenous Medicine 195
Part 7: Programmes to Develop Community Healthcare and Inter-Generational Healing 196
7.1 Community Health Care Pilot Project in Anuradhapura 197
7.2 *Hela Weda Gedera* 198
7.3 Preserving Vedda Culture and Medicinal Plants Cultivation .. 199
Conclusion 202

Chapter 5 205
Inter-Generational Healing and Loss of Culture
Introduction 205
Part 1: What is intergenerational healing? 206
1.1 *Visha Vaidya* (Poison healer) Rathnawathie 209
1.2 *Ansha Baga Vaidya* (Stroke and Paralysis healer) Sudu Banda 212
1.3 *Kadum Bidum* healer, Sunil Shantha 215
Part 2: Challenges for Inter-generational Healers 216
2.1 Limited employment opportunities 216
2.2 Secretive Knowledge 222
2.3 Inappropriate Treatment by the Government 223
2.4 Formal Education for Recognition 230

Part 3: Impacts of Government intervention on Inter-generational Healing: Assimilation and Loss of Cultural Diversity 232
3.1 Healers forced in Ayurveda.. 232
3.2 Competition and Tension between Western Doctors and the Inter-generational Healers 233
3.3 Assimilation of Vedda Community.. 235
3.4 Possibilities of protecting the diverse cultural heritage of inter-generational healing practice 239
Conclusion 241

Chapter 6 243
Conclusion
Introduction.. 243
Part 1: Summary of Findings 243
Part 2: Observations Based on Findings 247
2.1 Factors in Determining the Survival and Thriving of Traditional Knowledge Systems in Healing...................... 247
2.2 Loss of Cultural Heritage... 248
Part 3: The Main Concerns Relating to Protecting and Promoting Diverse Living Practices on Health and Wellbeing in Sri Lanka.. 251
3.1 Limited Legal Protection.. 251
3.2 Narrow Scope in Government Recognition........................... 251
3.3 Inappropriate treatment by the Government challenges the survival and traditional cultural aspect of inter-generational healing practices 252
3.4 Mixing Up of Terms... 253
3.5 Not Having Clarity on Terms 253
3.6 Issues in the Administration of Traditional Health Care 254
3.7 Ayurvedisation of Healing 254
3.8 Westernisation of Healing... 255
3.9 Socio-economic and cultural challenges that threaten the existence of Inter-generational healers 256
Conclusion 257

References 258
Secondary Sources 258
Government Material 280
Sessional Papers.. 281
International Material.. 282
International Law 285

Legislation – Sri Lanka 286
Foreign Legislations 287
Cases 287
Websites 287

Annex - List of Interviews Completed 289

SUMMARY

This book argues that the recognition, support and regulation by the Government of the Democratic Socialist Republic of Sri Lanka (hereafter known as Sri Lanka) of healing and wellbeing practices play an important role in determining, promoting, protecting or destroying the cultural aspects of healing. To make this argument this book looks into four aspects of healing and wellbeing in Sri Lanka. The first aspect the book examines is the diversity of healing and wellbeing practices in Sri Lanka. The second aspect is to consider how structured, formal healing systems, such as Western allopathic healing, Ayurveda, Siddha, Unani, Acupuncture and Homeopathy are more likely to be recognised, supported and regulated by the Government of Sri Lanka, while the informal healing systems such as inter-generational healing and cosmic healing practices are less likely to be recognised, supported and regulated. The third aspect this book focuses on is questioning the definitions of traditional knowledge in practical application in the Sri Lankan context, and, more broadly, the use of traditional knowledge as legal, social and cultural categories. The fourth aspect that is explored are the issues related to protecting the traditional cultural aspects of healing in the process of systematic regulation by discussing inter-generational and cosmic healing practices.

Taken together, this book highlights existing diverse forms of healing practices matter because of their value in health and wellbeing of the community. These practices also strongly contribute towards the intangible cultural heritage of the country. Yet, it is not always possible for the Sri Lankan Government to protect the traditional cultural aspects of all forms of healing practices by recognising, supporting and regulating the diverse forms of healing practices existing in the country. While recognising Government limitations in protecting some traditional cultural aspects of healing the book highlights the need of the existing regulatory mechanism to be sensitive to traditional cultural aspects of healing and broaden the scope of recognition and protection.

This argument is presented in 7 chapters. Chapter 1 examines the diversity of healing and wellbeing practices in Sri Lanka. Chapter 2 discusses the main regulatory frameworks, schemes and practices related to health and wellbeing applicable in Sri Lanka. Chapter 3 provides an overview of the research design and methodology used to answer the research question. My findings are presented in Chapters 4 to 6. Chapter 4 is an attempt to understand the complexities of living healing practices in Sri Lanka and questions the healing practices that are considered and used in Sri Lanka. Chapter 5 examines the history and nature of the Government recognition, support and regulation of traditional healing practices in the country. Chapter 6 examines inter-generational healing in Sri Lanka, and argues that this is facing the threat of loss of the cultural heritage aspects of healing due, in large part, to Government interventions in recognising, supporting and regulating healing practices. Chapter 7 is the conclusion of the book.

ACKNOWLEDGEMENTS

This book is based on my PhD research. Being born with an inquisitive mind and an inner need to better understand the world and to make a significant contribution towards knowledge systems and towards humanity, reading for a PhD has been one of my goals since childhood. Achieving this goal never came easy. There was a time being a single mother of a three-month-old infant, struggling to make ends meet, that I thought reading for a PhD was beyond my wildest dreams. It was thanks, however, to the support and encouragement that I received from so many special people who believed in me and stood by my side that I have managed to complete my PhD and this book.

It was with Dr. Sinharaja Tammita-Delgoda that I first discussed the research idea and developed the research proposal. Dr. Tammita-Delgoda was my External Supervisor for Griffith University and he patiently guided me through initial literature reviews, archival research/ historical research and field work in Sri Lanka. He rehearsed how I should behave and work in the field.

It was thanks to the generous scholarship I received from Griffith University (Griffith University International Post-Graduate Research Scholarship and the Griffith University Post-Graduate Scholarship) that I managed to pursue the research. I am eternally grateful to Griffith University for the generous support.

My first Principle Supervisor was Prof. Fiona Kumari Campbell. She was accommodative and understanding. She viewed me not only as her PhD student but a human being with human problems. I appreciate her understanding and the loving kindness that made it possible for me to pursue the PhD at the initial stage. There were many times that I felt 'theory' was beyond me. Prof. Campbell patiently introduced me from the very basic works to the complexities of theoretical debate. Before going into the field, she also gave me a strong grounding in research methods and research ethics. Prof. Campbell made me question things I have taken for granted and analyse knowledge from different perspectives.

From the beginning of my PhD, Prof. Jay Sanderson has played a vital role in guiding me, first as my Associate Supervisor, then as my Principle Supervisor and at the last stages as my External Supervisor. Regardless of the designation, he has been a great pillar of strength throughout. He made me focus, get the structure right and get started in writing. If Prof. Sanderson had ceased to supervise me when he left the University in January 2015, I don't think I would have had the courage to start all over with new supervisors. But Prof. Sanderson continued to closely supervise me and revise many drafts of the thesis.

I am grateful also to Prof. Afshin Akhtarkhavari and Prof. Kieran Tranter for being my saviours and acting as my Co-Principle Supervisors for my final year of the research. During this final year I re-wrote the whole thesis. Both of them reviewed at least three drafts of each chapter before finalising. Their attention to detail and commitment towards reviewing the chapters has continuously amazed me. They used to send me comments while they were abroad, on public holidays, early mornings and late at night. Many a times they pushed my boundaries in seeking for knowledge and opened my eyes to new ways of thinking. There are no words to thank Prof. Afshin Akhtarkhavari and Prof. Kieran Tranter for taking me on board and guiding me to complete the research.

Working with five supervisors on this research was not an easy task. But it was a blessing in disguise. The process of working with five supervisors has enriched my academic experience and shaped my knowledge in ways I never imagined. All my supervisors gave me space to be inventive and creative while guiding me to bring out the best. I am ever so grateful to all five of them.

Dr. Sanjay Garg, my Supervisor and Deputy Director of South Asian Association for Regional Cooperation (SAARC) Cultural Centre has also played an important role in encouraging me to pursue this research at a time when I had lost all my self-confidence. Understanding my personal plight and enthusiasm for knowledge, he was very accommodative throughout, permitting me to pursue my research while working at SAARC. He also encouraged me to co-convene a SAARC Regional Conference on Traditional Knowledge and Traditional Cultural Expressions of South Asia.

I am also grateful to the Ministry of Indigenous Medicine for granting permission to conduct the research, to interview any official under the purview of the Ministry and conduct participant observation in all of the institutions under the purview of the Ministry.

The support of Sanduni Warnasuriya and Navindra Gamalathge in attending to some of the administrative work involved in this research is also recognised.

I appreciate the services of Griffith University Library, for accessing for me the many books and articles from various institutions in Sri Lanka and in Australia. I also want to acknowledge the support from

Griffith Law School Administrative staff, Griffith IT support team and Griffith Ethics Committee in complying with procedures.

I humbly recognise the contribution of all the healers, academics, researchers and policy makers who allowed me to do the interviews and participant observation. I am grateful for their trust in me and for their valuable time.

With heart felt gratitude I acknowledge the unconditional love and support given by my parents throughout my life in all my pursuits. It was thanks to the values they instilled in me about hard work, persistence, facing challenges, being duty bound, independent and inquisitive; that I have managed to fulfil my dream of completing the research and this book. As always, they were a great source of energy for me giving their fullest support in whatever way possible, sometimes accompanying me in the field to babysit my son, Anuk; helping me identify my research material that I left in Sri Lanka while I was in Australia and always having time to listen to my stories and problems. I also appreciate love and encouragement of my brothers and the extended family.

I am failing my duties if I do not acknowledge a very special person, my son, Anuk Randev de Silva for all his support and sacrifice. Anuk has spent hours in libraries and in the University. He joined me in my field research, travelled all over Sri Lanka, and patiently stayed by my side till I completed my interviews. He also accompanied me to Australia and gave me love and a reason to continue my dream.

CHAPTER 1

LIVING PRACTICES IN HEALTH AND WELLBEING IN SRI LANKA

Part 1 Background

This book, 'Health and Wellbeing: Culture, Practices and the Role of Government of Sri Lanka,' examines healers and practices related to health and wellbeing in Sri Lanka. Living practices of health and wellbeing are vivid and diverse. To introduce the nature and diversity of healing practices that will be discussed throughout the book, this chapter begins by presenting four reflections on experiences and interviews of healing and wellbeing practices and practitioners in Sri Lanka.[1] These reflections bring to light not only the diverse forms of living practices in health and wellbeing in Sri Lanka, but also some of the themes and issues that are associated with the culture of healing and wellbeing practices in this country, such as, the role of religion, language, social systems,[2] customs, education, payment, organisation and duty. This chapter then briefly considers why Sri Lanka matters and why it is necessary to examine some of the traditional practices related to health and wellbeing in Sri Lanka in detail. Afterwards the chapter introduces the research question, the key terms and concepts used, and gives an overview of the book.

1.1 Reflection 1: Spirit Healer Ghana Manio[3]

In 1995, a young 15-year-old girl who was suffering severe headaches was taken to Ghana manio (mother Ghana) in Anuradhapura, the capital city of

---

[1] These reflections are based on the interviews and participant observations conducted with the healers (see Chapter 3 for the methodology adopted in conducting interviews and participant observation).

[2] For a definition of social systems see, Parsons (1970), (1977), (1978).

[3] Ghana Manio (# 60). (When referring to an interview, I have used the name of the healer and number of the reflection in brackets. These numbers refer to the number of the interview in 'annex – list of interviews completed.' Annex provides full details

the North Central Province in Sri Lanka. Without asking any questions, Ghana manio confidently stated to the girl: "I can cure your headaches." When the session started Ghana manio was in a trance. She applied a *hisa kudichchi* (medicinal pack) to the top of the girl's head for approximately 15 minutes, and then carried out a *nasana* (putting a few drops of herbal oil into the girl's nostrils), getting the girl to inhale forcefully as she did so. After only four visits with Ghana manio the girl has not suffered another severe headache. That young girl was me.

Returning to Ghana manio[4] in 2012, I was able to reflect on these treatments, particularly the importance of the trance to Ghana manio. Ghana manio said that entering into a trance allows the spirits to enter her body, and mediate the treatment process. In this way, it is the spirit (not Ghana manio) that controls her body; including her language, tone, accent and body postures. Furthermore, she explained that every individual has the protection of a particular spirit god such as Patthini, Kalu Bandara, Vishnu, Saman, Gana, Suniyam, Maha Kali (when she was treating my headaches it was the spirit of Badra Kali that entered her body and told her what treatment to use), and that it is always the spirit gods who diagnose the illness, prescribe the herbs and other remedies to be used. While the tone and accent of each spirit god is different, and some spirits talk in many languages, Ghana manio only talks in Sinhala (the native language of the Sinhalese people, who make up the largest ethnic group in Sri Lanka). In an interview with Ghana manio conducted on 14 July 2012 she explained:

> I have been practicing as a spirit healer for 30 years. I am a strong Buddhist from a humble background from Anuradhapura. We were living in a small mud hut. I always wanted to serve humanity. I used to work as an attendant in the Anuradhapura General Hospital. Very regularly I used to go to the

---

of the interview including name of the healer, designation, organisation if applicable, contact details, subject of the interview, date of interview and the place of interview. The process I have followed to conduct these interviews is given in Chapter 1, Part 6: Methodology.)

[4] Ghana manio (# 60). When conducting interviews with Spirit Healers, I was required to obtain the consent from the spirit. Only after the spirit approves can I speak to the spirit or the person who possess the spirit. I had to spend 12 hours on a Saturday at the Dewalaya to get my opportunity to speak to the spirit. There were 500 other people sitting under the trees waiting for their chance to be called by the spirit inside the hut where it consulted people. The spirit decides at what time it is going to call and to whom it would give an opportunity. When speaking to the spirit it said it was delighted about my study and granted me permission to do an interview with Ghana manio. On Monday afternoon I visited Ghana manio at her home to interview her.

> temple of Sri Maha Bodhiya (the sacred Bo tree) and worship. I would pray for the power and strength to be of service to others. The first time I went into a trance was at the temple of Sri Maha Bodhiya. I do not know what happens to me while in the trance as I am not conscious. The spirit takes control of my body. The spirit can predict the problems of other human beings and give solutions.[5]

Ghana manio does not see her healing activities as being under her own volition. Rather she is an agent. She says that:

> With the power of the spirit gods, I can answer any human problem. This includes treating physical illnesses by performing operations, addressing human needs (such as fertility treatment), finding partners for marriage, giving blessings for examinations and blessings for finding jobs, giving protections for people, houses and land, and exorcising malevolent spirits from the human body.[6]

Figure 1.1 and 1.2 below portrays Ghana manio in a trance consulting patients. Figure 1.3 contains some of the statues of spirits gods that are believed to use Ghana manio's body[7] for healing and for serving humans. Figure 1.4 represents offerings given by devotees for fulfilling healing and wellbeing wishes.

[5] Ghana manio (# 60).

[6] Ghana manio (# 60).

[7] Some healers believe spirits of gods cannot enter the human body as they are more supreme than humans and it is spirits of dead persons (mostly dead relatives) who do not possess sufficient merit to hold a peaceful existence who enter a human body and perform meritorious deeds to obtain good karma for a better existence. (W. S. Pushpakumara (# 61), B. A. Anoma Damayanthi (#62), K. G. K. Rasika Sumidimali (#71), Gallage Niroshan Dilantha Kumara (#73).

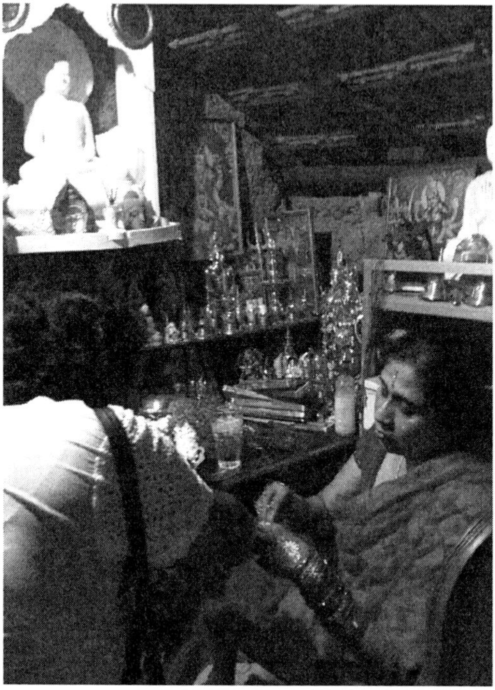

Figure 1.1 – Ghana manio blessing a patient for good health. Image taken by author.

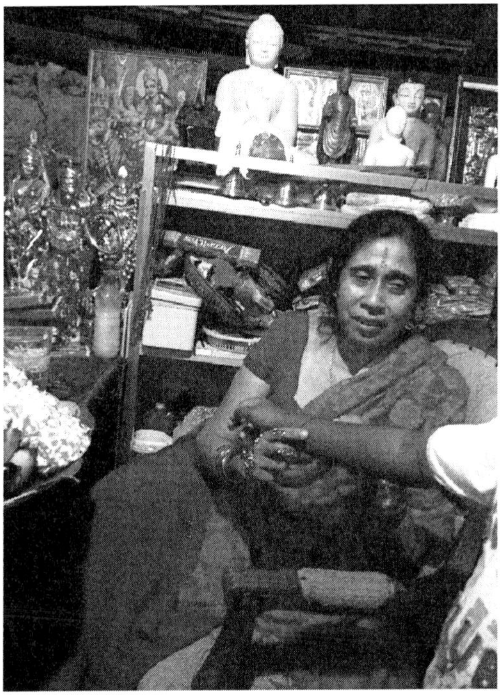

Figure 1.2 – Ghana manio tying a protection on a patient. Image taken by author.

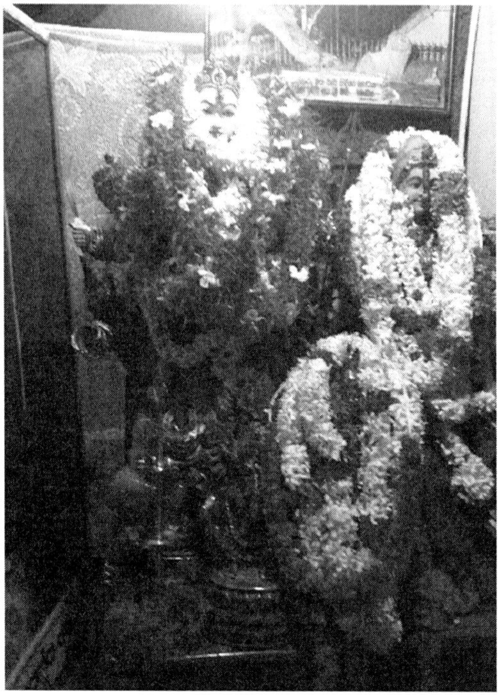

Figure 1.3- Garlands for the deva statues offered by the devotees/patients who have come for consultation with Ghana manio. Image taken by author.

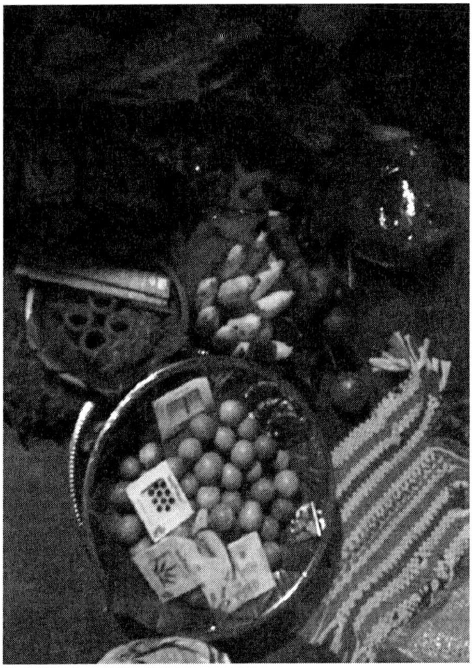

Figure 1.4 – Offerings for fulfilling healing and wellbeing wishes. Image taken by author.

The healing practice of Ghana manio is in great demand. She explains how she conducts her healing and is renumerated:

> Saturday*(s)* and Sunday(*s*) are the days of consultation. There are about 500 people who come each day, out of whom about 100 people are turned away. Tuesday is the day of treatment. When a person is treated or their wishes are fulfilled, they usually make an offering of fruits.[8]

Ghana manio is an example of spirit healing in Sri Lanka. Another popular healing system is spiritual healing, and an example of this is portrayed by the reflections on Venerable Wellawatthe Seelagawesi Thero's case described below.

---

[8] Ghana manio (# 60).

1.2 Reflection 2: Spiritual Healer Venerable Wellawatthe Seelagawesi Thero[9]

Venerable Wellawatthe Seelagawesi Thero is a Buddhist monk and a spiritual healer.[10] Despite not having systematic, formal training in healing Venerable Seelagawesi uses a form of healing based on *Karuna* (loving compassion) to treat a range of ailments.[11] As a young man, before taking robes and becoming a monk, he worked for a non-government organisation called the Socio-Economic Institute in Kandy.[12] He began by volunteering and later worked as a Health Extension Officer to eradicate malnutrition among the young children and mothers of Kandy. In order to address the issues associated with malnutrition, including neglectful and alcoholic fathers, he introduced and coordinated a mindfulness training programme for fathers. In this mindfulness training programme, the consultant trainer who convened the programme based it on *Maha Mangala Sutthraya*, which describes 38 qualities one should cultivate for a prosperous, happy and fulfilled life.[13] The first 20 qualities expressed in the *Maha Mangala Sutthraya* are based on different forms of virtue, the next 10 qualities are based on concentration, and the final 8 qualities are based on wisdom. Listening to the training, Venerable Wellawatte Seelagawesi became interested in exploring Buddhism for health and wellbeing. By the age of 26, he had taken robes and the name of Venerable Wellawatte Seelagawesi. *Figure 1.5* below portrays Venerable Seelagawesi meditating for spiritual development.

Since his time as a Health Extension Officer with the Socio-Economic Institute of Kandy, Venerable Seelagawesi has developed a range of healing techniques based on spirituality and understanding of the universe. Using the essence and meaning of Buddhism, and according to the personality traits of the client, and the form of diseases needing treating, Venerable Seelagawesi uses the name of the patient, the date of birth and their astral sign to 'access' patients. The specific techniques practiced by Venerable Seelagawesi include counselling, occupational therapy, telepathic healing, healing through sounds, healing through auras, neuro-

---

[9] Venerable Wellawatthe Seelagawesi (# 66).

[10] Venerable Wellawatthe Seelagawesi (# 66). His meditation centre is in the Central Province of Sri Lanka. Seelagawesi Thero travels widely within the country and overseas.

[11] Venerable Seelagawesi (#66) has reportedly healed cancer, meningitis, heart ailments, depression, and personality disorders.

[12] Kandy is a city in Central Province of Sri Lanka.

[13] For a discussion on the *Maha Mangala Sutta* see Soni and Khantipalo (2006).

psycho immunity, *Kem Krama*, and Pirith, and herbal and oil treatments.[14] *Figure 6* portrays Venerable Seelagawesi practicing healing.

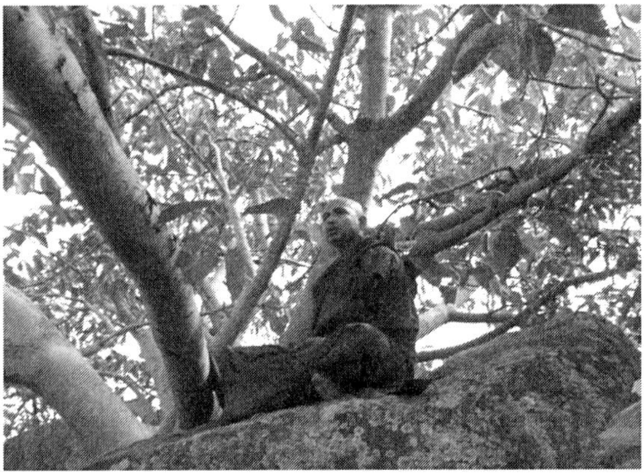

Figure 1.5- Venerable Seelagawesi Thero meditating; Image provided by Venerable Seelagawesi Thero.

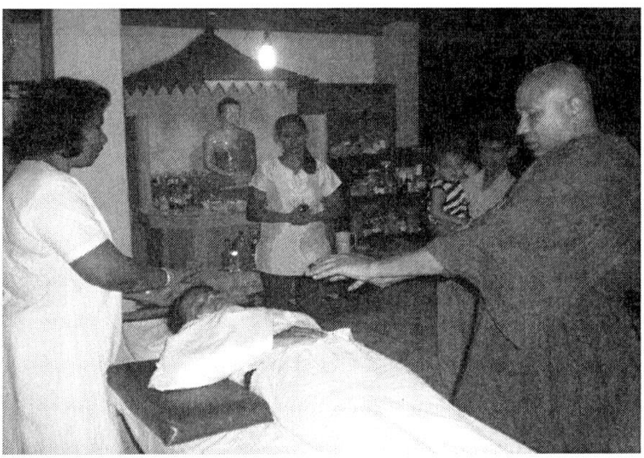

Figure 1.6- Venerable Seelagawesi Thero healing a cancer patient; Image provided by Venerable Seelagawesi Thero.

[14] To treat cancer patients there needs to be two healers -one healer to give positive rays and another healer to manage the rays in the body. The therapy sessions are 9 minutes long.

Venerable Seelagawesi's main objective in life is to attain enlightenment (*Nissarana Sapaya*) by developing self and by contributing towards the wellbeing of other human beings. He does not believe in claiming ownership over the healing methods or the medicine that he uses; nor does he want to develop a *guru kula* (a restricted group with authority). This means that anyone interested in healing and who has developed loving kindness (*Karuna)* qualities could practice his healing method.[15] According to Venerable Seelagawesi, the practitioner of spiritual healing does not need to be Buddhist. Venerable Seelagawesi's practice of spiritual healing is not advertised, nor does he put a price tag on what he does. With over 20 years of experience in healing Venerable Seelagawesi has created healing groups not only in Sri Lanka, but also in the United States of America, Denmark, England and Malaysia. Venerable Seelagawesi says, 'I don't have a license to practice as a doctor but I have a right to heal when someone comes to me for treatment.'[16]

1.3 Reflection 3: Inter-generational Healing Practice of Horiwila Kadum Bidum[17]

In Sri Lanka, one of the most famous (orthopaedic) schools for treating fractures, dislocations and wounds is *Horiwila Kadum Bidum.[18]* The current practitioners of *Horiwila Kadum Bidum* are descendants of the famous 'Horiwila' family of Ayurveda Vaidyas.[19] The methods and practices of *Horiwila Kadum Bidum* are still very much intergenerational and passed down amongst family members. Influenced by Buddhism, this traditional knowledge is passed down from fathers to their sons by mentoring from childhood. This traditional healing practice is written down on ola leaves

[15] Venerable Seelagawesi Thero does not claim ownership of his knowledge. He also portrays a desire to resist the formalization of healing practices and how knowledge is transmitted informally when compated with the written traditions of transmitting knowledge in more formalized systems of healing practices such as bio-medicine, Ayurveda, Siddha, Unani, Homeopathy and Acupuncture.

[16] Venerable Seelagawesi Thero (# 66).

[17] S. M. K. Nimal Karunarathne (# 93), R. A. Sudath Priyantha (# 94) and S. M. H. Seneviratne (# 95) Horiwila, Paalugaswewa in North Central Province.

[18] Treatment centres are located in Horiwila (North Central Province), Colombo (Western Province) and Ambalangoda (Southern Province).

[19]*Vaidya*s the Sinhala word for Medical Doctor (*Here it means an indigenous healing practitioner).*

(see Figure 1.7) or hand-made notes.[20] The way healing is learnt and practiced is perhaps best explained by a *Horiwila Kadum Bidum* healer:

> My father and my uncle used to practice *Horiwila Kadum Bidum* tradition under one roof. My uncle was the more famous one. We used to help them with finding and preparing the medicines when we were small. They taught us the secret traditional knowledge. I have been giving treatment by myself for 8 years now. Before starting on my own I used to work with my brothers. [21]

The same *Horiwila Kadum Bidum* healer explains how they learnt the tradition of healing:

> The first thing we used to do as apprentices in my uncle's home was identify and collect the medicinal herbs. Then we started (preparing) the oil refinery (*thel hindinna)*. We also had to identify different kinds of oils used for different forms of ailments, ie., for wounds, scars, inflammation, fractures, dislocations and spasm, the seven kinds of *patthu* (applications) and fourteen kinds of *mallum* (herbal packs). [22]

Figure 1.8 portrays a *Horiwila Kadum Bidum* healer preparing the oil for treatment while Figure 1.9 is a patient treated for a fracture based on the *Horiwila Kadum Bidum* healing method. In inter-generational healing practices, religion plays a vital role. In this next passage a *Horiwila Kadum Bidum* healer explains the role of religion in the *Horiwila Kadum Bidum* tradition of healing:

> Our religion (Buddhism), the Buddhist principles and values play an important role in our healing practice. We believe the healer should live by the principles of Buddhism and maintain high standards of moral values for the treatment to be effective.[23]

The statement above describes how religious beliefs and rituals have become an integral part of healing. This assertion is supported in Figure 10 below that portrays how vows are tied based on religious beliefs on behalf of the wellbeing and protection of the patients.

Despite being one of the most famous and recognised indigenous healing practices in Sri Lanka, *Horiwila Kadum Bidum* is not supported by the Sri Lankan Government, and is not formally organised or practiced in a

---

[20] The researcher was given access to the ola leaves and the hand written notes (12 July 2012).

[21] S. M. K. Nimal Karunarathne (# 93).

[22] S. M. K. Nimal Karunarathne (# 93).

[23] S. M. K. Nimal Karunarathne (# 93).

systemic way. As noted by a *Horiwila Kadum Bidum* healer S. M. K. Nimal Karunarathne:

> Although *Horiwila Kadum Bidum* healing practice is recognised as one of the most famous indigenous healing practices, we are not strong enough to systematically organise this knowledge and share the knowledge at the university level.[24]

The other reason that hinders the systematic organisation of the *Horiwila Kadum Bidum* healing system is that traditional healing is an honorary profession and not a livelihood. Healers often practice healing in conjunction with agriculture, and do not have fixed fees for the treatment. While some patients place money within the betel leaf many cannot afford to pay for the treatment. Perhaps more importantly, practitioners of *Horiwila Kadum Bidum* consider treating patients as their duty. Indeed, there are times when practitioners give complimentary treatment and medicine, and also feed the patient and give them the money needed for a bus ticket home.[25]

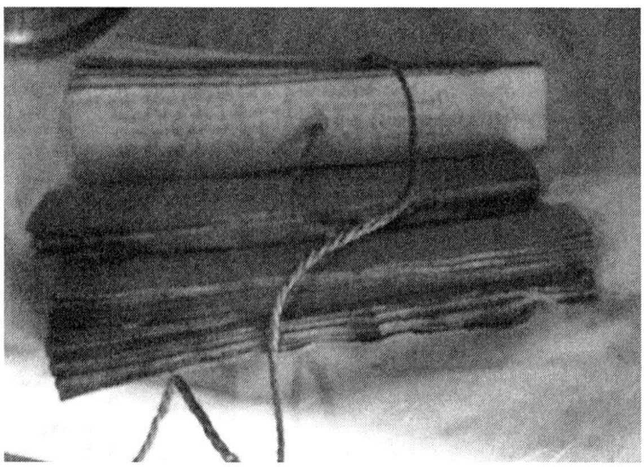

Figure 1.7- an ola leaf manuscript of Kadum Bidum healing. Image taken by author.

[24] S. M. K. Nimal Karunarathne (# 93).
[25] S. M. K. Nimal Karunarathne (# 93).

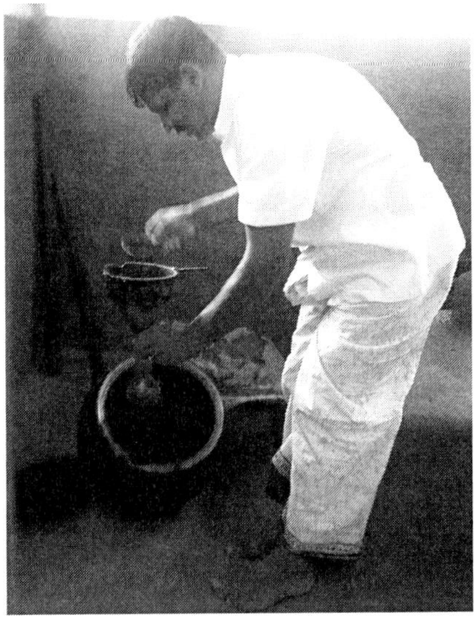

Figure 1.8- Horiwila Kadum Bidum healer preparing the oil for treatment. Image taken by author.

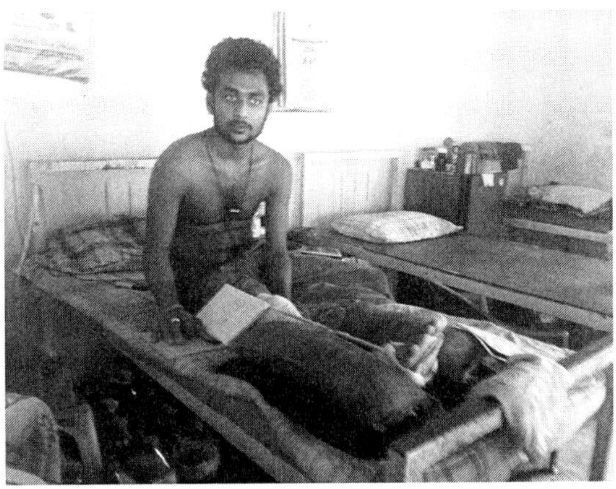

Figure 1.9 – A patient with a fracture in his right leg. Image taken by author.

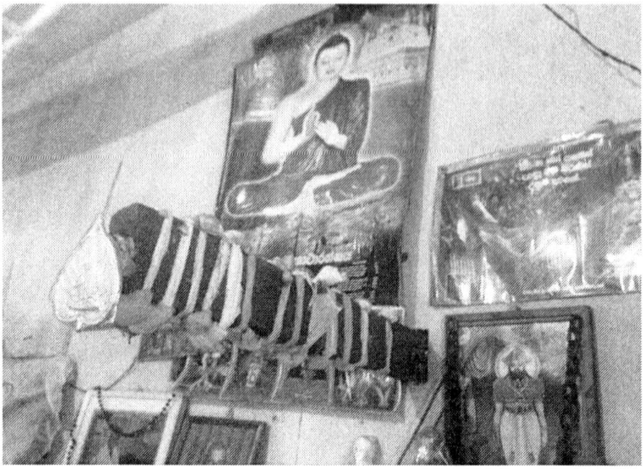

Figure 1.10 - The vows tied on behalf of the wellbeing and protection of the patients. Image taken by author.

1.4 Reflection 4: Traditional Siddha Doctor

For as long as she can remember, Dr Sarojini wanted to be a medical doctor and serve patients.[26] When she was in school, her ambition was to become a Western medical doctor, but as she did not obtain the required results for her G.C.E. Advanced Level examination she did not meet the entry requirements. Instead, she attended the Indigenous Institute of Medicine at the University of Colombo, where she studied Siddha Medicine. Siddha medicine is a system of healing of Dravidian origin, from southern India and is closely associated with Tamil civilisation.[27] The entire original literature on Siddha is in the Tamil language. The Siddha healers are called 'Siddhars:' individuals who achieved supreme knowledge in the field of medicine, yoga and meditation.[28] Almost all the students who joined the Siddha Department of the University of Jaffna, at the time Dr. Sarojini was studying, were of Tamil origin.[29] The ethnic tensions in Sri Lanka resulted in the Siddha Department being transferred to University of Jaffna in 1984. Dr. Sarojini was in the first cohort of students in the Siddha Department of University of Jaffna. Unlike the present Siddha degree that is offered in English, she studied Siddha medicine in Tamil, her mother tongue and

[26] Dr. Sarojini (# 98).
[27] Kandaswamy (1979).
[28] Narayanaswamy (1975).
[29] Dr. Sarojini (# 98).

found it easier 'to conceptualise and internalise the knowledge.'[30] Like the *Horiwila Kadum Bidum* healers, she does not come from a traditional healing background, and all of the knowledge she has acquired is from formal education. Dr. Sarojini states her experience with Siddha in the following way:

> When I got inducted to the subject, I found the Siddha principles interesting. Siddha principles are closely linked with our cultural beliefs and understandings. Also, I learnt and experienced the value of Siddha medicine. Now I feel my dream of being a doctor has been fulfilled. I am happy to be able to serve patients.[31]

Dr. Sarojini's statement illustrates how her becoming a Siddha doctor has become as rewarding to her as becoming a Western trained health professional.

These four experiences have contextualised the book by providing a background on the diversity of living practices of healing in Sri Lanka, including different kinds of healers with varying backgrounds located in different parts of the island. The reflections have presented a spirit healer, a spiritual healer, an inter-generational healing practice and a traditional form of healing formally recognised, supported and regulated by the Government. These reflections bring to light the diverse forms of living practices in health and wellbeing in Sri Lanka, as well as some of the themes and issues that are associated with the culture of healing and wellbeing practices, such as, the role of religion, language, social systems, customs, education, payment, organisation and duty which will be discussed in detail in the next part of this chapter.

Part 2: Living Practices in Health and Wellbeing in Sri Lanka

These four reflections of health and wellbeing show disparate practices and uses of diverse forms of knowledge and expression in Sri Lanka. From magical power, mind development, to Buddhism, these health and wellbeing practices are generally informed and sustained by a range of factors including religion, language and social systems. The reflections also highlight some of the themes and tensions that are evident in the debates and discussion about healing practices in Sri Lanka.[32] This part focuses on

---

[30] Dr. Sarojini (# 98).

[31] Dr. Sarojini (# 98).

[32] Reflection 1: role of faith in healing and use of language; Reflection 2: religious influence in healing practice; Reflection 3: Social systems and inter-generational

the role of religion, language, social systems in living practices in health and wellbeing in Sri Lanka[33] and the tension between 'Western' and traditional knowledge and expressions.[34]

In Sri Lanka especially, religion or belief systems influence the way of life of the community. Religion has always played a central role in Sri Lankan culture. It has significantly contributed in moulding the lifestyle and the diverse sources of knowledge of the Sri Lankans. Traditional practices related to health and wellbeing have mostly been influenced by Buddhism but also Hinduism and Islam. Religion, particularly Buddhism, Hinduism and its ideals play a key role in influencing the beliefs that the healing systems are based on and their rituals.

Language is the key tool in communicating and transmitting traditional practices related to health and wellbeing. Language specific terms and phrases used by a community in expressing their traditional practices are commonly indigenous to the particular community. The knowledge system could partly or completely die if a language dies.[35] While informal healing in the country is always practiced in the mother-tongue, there is a growing tendency to introduce the study of formal healing in universities in English.

Traditional social systems that were established based on values of the society to pass down the knowledge system and practices were the core mechanisms in place to systematically practice the traditional health and wellbeing related practices in the society. The two major social systems in pre-colonial Sri Lanka were the caste system and the *rajakariya* system. The Sinhala caste system[36] could trace its origins to India, but it had developed its own peculiar characteristics in Sri Lanka. The distinctive feature of the Sinhala caste system in contrast to the Indian model was that there were no religious sanctions from Buddhism for caste.[37] Most Sinhala castes had a service or occupational role. Traditional knowledge on occupation,

---

practice of healing; and Reflection 4: competition to become a Western doctors instead of a traditional doctor.

[33] The term 'Sri Lanka' was officially used in 1972. Yet for consistency and the purpose of this book I have used 'Sri Lanka' in the pre 1972 era.

[34] Simpson (1997) has argued how shifting social contexts have impacted in loss of communities of practice due to issues in transmission of ritual knowledge by ritual specialists among the Berava caste in Sri Lanka

[35] Kiene (2011), p 151.

[36] Caste is a system of social stratification. It is characterized by endogamy, hereditary transmission of a lifestyle including an occupation, ritual status in a hierarchy and customary social interaction and exclusion based on cultural notions of purity and pollution. (Scott, John and Marshall, Gordon (2005) p 66).

[37] De Silva (1981), p 41.

including healing, was passed down from generation to generation based on the caste system. The compulsory service system that prevailed in the ancient Sinhalese society is called the *rajakariya* system. The *rajakariya* was based on the caste system and the land tenure system.[38] It had two features, the personal service rendered to the 'king' or his agents by landholders who enjoyed land granted by him; and the liability of all landholders, irrespective of the nature of their tenure, to provide labour services on public works.[39] The *rajakariya* system contributed in sustaining the traditional knowledge of the community as it was a free compulsory service of a specific form of duty that had to be rendered to the king or public services.

The reflections in the previous section have also highlighted a number of contingent factors, such as formal and informal healing practices, customs passed down from generation to generation, level of education, economic factors, and tensions between Western knowledge and traditional knowledge and expressions.

As the previously presented reflections portray, there is a clear distinction between the formal[40] and informal[41] healing knowledge systems in Sri Lanka. The formal healing systems in the country are all adopted healing methods. These methods are available to anyone regardless of family heritage. It is the formal healing methods such as Western Allopathic healing, Ayurveda, Siddha, Unani, Acupuncture and Homeopathy that have received government recognition as cultural heritage and legal protection. These methods are systematically promoted by the government through the provision of full sponsorship for education and research, the employment of doctors who have completed degrees in Ayurveda, Siddha and Unanai healing, and the facilitation of the provision of free medical consultations and treatment all over the island. The informal healing methods are the methods that have originated within the country. These healing methods are diverse and unsystematic.

The informal healing methods can be acquired from family lineage,[42] by self-learning,[43] or the power of external forces.[44] These informal

[38] Lowe (2007), p 69.

[39] De Silva (1981), p 244.

[40] Reflection 4 on Siddha Doctor refers to a formal healing system in Sri Lanka.

[41] Reflection 1 on Ghana manio (spirit healing); story 2 on Venerable Wellawatthe Seelagawesi Thero (spiritual healing); and reflection 3 on *Horiwila Kadum Bidum* (inter-generational healing) refers to informal healing systems in Sri Lanka.

[42] Reflection 3 on *Horiwila Kadum Bidum.*

[43] Reflection 2 on Venerable Wellawatthe Seelagawesi Thero.

[44] Reflection 1 on Ghana manio.

healing methods are not systematically coded, documented or taught in formal educational institutes. There are no standards for the treatment methods followed.

In the pre-colonial era, knowledge was transmitted through generations based on the caste system or the *rajakariya* system. Although the social system in place significantly changed after European colonisation, as was seen in the reflection about the *Kadum Bidum* healers, inter-generational passing down of knowledge and customs still exists.[45] In addition to *Kadum Bidum* (orthopaedics), there are a significant number of healing systems that exist in the country, such as healers practicing treatment for *Sarvanga* (physicians), *Ass* (eye), *Ansha Baga* (paralysis) and *Visa* (poison), based on family lineage. Indigenous healing systems are passed down from generation to generation by observing, getting involved in the process by assisting the adult healer, memorizing the teachings taught verbally and referring to ola leaf manuscripts or hand written notes which are used to store and transmit knowledge.[46]

A feature of informal (indigenous/local) healing which were evidenced in the reflections is that it is not heavily influenced by the prevailing education system (most healers have not been to school or have been to only primary school); as a result, their view of the world is not based on Western thinking. Most of the informal healers still live in the rural areas and have not adopted an urban lifestyle. In contrast, traditional healers who have obtained a formal education in healing, such as Dr. Sarojini, have gone through the current formal education system in the country. They have fulfilled the academic requirements to enter a traditional healing course at university and have undergone formal rigorous academic training.

A strong message from the stories was that indigenous healers practiced healing as an honorary profession for the purposes of healing, performing duty towards fellow human beings and acquiring merit. Historically, granting a monetary value for healing was not part of the agenda of a healer: 'Although we practice healing wholeheartedly, our economic conditions significantly hinder our ability to systematically and effectively organise and share the knowledge system.'[47]

Finally, the four stories point (albeit implicitly) to tensions between 'biomedical' and traditional knowledge and expressions in healing. The biomedical structure is the dominant medical system of the country due

---

[45] Based on interviews with healers. ie, S. M. K. Nimal Karunarathne (# 93), B. A. M. N. D. S. Thejasuya (# 14), S. Shantha (# 25), S. K. Liyanarachchi (# 27), W. A. Kusuma Wijesekera (# 32), S. D. M. Mahipala (# 51).

[46] Ministry of Education, p 1.

[47] S. M. K. Nimal Karunarathne (# 66).

to the extensive government patronage, systematic domination by the professional bodies, and public preference. The government has even adopted a biomedical framework to safeguard traditional healing, with the administrative structure, the training system, and the treatment system all in accord with the biomedical framework.

This part of the chapter has discussed the living practices in health and wellbeing in Sri Lanka. Here it has portrayed living practices in health and wellbeing as informed and sustained by a range of factors including religion, language and social systems. It has also highlighted the tensions between 'Western' and traditional knowledge and expressions that affects in determining the living practices in health and wellbeing in Sri Lanka. The next part of the chapter focuses on why Sri Lanka's living healing and wellbeing practices matter.

Part 3: Why Sri Lanka matters

A wealth of local knowledge has been produced by the inhabitants in Sri Lanka throughout its long history and used effectively for development in the country. This local knowledge, which is also known as traditional knowledge, is based on opinions, beliefs and customs which are handed down from generation to generation.[48] Some of the traditional practices related to health and wellbeing have been proven to be effective by biomedical parameters, while many others have not been evaluated at all.[49] With the extensive reliance on scientific knowledge, trends in globalisation and homogenisation, traditional knowledge is facing the threat of extinction. In order to better safeguard traditional knowledge structures, current measures adopted are to, mark the parameters of traditional knowledge structures. This is done by surveying the origins, sources, and causes of its evolution and forms in health and wellbeing practices. The section below is an historical analysis of healing and wellbeing practices in Sri Lanka to understand the parameters of traditional knowledge in healing and wellbeing in Sri Lanka. Chapter 5 and 6 of the book portray how these exact measures adopted to protect traditional knowledge can threaten the cultural aspects of traditional knowledge.

The history of Sri Lanka is important for understanding why healing practices are important. While a detailed history of Sri Lanka can

---

[48] Based on the definition given for Tradition in Uragoda (2000), p 1.

[49] Uragoda (2000), p 1.

be accessed from other sources,[50] this part of the chapter focuses on the history of Sri Lankan health care system, the scholarly work on Sri Lankan healing practices, the historical challenges for traditional forms of healing practices in Sri Lanka. The last section of this part focuses on why and how diverse healing practices in Sri Lanka could be safeguarded.

Organised systems of health care in ancient Sri Lanka can be traced to the 4th century BC.[51] Prematilleke and Aluwihare argue historically that Buddhism has played a major role in the socio-cultural upliftment and physical wellbeing of people.[52] They also argue that the long line of Sinhalese Buddhist rulers in Sri Lanka since the 3rd century BC were responsible for promoting healing and wellbeing in Sri Lanka.[53] The first historical books of medicine in Sri Lanka were written about 5 000 years

---

[50]The history of traditional knowledge and practices in Sri Lanka is very dependent on the Pali and Sinhalese chronicles. The earliest chronicle is the *Dīpavaṃsa* (History of the Island) which was composed in the 5th Century A.D, (edited and translated to English by Oldenberg (1879)). The *Dīpavaṃsa* incorporates traditions from earliest times to the end of the region of Mahāsena (278-302 A.D.). *Mahāvaṃsa* is known as the principle chronicle which aims to give a connected history of Sri Lanka up to recent times (English translation by Geiger (1908)). *Cūlavaṃsa,* (edited by Geiger, translated from German to English by Rickmers (1953)) known as the lesser chronicle, is the continuation of *Mahāvaṃsa*, written by different authors from time to time. A valuable and unique history is provided through these chronicles. Yet, these chronicles were written by Buddhist monks and it tends to report events that were of interest to Buddhism and the chronicles record events that occurred hundred years before they were set down. Yogasundram (2006), p xii. K. M. De Silva's *A History of Sri Lanka*. Colombo (Vijitha Yapa Publications: 2006, 2nd print) is a well-researched and deeply analysed publication on Sri Lankan history from the earliest times to 1981. The book provides comprehensive historical coverage of political, economic, social, artistic, religious, architectural, literary developments and international relations of Sri Lanka. Sri Lanka's historical developments from earliest recorded historical invasion of Vijaya, and formation of a classical Buddhist society and irrigation economy, to its emergence as a tropical colony producing for export market, and finally as an Asian democracy is very clearly documented. Some other sources that portray history, culture and politics in Sri Lanka include, Holt, J. (ed.) (2011), Hussein, A. (2009), Jayawardena, K. (2012), Kannangara, A. P. (2011), Samaraweera, V. (1997), Uragoda, C. G. (2000), Uyangoda J. (1998) Walpola, R. (1956), Wickramasinghe, N. (2006), Wickremasinghe, N. (2014).

See also, Holt (ed) (2011); and Spencer (ed) (1990).

[51] Prematilleke and Aluwihare (2012), p 84.

[52] Prematilleke and Aluwihare (2012), p 84.

[53] Prematilleke and Aluwihare (2012), p 84.

ago by King Ravana.[54] His best known books are, *Arkaprakasaya, Nadivignananaya, Kumarathanthraya* and *Udishasasthraya.*[55] Some forms of indigenous medical treatments have existed in Sri Lanka long before the arrival of Vijaya and the Indians.[56] These healing systems include healing by Mother Goddess, ancestral worship, like the Nee Yakku of the Veddhas, and tree worship which has been part of the treatment for ailments in pre-history.[57] The wealth of local knowledge that has been produced by the inhabitants in Sri Lanka throughout its long history has been used effectively for the human and socio-economic development of the country.

There have been numerous achievements in traditional practices related to health and wellbeing in Sri Lanka. According to the Mahavamsa,[58] the concept of hospitals was established in Sri Lanka during the reign of Pandukabaya, in the fourth century BC.[59] The literature suggests that there were four types of hospitals in ancient Sri Lanka: '(a) monastic hospitals where in-house treatment was provided for ailing monks for short or long periods; (b) hospitals for laymen where in-house treatment was provided (c) maternity homes and (d) hospitals where only outdoor treatment was provided.'[60]

Arjuna Aluvuhare highlights that surgical instruments found during excavations show a tendency towards high standards of technology and a similarity with the surgical instruments in the modern Western science.[61] The Sarartha Sangrahaya, a comprehensive manuscript which Sri Lankan physicians still use today for reference was written by King Buddhadasa in 398 AD.[62].

---

[54] Uragoda (1987), p 5.

[55] Uragoda (1987), p 5.

[56] Arrival of Vijaya from India to Sri Lanka in 543 BCE is a landmark event in Sri Lankan history as the written history of Sri Lanka began since the arrival of Vijaya. The earlier period in Sri Lanka is known as pre-history.

[57] Dissanayake (2009).

[58] The Mahavamsa is known as the single most important work of Sri Lankan origin (written in Pali language). It describes the life and times of the people who forged Sri Lanka, from the coming of Vijaya in 543 BCE to the regin of King Mahasena (334-361) (6th Century BC to 4th Century AD). The book could be downloaded from http://mahavamsa.org/ (last retrieved 19 February 2019).

[59] Mahavamsa, p 102.

[60] Siriweera, W. I. (21 July 2011) Hospitals in Ancient Rajarata as an Aspect of Cairing. Daily News. http://archives.dailynews.lk/2011/07/21/fea04.asp?&session-id=a0e8b0f846b1d0c4c487c2c21c94b349 (last retrieved 19 February 2019)

[61] Aluvihare (2012)

[62] IAAM Historical Perspective

References to healthcare in ancient Sri Lankan literature display an awareness of medical treatment methods as well as the performance of surgery on humans and on animals. Some examples are Sadharmaratmavaliya that prescribes first aid for many sicknesses; the Butsarana mentions that a mother would take medicine herself when her baby was sick; the Sivi Jataka refers to donation of an eye.[63] The Culavamsa refers to performing surgery on a snake by King Buddhadasa (337 – 365 AD) and King Parakramabahu I (1123-1186 AD) treating a crow[64] suffering with an ulcer that had formed in her cheek.[65]

Texts on traditional practices related to health and wellbeing were mostly written in Sanskrit *puskola poth* (Palm leaf manuscripts). Buddhist monks were fluent with the language.[66] As poetry was easier to comprehend, some medical books were written in poetry. History records incidents of royal invitation to translate medical books. For instance, Venerable Valivita Sangarajah translated a medical book, *Hesajja Manjusa* from Pali to Sinhala, based on King Narendrasinha's invitation.[67]

The pluralistic nature of Sri Lankan medical practices has been studied by many scholars. Waxler-Morrison argued the two formally structured systems of medicine, namely Ayurveda and Western medical practice, persist in Sri Lanka because the practitioners provide distinctly different services.[68] The Western influence and changes in traditional practitioner's behaviours was analysed by Ivan Wolffers to argue Western medicine has found a place in people's conceptual framework.[69] Kalinga Tudor Silva examined how indigenous herbal traditions existed in Sri Lanka to cope with malaria.[70]

---

http://www.instituteofayurveda.org/english/history.htm (last retrieved 19 February 2019).

[63] The Sivi Jataka story where the physician Sivaka transplants the King Sivi's eye to a Brahman could be found on the following link – http://jathakakatha.lk/english/index.php?option=com_content&view=article&id=300:485-sivi-jataka&catid=51:451-500&Itemid=99 (last retrieved 19 February 2019).

[64] Dissanayake (2012) argues whether the '*kaka*' (the Sinhala word for crow), meant the bird-crow or a resident of the crow island in the north.

[65] Culavamsa (1953) (Culavamsa is known as the 'lesser chronicle.' It is the more recent part of the Mahavamsa).

[66] Central Cultural Fund (1998), p 226.

[67] Quoted from Jayathilaka (1934) (1998), p 223.

[68] Waxler-Morrison (1988).

[69] Wolffers (1985) (1987), (1989).

[70] Silva (1991).

Sagara Kusumaratne adopted a medical sociological approach to study indigenous medical practices in Sri Lanka. He traced the origins and development of Ayurveda and other indigenous medical traditions based on field research conducted in Homagagama, on the significance of indigenous medicine in the treatment seeking behaviour of people in a semi-urban setting.[71] C. G. Uragoda traces the history of medicine in Sri Lanka from the ancient history to 1948. The study has emphasised the medical history in the colonial period and portrays both good and bad colonial influences on Sri Lanka's medical history.[72]

Gananath Obeyesekera has worked extensively on psychological medicinal practices in traditional healing systems in Sri Lanka. Obeysekera has applied the classical metaphysical base to understand contemporary healing practices of Sri Lanka. That is, Obesyeskera has applied the Ayurveda concept of mind and theory of psychological medicine in ancient Sanskrit texts to interpret and make sense of contemporary healing practices of Sri Lanka. Obeysekera's work, 'The Idiom of Demonic Possession,'[73] and 'Psycho-cultural Exegesis of a Case of Spirit Possession in Sri Lanka'[74] deal with exorcism or the practice of spirit healing. The role of religious rituals in healing is discussed in 'The Firewalkers of Kataragema: the Rise of *Bhakti* Religiosity in Buddhist Sri Lanka.'[75]

Historical studies show that Sri Lanka possesses diverse forms of practices related to health and wellbeing for all forms of diseases including viral, bacterial and fungal diseases, all forms of surgeries and mental illnesses. They also show that the Sri Lankan people possess rich knowledge on healthy living and wellbeing of individuals and communities.

While traditional beliefs, knowledge and practices have been, and continue to be, socially and economically important there are a number of challenges for traditional beliefs and practices. Indeed, Sri Lanka's is a complex social, religious and political history that mixes Sinhalese, Tamil, Muslim, Buddhist, Islam, Hindu beliefs, as well as colonial influences. Although the long history of foreign influences including settlement and trade in Sri Lanka can be dated back to 543 BCE,[76] it was only the Europeans who directly colonised the island. Sri Lanka was occupied by

---

[71] Kusumaratane (2005).
[72] Uragoda (1987).
[73] Obeysekera (1970).
[74] Obeysekera (1977).
[75] Obeysekera (1978).
[76] Geiger (tr.) (1960) notes that as recorded in Mahavamsa, Sri Lanka's written history begins with the Indo-Aryan immigration of Vijaya and his 700 followers in 543 BCE.

European colonial powers from 1505 to 1948.[77] The colonial impact in controlling the resources and the ideological influence in socio-political decision making eroded the traditional beliefs, knowledge and practices of the country.[78]

In colonial and post-colonial era reliance on scientific knowledge, trends in globalisation and the homogenisation of cultures, has meant that traditional practices related to health and wellbeing are facing potential extinction.[79] Furthermore, the influence of Western medical systems and the impact of multi-national corporations and media in marketing global medical and wellbeing products and services has become a threat to traditional practices related to health and wellbeing.[80] Obtaining intellectual property such as patents for traditional knowledge in health and wellbeing practices and medicine by third parties and sharing very little with the original bearers of traditional knowledge is another impact of globalisation.[81] The influence of information technology in creating a homogenisation of culture[82] is also threatening traditional knowledge.[83] If the rich and diverse traditional practices related to health and wellbeing are not safeguarded from the influences of globalisation, Sri Lankans will not be able to pass down this heritage, which Sri Lankans are currently enjoying thanks to their forebears, to their next generations.[84] Colonisation of the country, trends in globalisation, and extensive reliance on Western scientific knowledge, has resulted, therefore, in the threat of extinction of the traditional practices related to health and wellbeing.

---

[77] For a detailed discussion of colonial history of Sri Lanka see De Silva (1981)

[78] Coomaraswamy (1946).

[79] Historical influences including Colonisation of Sri Lanka and socio, political, cultural, economic changes discussed above in this Introduction have root causes for the threat of extinction of traditional knowledge.

[80] R. L. Kularatne (# 110), Dr. S. Sivashanmugarajah (# 99), Dr. B. Kotawalagedera (# 39).

[81] Prof. Piyal A. Marasinghe (# 41). Also, Twarog (2003), Twarog and Kapoor (2004) argue concerns such as use of traditional knowledge with little or no benefit sharing with original traditional knowledge holders and/or inappropriate patenting has raised increasing attention on the international agenda in the past decade.

[82] Firouzeh (2004) portrays the role mass media play in globalisation and homogenization of culture in developing countries.

[83] Information technology formalises, mainstreams and promotes homogenisation of traditional healing practices threatening the diverse and informal nature of traditional forms of healing practices.

[84] Traditional practices related to health and wellbeing survived and thrived due to organised social system, individual commitment and the recognition by the state and community.

An enormous share of the traditional practices related to health and wellbeing has been lost during the colonial period due to some policies of colonial administration.[85] Although the revival efforts have reactivated some aspects of traditional practices related to health and wellbeing, they still face the threat of extinction. Reasons for this include, political pressures, social and economic pressures, territorial pressures, exploitation of traditional knowledge, development policy and globalisation and trade liberalisation.[86]

Protecting traditional practices related to health and wellbeing would improve the lives of traditional knowledge holders and communities who depend on traditional knowledge for their livelihoods, health and wellbeing. The World Health Organisation estimates the percentage of the world's population depending on traditional medicine for their primary health needs to be 80%.[87] Eleven percent of the Sri Lankan population seeks treatment in Government Ayurveda hospitals.[88] The percentage of the population seeking treatment from traditional healers or the population that depends on traditional medicine for primary health needs in Sri Lanka is not known due to the informal nature of the practices. For the survival of traditional practices related to health and wellbeing, it is important to adapt to current socio-economic trends, protecting the very nature and traditional cultural aspects associated with healing practices. An increased use of traditional knowledge-based technology could increase performance by enabling commercial utility of the biological knowledge and enhancing exports of traditional health and wellbeing related products.[89] Traditional products and services in health have a strong role in boosting the identity of traditional knowledge bearers, which in turn contribute towards their

---

[85] Prof. Piyal A. Marasinghe (# 41).

[86] Kelly (2005), p 25. This Report on Threats to the Practice and Transmission of Traditional Knowledge Regional Report: Asia and Australia is produced by Australian Institute of Aboriginal and Torres Strait Islander Studies is produced as Phase II of the Composite Report on the Status and Trends Regarding the Knowledge, Innovation and Practices of Indigenous Peoples and Local Communities relevant to Conservation and Sustainable Use of Biodiversity. http://aiatsis.gov.au/sites/default/files/products/research_outputs_submission/2006-convention-on-biological-diversity.pdf (Last retrieved 19 February 2019)

[87] WHO (1993).

[88] About Us. Ministry of Indigenous Medicine. http://www.indigenousmedimini.gov.lk/About_us.html (Last retrieved 19 February 2019).

[89] Dutfield (2006) p. 12.

wellbeing.[90] Safeguarding traditional practices related to health and wellbeing against globalisation and cultural hegemony, industrialisation and green revolution, bio-pirates and copyright infringements will ensure cultural diversity and the wellbeing of local communities.

The start of this section focused on the history of the Sri Lankan health care system. Analysis of its history of health and wellbeing practices has portrayed the rich and diverse forms of practices related to health and wellbeing that exist in Sri Lanka. The examination of scholarly work on Sri Lankan healing practices has covered a wide ambit: history of medicine in Sri Lanka from ancient history,[91] the origins and development of Ayurveda and other indigenous medical traditions in Sri Lanka,[92] psychological medicinal practices in traditional healing systems in Sri Lanka,[93] indigenous herbal traditions existed in Sri Lanka to cope with malaria,[94] the pluralistic nature of Sri Lankan medical practices,[95] and the Western influence and changes in traditional practitioner's behaviours.[96] Yet the diverse scope of scholarly work does not address how the Government of Sri Lanka's recognition, support and regulation have impacted the healing practices and traditional cultural aspects of healing.

Challenges for traditional beliefs and practices identified above include the European colonial influences in socio-political decision making; the trends in adopting and following new systems introduced by the colonisers that prioritised Western education, religion and culture through state laws and policies, state administration and sponsorship; the adoption of a capitalist economy, reliance on scientific knowledge, trends in globalisation and the homogenisation of cultures. These challenges have threatened the existence of diverse forms of healing and wellbeing practices and the associated traditional cultural aspects to protect the traditional practices related to health and wellbeing including the cultural aspects, in Sri Lanka, it is necessary to understand these living practices and the role of the Government in recognising, supporting and regulating traditional

---

[90] Vishwakeerthi Vanaspathi Uru Walige Wanniya Attho (# 18) explains the importance of engaging in traditional practices related to health and wellbeing and how such engagements contribute towards the wellbeing of the traditional knowledge bearers.

[91] Uragoda (1987).

[92] Kusumaratane (2005).

[93] Obeysekera (1970).

[94] Silva (1991).

[95] Waxler-Morrison (1988).

[96] Wolffers (1985) (1987), (1989).

practices related to health and wellbeing. In the next part this chapter explores the resultant research question of this book in this regard.

Part 4: Research Question

The research question behind this book is: what role does the recognition, support and regulation by the Government of Sri Lanka of healing and wellbeing practices play in determining, promoting, protecting or destroying the cultural aspect of healing? Traditional knowledge is a disparate set of knowledges, practices and beliefs, too often spoken about collectively as a singular traditional knowledge. In order to understand traditional knowledge, we must therefore examine specific contexts, places and practices. In examining traditional knowledges, expressions and practices in health and wellbeing in Sri Lanka, this study will consider current practices of traditional knowledge and traditional cultural expressions in health (mental and physical) and wellbeing in Sri Lanka. Determining current traditional knowledges and traditional cultural expressions is important because it enables researchers and policy makers to identify the traditional knowledge holders of health and wellbeing in Sri Lanka and the main forms of traditional knowledge.

To answer this question this work argues that we must understand the rich diversity of existing traditional knowledge and intangible cultural heritage, the current status of this heritage and how to overcome the threats of extinction. In order to understand the current status of traditional knowledge, expressions and practice, this book has considered the role of the government in recognising, supporting and regulating traditional knowledge. The regulation of traditional knowledge and traditional cultural expressions is done through a complex mix of international and national measures. In order to understand the role of regulations and its impact on society, it is necessary to examine the role of the government in implementing those regulations. Specifically, it is necessary to address questions about how the Sri Lankan government has adopted international measures and developed national measures to protect the traditional knowledge and traditional cultural expressions. In doing so it is important to consider why (or why not) the Sri Lankan government has protected specific traditional knowledge and traditional cultural expressions.

Part 5: Key Terms and Concepts

It is important to be clear of the meaning of key terms and concepts used in this book. This part presents the complexities of the definition of traditional knowledge and traditional cultural expressions. Then the terms traditional practices related to health and wellbeing, traditional health, traditional doctor, healer and wellbeing are defined.

There is not, at this time, an agreed legal definition of traditional knowledge and traditional cultural expressions. In the context of cultural, traditional and indigenous knowledge Peter Drahos in *Intellectual Property, Indigenous People and their Knowledge* refers to the problems of lawyerly definitions as the 'quicksands of definition.'[97] Indeed, there have been numerous definitions of traditional knowledge and cultural expression advanced in the literature and discussion in the area.[98] Over the years, various terms have been used by policy makers to describe the subject matter of this book, such as healing practices, healing rituals, dance, performances, and story-telling. These terms include, but are not limited to 'folklore;'[99] 'indigenous heritage;'[100] 'traditional cultural heritage;' 'cultural expressions,'[101] 'knowledge, innovation and practices of indigenous and

---

[97] Drahos (2014), pp 23-27.

[98] There are many definitions of traditional knowledge in literature and draft legislation; see for example Anton's summary of the different definitions in Christoph Antons, 'Introduction,' in Traditional Knowledge, Traditional Cultural Expressions and Intellectual Property Law in the Asia-Pacific Region, Antons, (ed.) (2009), pp 1–36, pp 1–4.

[99] *UNESCO Recommendation on the Safeguarding of Traditional Culture and Folklore (1989), A,* defines folklore as 'the totality of tradition-based creations of a cultural community, expressed by a group or individuals and recognized as reflecting the expectations of a community in so far as they reflect its cultural and social identity; its standards and values are transmitted orally, by imitation or by other means. Its forms are, among others, language, literature, music, dance, games, mythology, rituals, customs, handicrafts, architecture and other arts.' http://portal.unesco.org/en/ev.php-URL_ID=13141&URL_DO=DO_ TOPIC&URL_SECTION=201.html (last retrieved 19 February 2019).

[100] *Draft Principles and Guidelines for the Protection of the Heritage of Indigenous People* (2000), A 12, 13, 14 defines the heritage of indigenous people. See Economic and Social Council (2000) Annex I, p 13.

[101] *UNESCO Convention on the Protection and Promotion of the Diversity of Cultural Expressions (2005) A 4 (3)* defines cultural expressions as 'those expressions that results from the creativity of individuals, groups and societies and that have cultural content.'

local communities,'[102] 'indigenous knowledge'[103] and 'traditional knowledge.'[104] For example, as detailed further in chapter 2, the World Intellectual Property Organization's Intergovernmental Committee on Intellectual Property and Genetic Resources, Traditional Knowledge and Folklore (IGC) produced draft legal instruments to protect traditional knowledge, traditional cultural expression and folklore.[105] In so doing, they have proposed a number of definitions of traditional knowledge that includes a range of alternatives.

In 2014, the IGC prepared new draft articles on the protection of traditional knowledge[106] and the protection of traditional cultural expressions.[107] The square brackets indicate that the text is far from finalised and will be resolved at a later date. The IGC draft articles in defining traditional knowledge and traditional cultural expressions have said that:

> "traditional knowledge" [refers to]/ [includes]/ [means], for the purpose of this instrument, know-how, skills, innovations, practices, teachings and learnings of [indigenous [peoples] and [local communities]]/[or a state of states]. [108]

---

102 *Convention on Biological Diversity (1992), A 8 (j)*

103 WIPO (2001), p 23 defines indigenous knowledge in two ways: (i) it is used to describe knowledge held and used by communities, peoples and nations that are "indigenous;" (ii) is also used to refer to knowledge that is itself "indigenous."

104 Various forms in which traditional knowledge may be found is discussed in WIPO Intergovernmental Committee on Intellectual Property and Genetic Resources, Traditional Knowledge and Folklore. Seventeenth Session (WIPO/GRTKF/IC/17/INF/9) http://www.wipo.int/edocs/mdocs/sct/en/wipo_grtkf_ic_17/wipo_grtkf_ic_17_inf_9.pdf (last retrieved 19 February 2019).

105 WIPO, Traditional Knowledge - http://www.wipo.int/tk/en/ (last retrieved 19 February 2019).

106 *WIPO-IGC, Draft Article -. The Protection of Traditional Knowledge* (WIPO/GRTKF/IC/27/REF/FACILITATORS DOCUMENT REV.2) was agreed at the IGC 27 on 28 March 2014. Draft Article available at http://www.wipo.int/meetings/en/doc_details.jsp?doc_id=270556 (Last retrieved 19 February 2019).

107 WIPO-IGC, *Draft Article* -. The Protection of Traditional Knowledge (WIPO/GRTKF/IC/27/REF/FACILITATORS TCES DOCUMENT REV.2) was agreed at the IGC 27 on 4 April 2014. Draft Article available at http://www.wipo.int/meetings/en/doc_details.jsp?doc_id=271146 (last retrieved 19 February 2019).

108 Use of Terms, Traditional Knowledge in The Protection of Traditional Knowledge: Draft Articles Rev. 2 (March 28, 2014), WIPO/GRTKF/IC/27/REF/FACILITATORS DOCUMENT REV.2.

> [Traditional knowledge may be associated, in particular, with fields such as agricultural, environmental, healthcare and indigenous and traditional medical knowledge, biodiversity, traditional lifestyles and natural resources and genetic resources, and know-how of traditional architecture and construction technologies.][109]

The proposed definition for traditional cultural expression is as follows:

> [Traditional] cultural expression means any form of [artistic and literary], [creative and other spiritual] expression, tangible or intangible, or a combination thereof, such as actions,[110] materials,[111] music and sound,[112] verbal[113] and written [and their adaptations], regardless of the form in which it is embodied, expressed or illustrated [which may subsist in written/codified, oral or other forms].[114]

Too often, traditional knowledge is conceived unsophisticatedly as a reflection of mainstream knowledge, in particular, science.[115] Importantly, indigenous groups claim that their rights extend to defining (for themselves) the extent and characteristics of the intellectual property.[116] In general terms, traditional knowledge has been described as the 'understanding or skill possessed by indigenous peoples pertaining to their culture and folklore, their technologies, and their use of native plants for medicinal purposes.'[117] Put another way, traditional knowledge is the cumulative and dynamic body of knowledge, know-how, practices and representations

---

[109] Use of Terms, Traditional Knowledge in The Protection of Traditional Knowledge: Draft Articles Rev. 2 (March 28, 2014), WIPO/GRTKF/IC/27/REF/FACILITATORS DOCUMENT REV.2.

[110] [Such as dance, works of mask, plays, ceremonies, rituals, rituals in sacred places and peregrinations, games and traditional sports/sports and traditional games, puppet performances, and other performances, whether fixed or unfixed.]

[111] [Such as material expressions of art, handicrafts, ceremonial masks or dress, handmade carpets, architecture, and tangible spiritual forms, and sacred places.]

[112] [Such as songs, rhythms, and instrumental music, the songs which are the expression of rituals.]

[113] [Such as stories, epics, legends, popular stories, poetry, riddles and other narratives; words, signs, names and symbols.]

[114] Use of Terms, Traditional Cultural Expressions in The Protection of Traditional Knowledge: Draft Articles Rev. 2 (April 4, 2014), WIPO/GRTKF/IC/27/REF/FACILITATORS TCES DOCUMENT REV.2

[115] Unesco. Bureau of Public Information (2006) Traditional Knowledge. http://www.unesco.org/bpi/pdf/memobpi48_tradknowledge_en.pdf (last retrieved 19 February 2019).

[116] Fecteau (2001), p 84.

[117] Munzer and Rustiala (2009), p 38.

possessed by peoples with long histories of interaction with their natural milieu.[118] Traditional knowledge is intimately tied to language, social relations, spirituality and worldview, and is generally held collectively.

In Sri Lanka, existing systems of traditional knowledge include traditional administrative systems, traditional social systems (caste systems), irrigation systems, traditional legal system, architecture including traditional village planning, art, religions- Buddhism, Hinduism, Islam, literature, rituals, etc. Traditional knowledge is an intangible cultural heritage of human beings that portrays the rich civilisation and diversity of the community. By recognising traditional knowledge, cultural diversity can be promoted. Pluralistic and multi-cultural societies give an opportunity to their members to maintain their own identity which contribute towards satisfaction and self-fulfilment. Due to traditional knowledge's impact on culture, sustainable development, environmental conservation, food security, agriculture, traditional healing and wellbeing the importance of protecting traditional knowledge internationally and nationally has been repeatedly emphasised.

This book is not a doctrinal or legal analysis of traditional knowledge and cultural expression. Yet the terms 'traditional knowledge' and 'traditional cultural expressions'; are used based on context where Sri Lankan institutions have adopted these concepts. The most commonly used phrase in this book is 'practices related to health and wellbeing.' More specifically I use:

> *Traditional practices related to health and wellbeing* – is utilised in a general sense and is deployed in this book to comprise traditional know-how, skills, innovations, practices, teachings, expressions and learnings of that has been originated or adopted in Sri Lanka from other countries.

Importantly this term is not exclusionary, but is used to reflect the broad range of practices used in Sri Lanka to promote and protect health and wellbeing. The concepts of health and wellbeing are also central to this book. These terms as used in this book are defined in the following way:

- *Traditional health* - is providing health care guidance and treatment by using herbal, animal and mineral substances, spirituality and certain other methods based on the social, cultural and religious background, and the knowledge, attitudes and belief that are

[118] Talaat, Asma, Mohd and Lokman (2012)

prevalent in the community regarding physical, mental and social wellbeing and the causation of diseases and disability.[119]

- *A traditional doctor* is a person who has obtained a formal university education (Bachelors degree or above) in traditional medicine (Ayurveda, Siddha and Unani).
- *A healer* is a person who contributes towards another person's mental, physical, spiritual and emotional health and wellbeing and is recognised by the community as a healer.
- *An indigenous healer* is a person who is recognised by the community in which he lives as competent to provide traditional health care.
- *Wellbeing* can refer to, (a) a positive state of being; (b) a person's overall sense of health and wellbeing; (c) a person's feelings of happiness or general satisfaction with his/her quality of life; (d) the experience of contentment and fulfilment with one's life circumstances.[120] Wellbeing is said to be experienced when a person's individual, relational, and collective needs are fulfilled[121]. Wellbeing is a dynamic concept, and individuals work towards achieving a state of wellbeing by fulfilling their needs. The achievement of wellbeing is determined by psychological and social dimensions, that is, the individual efforts and the social context in which the individual is placed.[122]

For the purpose of this book, then, the terms health and wellbeing are taken to include four clusters or 'kinds' of health and wellbeing:

(i) healing – treatment of patients by using oral medicine or application of medicine,
(ii) rituals – treatment of patients using music, sounds, dance, drama or any other forms of ritualistic practices and,
(iii) forecasting – predicting the future by using astrology, body traits or power of spirits for mental and physical wellbeing and,
(iv) spiritual – ensuring healing and wellbeing of individuals by personal spiritual development.

[119] Adopted based on Jan Stephan's definition of a traditional healer (1983), p 292.
[120] Definitions are based on PADHI definitions on Wellbeing (2009), p 19.
[121] Prilleltensky (2005) quoted in PADHI (2009), p 19.
[122] PADHI (2009), p 19.

Traditional healing practices, traditional knowledge and cultural heritage, are linked to the identity[123] of a person or a community and are tied up with the concepts of 'indigeneity', 'authentic' and 'traditional culture.' Indigeneity is claimed by self-consciously recognising and mobilising certain cultural ''traits'' (such as language, religion, ancestry) that are considered important to represent one's self, and contribute towards belonging.[124] Notions of 'authentic'[125] and 'traditional' cultural expressions are recognised as core features in defining indigenous identity.[126] Harris, Carlson and Poata-Smith (2013), argue that indigenous identities change and emerge in response to changing social and cultural circumstances.[127] Due to the identity of healers and practitioners evolving and changing overtime, it is questionable what is meant by an authentic indigenous identity. What it means to be an authentic indigenous healer changes over time. Can changing and evolving traditional (ancient) cultural expressions overtime still be called authentic identity?[128] The book recognises that the concepts of indigenous identity authentic culture and traditional culture change and evolve. This means that traditional healing practices, traditional knowledge and cultural heritage as continuously evolving and changing phenomena based on social, cultural and political influences.

Part 6: Methodology

This book seeks to answer the question 'What role does the recognition, support and regulation of the Government of Sri Lanka in healing and wellbeing practices play in determining, promoting, protecting or destroying the cultural aspect of healing?' This part provides an overview of the research design and methodology used to answer this research question. The research tools adopted to conduct the study, the data analysis method, ethical considerations and the limitations of this study are discussed.

---

123 Identity is '...a socially constructed, variable definition of self or other, whose existence and meaning is continuously negotiated, revised and revitalized.' Nagel (1993), p.2.

124 Dean and Levi (2003).

125 Particularly biological and/or cultural authenticity that is deeply-rooted in institutional practices and public consciousness. Harris, Carlson and Poata-Smith (2013), p. 6.

126 Harris, M. (2013) pp. 10-11.

127 Harris, Carlson and Poata-Smith (2013), p. 6.

128 Harris, M. (2013) p. 16.

Research Tools

This research utilised three research tools to gather data and information on traditional knowledge and cultural expressions in Sri Lanka: archival research; interviews; and participant observation. Each of these will be discussed separately in the following sections.

Archival Research

Archival research involves pursuing and extracting information and evidence from original archival records.[129] It is a process of locating, evaluating, and systematically interpreting and analysing sources found.[130] Archival research enables researchers to 'ask new questions of old data, provide a comparison over time, verify or challenge existing findings, or draw together evidence from disparate sources to provide a bigger picture.'[131] Archival material includes official sources (such as government papers), organisational records, medical records, personal collections, other contextual materials, unpublished manuscripts, and associated correspondence.[132]

The archival research included a historical review of the development and transformation of traditional knowledge in health and wellbeing, and an integrative review of the current status of knowledge and the new findings of researchers. Archival research was conducted in a number of Sri Lankan libraries and depositories.

Field Research

Following the archival research, extensive field research was conducted. The field research included interviews and participant observation. These focused on three main themes: the government recognised, supported and regulated traditional medical system; traditional living practices related to physical healing and wellbeing; and traditional living practices related to mental health and wellbeing. Categorising the interviews in this way meant that understanding and analysing the prevailing diverse forms of healing and wellbeing practices in the country and the state sponsorship received was simplified by focusing on formal, semi-formal and informal healing

---

[129] Gaillet (2012), p 30 explains archival research as primary sources of creating knowledge.

[130] Hill (1993).

[131] Corti (2004), p 21.

[132] Hill (1993).

categories existing in Sri Lanka. Each of these categories will be discussed in turn.

The first theme is the *Government traditional medical system*: The Sri Lankan government structure for traditional medical systems comes under the auspicies Ministry of Indigenous Medicine. The two arms of the Ministry are the Department of Ayurveda and the Ayurveda Drug Corporation. Figure 1.11 portrays the main organs of the Ministry.

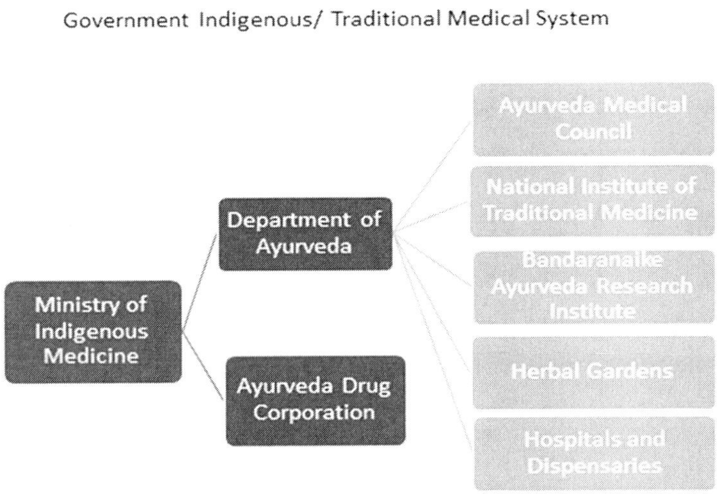

Figure 1.11– Government indigenous/ traditional medical system

Government traditional medical structure covers administration, community health care services, curative services, education, legislation, medicine and research. I conducted participant observation in institutions listed in Figure 1.11, in order to understand how government mechanisms work. My interviews covered officials belonging to the following institutions/ programmes-

Administration	- Department of Ayurveda - Provincial Administration of Indigenous Medicine - Sri Lanka Ayurveda Medical Council
Research	- Ayurvedic Research Committee - Bandaranaike Memorial Ayurveda Research Institute
Education	- Ayurveda Education and Hospital Board - National Institute of Traditional Medicine - Institute of Indigenous Medicine, University of Colombo - Gampaha Wickramarachchi Ayurveda Institute, University of Kelaniya - Department of Siddha, University of Jaffna - Samastha Lanka Paramparika Ayurveda Vaidya Vidyalaya of Keraminiya - Pirivena Ayurveda Medical Institutes
Curative Services	- Borella Ayurveda Teaching Hospital – Colombo 8 - Kaitady Siddha Teaching Hospital – Jaffna - Gampaha Wickramarachchi Ayurveda Teaching Hospital – Yakkala - Government Homeopathy Hospital - District Ayurveda Hospitals - Rural Ayurveda Hospitals - Central Dispensaries
Ayurveda Medicine	- Formulary Committee - Sri Lanka Ayurvedic Drug Corporation - Herbal gardens - Development programme of the Ministry medicinal plant cultivation
Community Health Care Services	- Medicinal plant cultivation - Poshana Mandira - Hela Veda Gedera - Preserving Vedda culture and medicinal plant cultivation

Figure 1.12 – Mechanisms of Government traditional indigenous medical structure

In regards to Ayurveda education, I visited all the major institutions in the country that provide formal Ayurvedic education.[133] I interviewed the administrative staff, academics and convened informal group interviews with the students (the informal interviews are not accounted for in my interviewing list). The curative services structure is widely spread in Sri Lanka. I visited all the three major teaching hospitals[134], district hospitals[135], rural hospitals and central dispensaries. At these institutions, in addition to the formal interviews with the hospital staff, I had informal discussions with the patients and the auxiliary staff of the hospital.

The second theme concerned the *Traditional practices related to healing*. My field work on traditional healing practices included an orientation for each of the healing items listed below in order to obtain an understanding of the healing practice, the beliefs attached to the practice and perspectives and acceptance by different stakeholders. For each healing practice listed in Figure 1.13, I interviewed up to 10 healers, conducted informal interviews with the patients and carried out participant observation. The difference in the number of interviews in each group was due to some healing practices being very common and practiced all over the country, but with significant diversity within the practice according to family lineage. Some healing systems are very unique and are practiced by only a very few healers. As the study was explorative research, and as I was trying to identify the diversity and similarities of the practices all over the island, the number of interviews for each category varied significantly.

---

[133] National Institute of Traditional Medicine (NITM), Institute of Indigenous Medicine, University of Colombo, Gampaha Wickramarachchi Ayurveda Institute, University of Kelaniya, Department of Siddha Medicine, University of Jaffna, Samastha Lanka Paramparika Ayurveda Vaidya Vidyalaya of Keraminiya, Sri Vajira Ghanodaya Pirivena, Sri Mahinda Pirivena.

[134] Borella Ayurveda Teaching Hospital – Colombo 8, Kaitady Siddha Teaching Hospital – Jaffna, Gampaha Wickramarachchi Ayurveda Teaching Hospital – Yakkala.

[135] In Matara, Trincomalee, Kurunegala, Pallakelle.

Traditional Practices Related to Healing	- Ayurveda - Siddha - Unani - Homeopathy - Acupuncture - Vedic Alchemy - Physicians (*Sarvanga*) - Orthopedics (*Kadum Bidum*) - Eye Treatment (*Ass Vedakama*) - Cancer Treatment (*Pilika*) - Stroke and Paralysis (*Angshabagha*) - Poison (*Visa*) - Headache (*Iru Rudawa*) - Indigenous Healing of the Vaddha Community

Figure 1.13 – Traditional practices related to healing

The third category of field work concerns *Traditional practices related to mental health and wellbeing*. In this category I focused on spiritual healing, spirit healing, rituals, and forecasting methods as listed in Figure1.14. Rituals and forecasting methods are integral part of Sri Lankan culture. These practices play an important role in cultural identity and mental wellbeing of a community. The methods listed are not an exhaustive list, but for the purpose of this study I have examined the practice of each ritual and forecasting method, including the traditional beliefs attached to the practice and the current impact in the society, by conducting interviews with the traditional healers/ ritual performers, participant observation and informal interviews with patients.

Rituals	- Bodhi Pooja - Pahan Pooja - Protection from Evil Eyes, Evil Mouth (*Ass Vaha Kata Vaha Mathirima*) - Vows - Shanthi Karma - Amulets and Charms (*Yanthra Manthra*) - Psycho Drama (*Thovil*) - Hethme Ritual - Kem Krama - Sound Therapy (*Seth Kavi*, Beating of Drums - Pirith - Yoga - Religious Possessions (*Perahara*)
Spirit healers	- Exorcist
Forecasting	- Astrology (*Jothishaya*) - Power of Spirits - Palm Reading (*Hastha Rekha*) - Biological Indicators
Spiritual	- Meditation - Telepathic Healing - Healers using their spiritual powers to heal

Figure 1.14 - Traditional practices related to mental health and wellbeing

In total there were 117 interviews conducted with a range of healers, shamans, monks, academics, lawyers and policy makers. (For a full list of participants see Annex). At the designing phase of the study, I did not anticipate undertaking extensive field interviews. However, as it became clearer, when conducting archival research, that there was no comprehensive and reliable account of existing indigenous healing systems in Sri Lanka, the field interviews became necessary. The interviewees were recruited using the snowball cluster sampling method[136], where an interview with one healer led to a recommendation and invitation to talk with another healer. It was through this process that I was able to gain access to healers whose forms of healing were not officially recognised. I also wanted to cover the traditional healing systems that were officially recognised by the Government of Sri Lanka and the state mechanism in place, this process

136 Neuman (1994), p 199.

also led to interviews with officials in government institutions all over the country. To supplement the interviews, participant observation was carried out in government institutions on traditional healing, traditional practices related to healing and traditional practices related to mental health and wellbeing.

Participant Observation

Participant observation aims to generate practical and theoretical truths about human life grounded in the realities of daily existence, by focusing on human meaning and interaction from the perspective the insiders or members of particular situations and settings.[137] Participant observation is located in the here and now of everyday life situations and settings as the foundation of inquiry and method.[138] In participant observation, the researcher performs a participant role that involves establishing and maintaining relationships with the subjects in the field; and uses direct observation along with other methods of gathering information. The process of inquiry is open-ended, flexible, opportunistic, and requires constant redefinition of what is problematic, based on facts gathered in concrete settings of human existence. Participant observation is used as a research tool in this study as it is an exploratory study[139] that examines healing and wellbeing practices, associated cultural attributes and the role of the Government of Sri Lanka.

In carrying out the participant observations, I observed and systematically recorded naturally occurring events as field notes, videos, or photos in order to later develop a hypobook about why they occured.[140] The following figures 1.15 to 1.20 are some examples of traditional knowledges, practices and expressions on healing and wellbeing I observed.

---

[137] The definition of participant observation is based on Jorgesen's features of Participant Observation. Jorgesen (1989), p 14.

[138] For purpose and techniques of participant observation, see- Lofland (1974); Lofland and Lofland (1995); Neuman (2000); Smith (1978).

[139] Jorgesen (1989), p 12 describes how participant observation is appropriate for exploratory studies, descriptive studies, and studies aimed at generating theoretical interpretations.

[140] Based on naturalistic observation definition in Graziano and Raulin (2004), p 125.

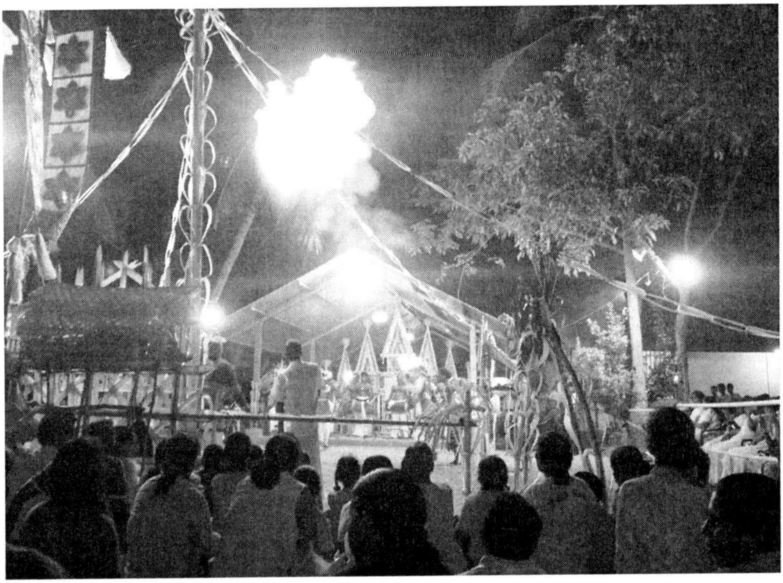

Figure 1.15 - Observed over-night Gammadu Shanthi Karma in Allen Mathiniyarama on 4 August 2012. Image taken by author.

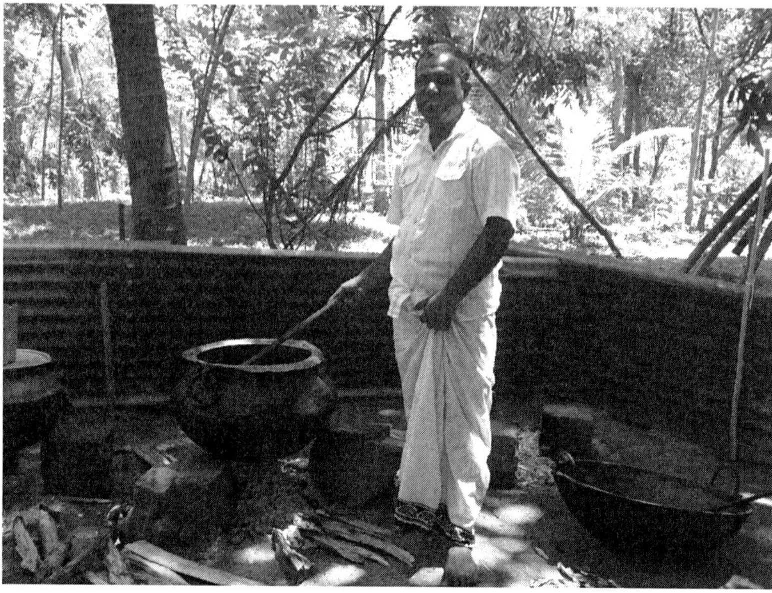

Figure 1.16 - Observed sacred methods of preparing medicine at Horiwila Medical Centre (for Kadum Bidum Wedakam/ Fractures and Dislocations) on 1 May 2013. Usually, indigenous medicine is not prepared in front of an outsider as they believe evil will affect the quality of the medicine. The healer who prepares the medicine avoids killi[141], bathes, dresses in clean clothes and worships before preparing medicine. Image taken by author.

[141] *Killi* is impurity. To avoid *killi* one becomes vegetarian, avoids funerals and homes of girls who have got their first menstruation. Daya Dissanayake (# 87).

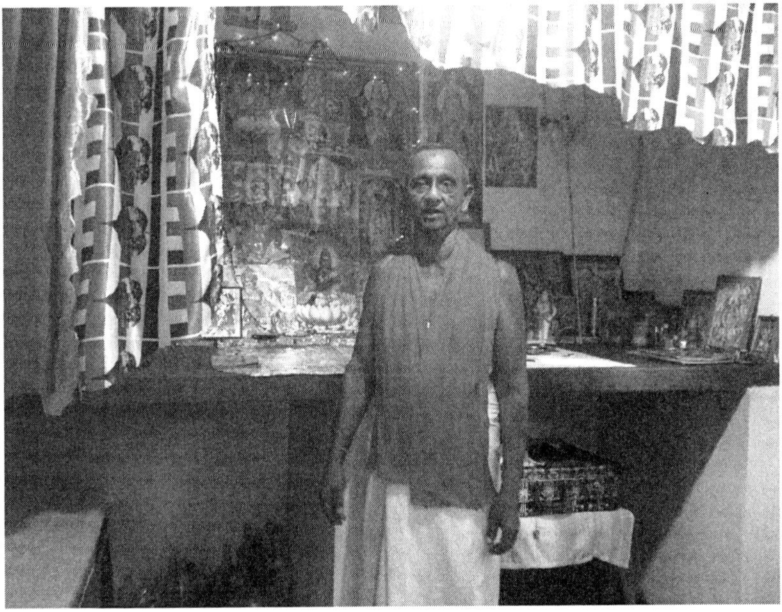

Figure 1.17 - Observed Astrologer and Ritual Healer P. D. Premachandra in 'Shanthi Sevana' Kurunegala, reading astrological predictions and performing rituals for the God on 8 August 2013. Image taken by author.

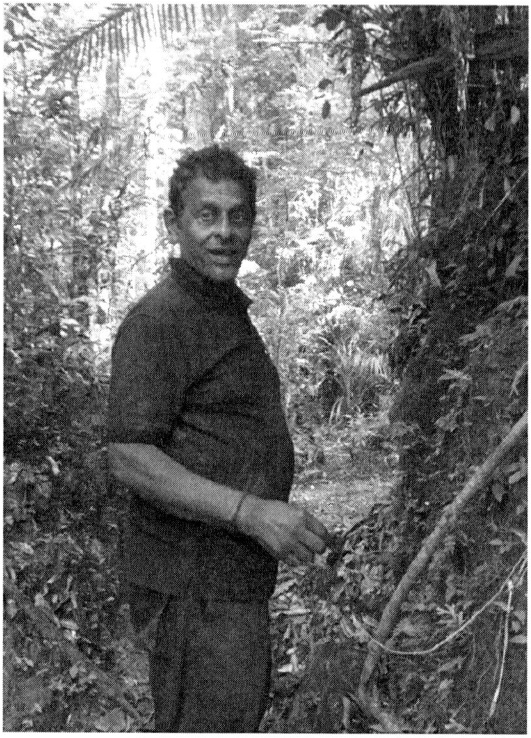

Figure 1.18 - Kalu mama, Indigenous Healer, Jungle Dweller, Guide to Sinharaja Forest Reserve. I went on a two-day hike in the Sinharaja forest reserve with Kalu mama, understanding traditional medical value of different plants and listening to stories of indigenous healing and the role of nature in healing. Image taken by author.

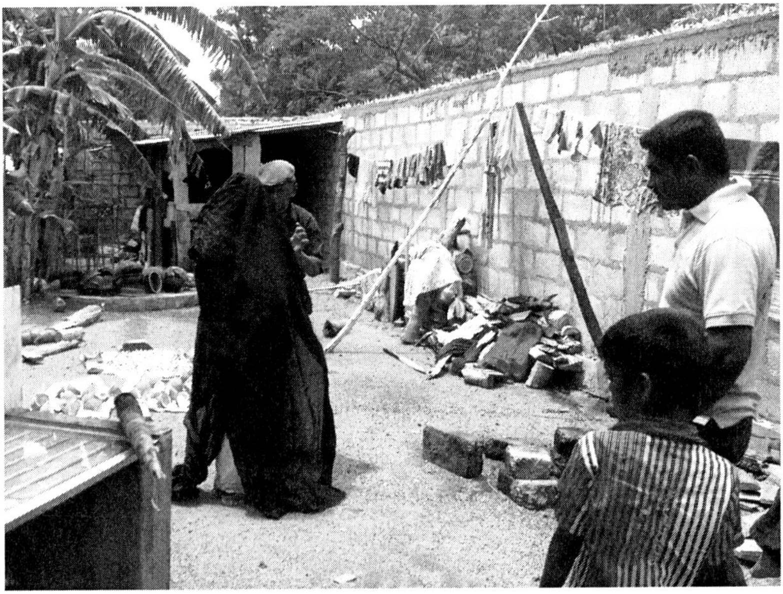

Figure 1.19 - Observed Mr. W. S. Pushpakumara performing various forms of exorcism in Anuradhpura full day on 30 July 2012. Before starting to observe, I had to obtain permission from the power of the spirit that helps him in performing exorcism. Image taken by author.

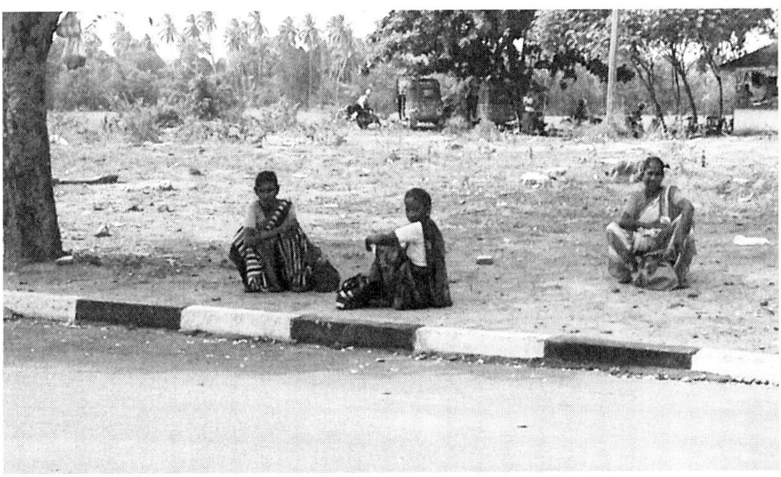

Figure 1.20 - Observed Thelangu Palm Readers, in Sri Maha Bodhiya, Anuradhapura. Image taken by author.

Participant observation on the government structure (all institutions and programmes mentioned above) were conducted to understand how the government mechanism works, from national to rural level, types and quality of services offered, power structures, community response towards government traditional health care services offered. Participant observation on healing practices and rituals (all practices documented in this book) were conducted to obtain a thorough understanding of the practice, its significance and impact on individuals and communities, and the strengths, weaknesses, opportunities and threats of such practices.

Interviews

The forms of interviews conducted can be categorised as key informant interviews and semi-structured interviews. Key-informant interviews are qualitative, in-depth interviews conducted with wide range of people who know what is going on in the community, and who could provide insight on the nature of problems and recommendations for solutions.[142] Key-informant interviews[143] were conducted to gather qualitative and background data from stakeholders, such as academics, policy makers, lawyers, who have an understanding of traditional knowledge systems in the country, traditional healing systems, government mechanism and relevant laws. Interviews were based on a framework of inquiry that was influenced by others, particularly Dutfield.[144]

Semi-structured interviews are qualitative informal interviews conducted by the interviewer in a conversational manner to elicit information from the interviewee on a list of pre-determined questions,[145] but the conversation is free to vary and is likely to change substantially between participants.[146] This technique was used to collect qualitative data from all the willing traditional knowledge bearers in healing and wellbeing. The focus of the semi-structured interviews was to gather information, source materials, opinions and references on traditional knowledge in health and wellbeing specific to Sri Lanka; and to understand subjective perspectives on the status of traditional knowledge. Open-ended questions without any

---

[142] UCLA Centre for Health Policy Research. Section 4: Key Informant Interviews. http://healthpolicy.ucla.edu/programs/health-data/trainings/documents/tw_cba23.pdf (last retrieved 19 February 2019)

[143] For more information on conducting interviews, see Neuman (2000), pp 344-380.

[144] Dutfield (2006).

[145] Longhurst (2010), p 103.

[146] Fylan (2005), p 65.

particular order were used to gather information.[147] Based on the answers given by the respondents, leading questions were asked giving them an opportunity to express their own worldview and to play an active role in the interview. Semi-structured interviews were used to allow the researcher flexibility to omit questions, change the order depending on the flow of conversation and to include additional questions when exploration of topics raised by participants was required.[148] The sensitive nature of the research, healers being sceptical of the kind of research and in some cases being unwilling to participate, were also some reasons to adopt semi-structured forms of interviews as this form allowed the freedom to adapt the interview structure to suit the situation.

Selection of interviewees

For both key-informant and semi-structured interviews I selected the sample by using a snowball cluster sampling method. This is a sampling method of collecting data from a subject/ or subjects of the target population that the researcher can locate, then asking those subjects for information to locate other members of that population whom they know. This technique was used as it was difficult to locate the members of the indigenous/ traditional healing population. I used the key- informant interview to gain a background understanding of the traditional healing system in Sri Lanka. The first set of interviews concentrated on academics/researchers, who have worked in the field of health, traditional healing, intellectual property, Sri Lankan history, culture, and senior government officials attached to Ministry of Indigenous Medicine at the national level. The sample for key-informant interviews was identified by web search and references from the persons I interviewed.

In order to identify my sample of healers for semi-structured interviews, I used the definition of healer as a person who contributes towards another person's mental, physical, spiritual and emotional health and wellbeing and is recognised by the community as a healer. I was given access to the database of traditional/ indigenous healers registered with the Ministry. This database was not properly updated and most addresses given in the database were wrong. In this database only very few phone numbers were available and, in most cases, given numbers did not work. I did not want to limit my sample to the healers registered in the Ministry as it did not cover the wide spectrum of indigenous/ traditional healers. Only the

---

[147] The Framework of Inquiry used is given in Appendix C.

[148] Eg, Saunders et al. (1997).

healers who passed the assessment conducted by the Ministry and who belonged to the clusters of healing identified by the Ministry were able to register as a healer. I realize there were many forms of rituals and healing methods in the country that have not been officially acknowledged. Rather than depending only on the references received from key-stakeholder interviews or the Ministry database, in each district, I spoke to the three-wheeler drivers, shop keepers in the area and the villagers to identify local healers. I also got references from the healers I interviewed. Figures 1.21 to 1.28 portray the diverse types of healers interviewed for the purpose of this study.

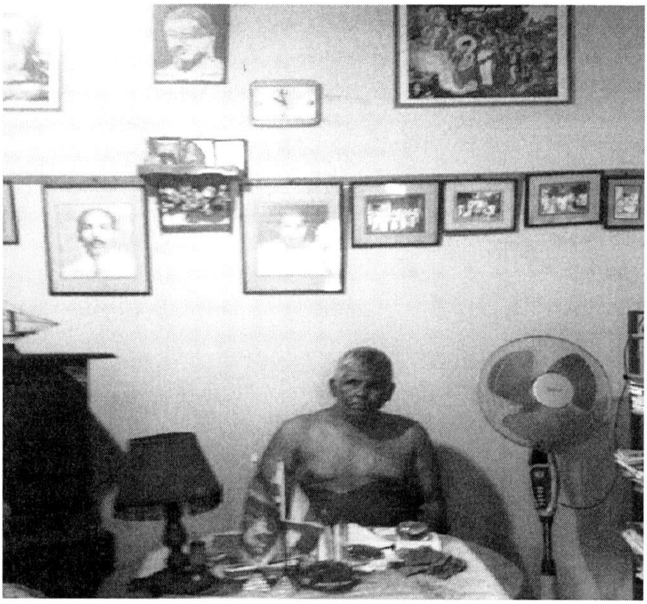

Figure 1.21 – Interviewed Mr. S. D. M. Mahipala, Inter-generational healer – Jalabithika and Sarpavisha, No. 221, Kandy Road, Aluthgama, Bogamuwa, Yakkala. He was explaining the difficulties of practicing indigenous healing due to the aspects of capitalization and extensive reliance of western scientific knowledge.

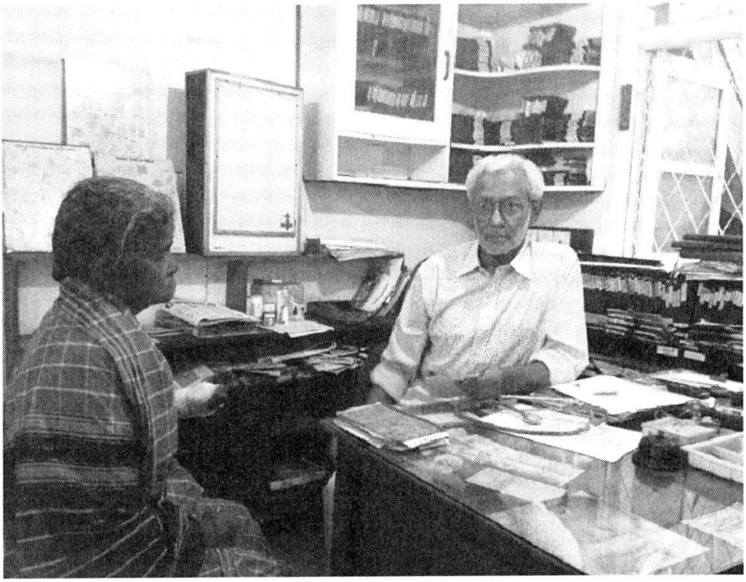

Figure 1.22 - Dr. Hameed A. Azeez, Visiting Lecturer, IIM University of Colombo and Azeez Medical Centre, Kandy Road, Mawanella (Unani, Ayurveda, Homeopathy) Interviewed Dr. Hameed about the medical system, observed how he manufactures medicine and treats patients.

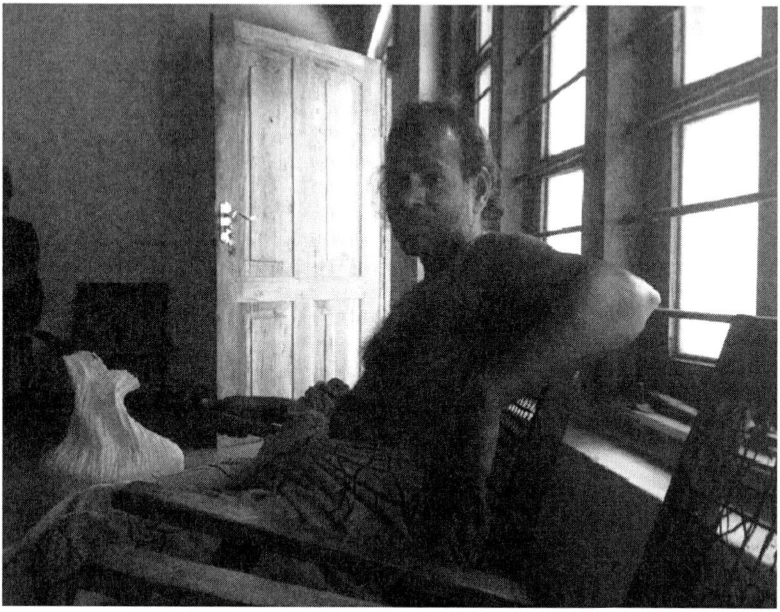

Figure 1.23 – Interviewed Mr. Dambane Gunawardena, First Vaddha Graduate and the Principal of Dambana Kanishta Vidyalaya, Dambana. He was explaining how the long history of efforts in mainstreaming the Vaddha population and integrating to the Sinhala and Tamil communities have affected the maintenance of the cultural diversity and the distinctive rituals in health and wellbeing.

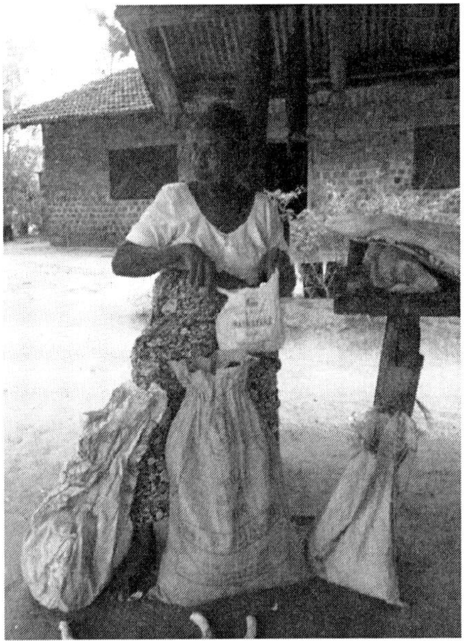

Figure 1.24 – Interviewed Mrs. W. M. Anulawathie, who lives in a very rural location in Meegahapitiya, Mahiyanganaya. She is an indigenous healer 'Kadum Bidum' (Traditional Orthopaedics) and 'Iru Rudhawa' (Headaches due to the effects of the Sun). The parcels in the ground and what she is holding are herbs she has collected from the jungle, that she uses as ingredients to prepare medicine.

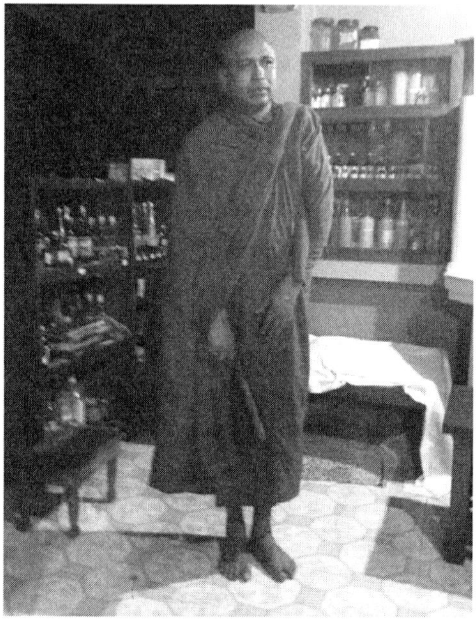

Figure 1.25 - Ven. Wellawatte Seelagawesi Thero, Sri Sumedha Meditation Centre, Gomaraya Road, Thawalanthanna (Physical and Mental Healing through Spirituality). Being a very popular healer with an extremely busy schedule, it was very difficult to obtain an appointment. I had to stay for three hours to meet the Rev monk. Then after fifteen minutes, Rev had to go for a protection in a house and he invited us to join. After the protection, Ven. introduced me to several patients he has healed. For the interview with the monk afterwards, we went to the place Rev was staying the night and the interview lasted for three hours. It was past midnight when we finished the interview. Rev explained about all forms of spiritual healing he performs.

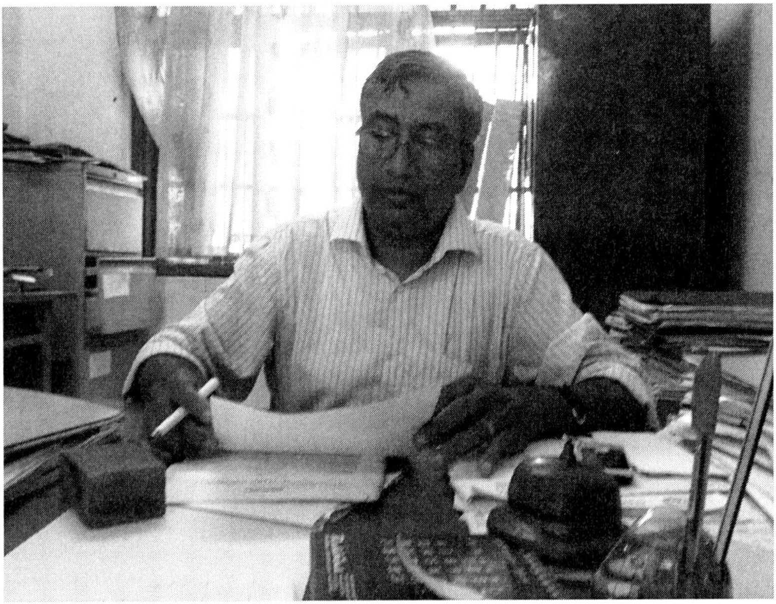

Figure 1.26 - Interviewed Dr. S. Sivashanmugarajah, Head, Department of Siddha Medicine, University of Jaffna on academic administration of traditional healing.

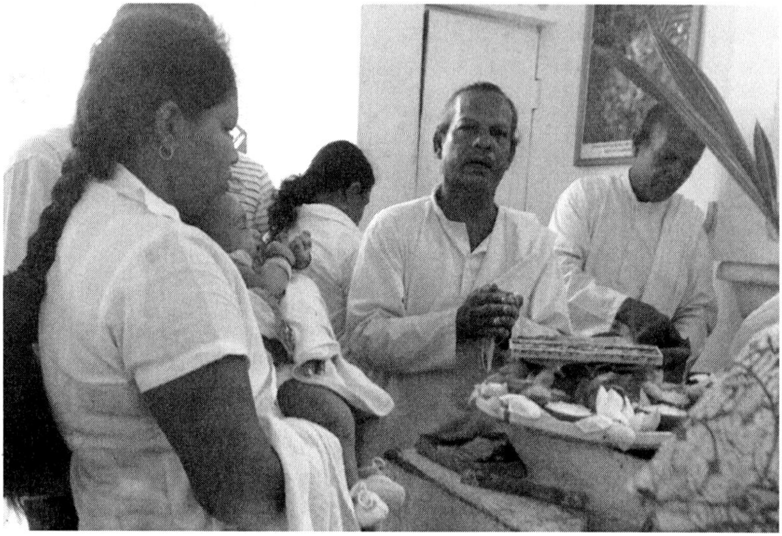

Figure 1.27 – Interviewed Mr. R. P. Udayapala, Kapu Mahaththaya, Sri Maha Bodhiya, Anuradhapura. He explained the historical role of the Kapu Mahathaya and current day practices in making vows on behalf or devotees and performing rituals for mental and physical wellbeing.

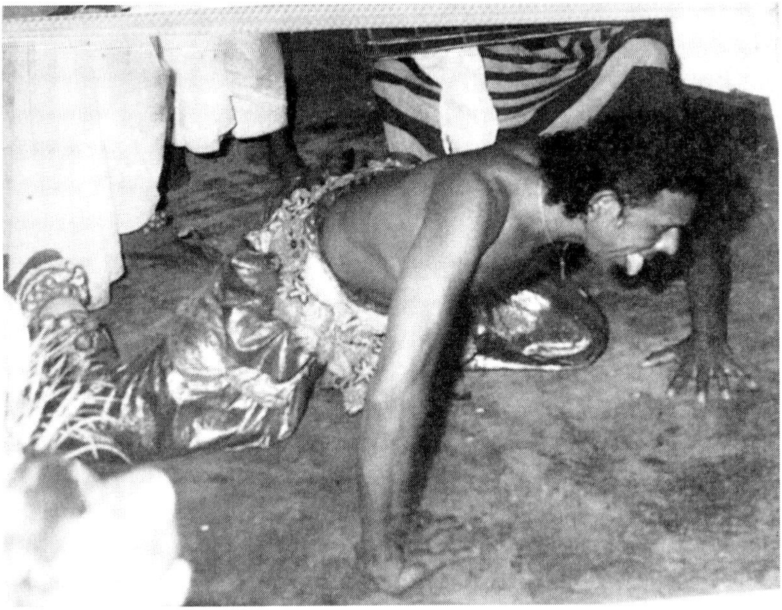

Figure 1.28 – Interviewed Ambalangoda Kapu Mahathaya, Sri Murthi Devalaya, Devalaya Gedera, Theriyagama, Kataragama; who predicts the problems from the power of spirits and performs rituals for protection.

Method of conducting interviews

I conducted all the interviews in person, face-to-face. Most of the key-informant interviews were conducted after I had contacted the interviewee by calling or emailing, explained the research and scheduled an appointment. Even with prior scheduled appointments, on many occasions I had to wait for hours before I could get the opportunity to interview government officials.

As I did not have any contact details for the indigenous and traditional healers outside the Sri Lankan government structure, I had to visit them in person to get an appointment. Some healers lived in very remote, rural locations that were 5-10 kilometres away from the nearest accessible place for public transport. In some cases, I had to walk a few kilometres, as there was no vehicular access. When I visited the places of healing, I stayed in the queue for my turn to speak to the healer. I also observed the practices and rituals conducted in the treatment centre.

It was extremely difficult to get an opportunity to meet popular, traditional/ indigenous healers. There were instances where I went four or five times (sometimes joining a queue that did not eventuate in an appointment, other times being told that the healer was too busy and sent home) before I got an opportunity to interview. Then some days I would spend a whole day in the treatment centre before I managed to talk with the interviewee. Traditional healers are much respected in Sri Lankan society. This respect and honour are the greatest tributes to the healer[149] and are based on the trust and faith in the healer, due to their skills, morality, ethicality, divine ability and connection, holistic approach to treatment and kindness.[150] Most of them did not specify any fees for their treatment. I wanted to give my due respect, but I also did not want to intrude on their practice.

Most of the time, I went without any introductions or references. I had to do a self-introduction to the healer. I wanted to be as humble as possible and develop a positive relationship with them. It is interesting that when it came to interviewing spirit-healers, I had to obtain permission not only from the healer him/ herself, but also from the spirit power. I did not make any financial payments for the time they spent with me.

Recording and Transcribing Interviews

The answers given by the respondents were recorded in their own words. I took free-form notes of the interviews and also audio or video recorded the interviews on an Apple tablet using the Evernote app[151] or audio recorder. In most instances, when a traditional or indigenous healer was interviewed, the person interviewed and his/ her form of healing practices were photographed and/or videoed.

The digitally recorded interviews were uploaded to the author's computer and then transcribed. All interview data were transcribed within a week of being recorded, when the memory of the interview was still clear. After transcribing the interviews, I went through the transcription and the recording to ensure I had not missed important information. When I discovered there was missing information, I had to re-visit the healer to clarify the data. There were also times when I ran out of battery or memory

---

[149] Interview with H. D. Karunawathie (# 53), P. Weerasinghe (# 52), R. M. D. J. Gunasekera (# 58), Ghana Manio (#60).

[150] Interview with Ven. Wellawatte Seelagawesi (#66), H. N. Nandasena Herath (#68), P. Weerasinghe (# 52), W. S. Pushpakumara (# 61), Je Jeyalan (# 100).

[151] Evernote https://evernote.com/ (last retrieved 19 February 2019).

space in the recording device and at such interviews I had to depend on my unstructured notes.

Transcription was verbatim and completed only by myself to ensure accuracy and security of data. In addition, the process of transcription or the process of validating transcripts by listening to the recordings and verifying the transcripts provided me with the opportunity to undertake the first analysis of the interview data. Patton suggests that analysis is an iterative process beginning with transcription[152] and the process of listening. The process of listening, typing, listening again and checking the transcription is one in which the researcher becomes familiar with the phrasing, ideas, and nuances of what is being said as well how it is said, which is an important aspect of qualitative analysis. During transcription, I noted, and highlighted trends and themes. Following transcription, the data were checked for accuracy by listening to the digital recording while simultaneously reading the transcription.

Interview Schedule

July 2012 to February 2013 was spent on field research. I started from Trincomalee, Eastern Province of Sri Lanka. When trying to interview government registered officials, I realised I could not proceed till I obtain permission from the Ministry of Indigenous Medicine. As a result, I had to come back to Colombo. It took 3 weeks to obtain the required clearance from the Ministry of Indigenous Medicine. I then covered the North Central Province which included Habarana, Polonnaruwa, Sigiriya, Dambulla, Horiwilla and Anuradhapura (I made more than 4 visits to Anuradhapura alone during 2012 - 2013. Each visit lasted a minimum of one week. Being the ancient capital in Sri Lanka, there are many forms of indigenous knowledge on healing practiced in Anuradhapura. I also covered Galle, Matara, Hambantota and Kataragama in the Southern Province and Kitulgala and Rathapura in the Sabaragamuwa Province during this period.

As I did not want to rely only on official and known sources to identify traditional healers and healing practices, I was keen on finding out various forms of healing that were not recognized officially. In order to identify these healers, I depended on three-wheeler drivers, the local community and references by the traditional healers themselves. Most of the healers were located in very rural, remote locations. Negotiating access to these healers was a very time-consuming process. The quality of data and time they would allocate for an interview would depend on their trust and

---

[152] Patton (2002).

liking of me. I was aware of the impacts of being a female researcher trying to enter and interview a domain dominated by males (most indigenous healers I came across were men), and not having any influence among the traditional healers. I used public transport (buses, trains), walking and three wheelers to travel and patiently waited with the other patients for my turn to introduce myself and to interview the healer. As I did not have access to their telephone numbers, it was not possible for me to obtain prior appointments. Being able to talk in the same language as the healers, and being able to relate to their religious orientation and cultural practices facilitated in interacting with the healers.

Sometimes, I spent several days interviewing one healer. The time spent with the interviewer was never limited for the sake of interviewing. Sometimes I spent days and nights observing one healing practice and trying to grasp its effects and the healer's relationship with the community.[153] The worldviews of the indigenous healers were varied, diverse and different from Western expectations. Being a person trained in Western education and worldview, I was keen to see the world through their lenses.

After the initial phase of field research, I realised there are many more hidden traditional/ indigenous knowledge systems in the country that are not recognized anywhere. I felt that I had only found the tip of the iceberg of traditional healing and wellbeing methods. I came to Australia in February 2013 for my early candidature presentation and then returned to the field.

The next phase of field work started with trying to understand the existing government structure in indigenous healing and wellbeing (March to June 2013). This included the Ministry of Indigenous Medicine, the Department of Ayurveda, Ayurveda Drug Control Board, Ayurveda Medical Council, Provincial Ayurveda Departments, Bandaranaike Ayurveda Research Institute, Ayurveda Teaching Hospitals, District Ayurveda Hospitals, Rural Ayurveda Hospitals, the National Institute of Traditional Medicine, the Indigenous Institute of Medicine, Wickramarachichi Institute of Siddha Medicine, Kereminiya School of Ayurveda, Pirivena Ayurveda Schools, Herbal Gardens, etc. The key institutions of the government structure are based in Colombo and the outskirts (Western Province). From July to September 2013, my focus was primarily indigenous and traditional healing methods that are not associated with the Government, but of course I visited the government institutes in the cities I covered during this period. Field locations covered during the period include, North Western Province

[153] For example, Gammadu Shanthi Karma, Devol Madu Shanthi Karma, overnight Pirith Ceremony, Protection Ceremony for houses, Tovil and Exorcism rituals.

(Chillaw, Puttlam), Central Province (Kandy, Peradeniya, Pallakelle, Bandarawela), Uva Province (Badulla, Mahiyanganaya, Dambana) Eastern Province (Maduru Oya, Ampara, Batticaloa).

I returned to Sri Lanka in mid-November 2013 to complete the archive research and field work in the Northern Province.

In order to clarify some information, I had gathered through interviews, I had to revisit some sessional papers, historical legal documents in the National Archives and the National Library. It was frustrating in many instances to find out many of the records of sessional papers I was looking for after a manual search were not released to the public as the volumes were not in good condition. Also, I tried to refer to original manuscripts including palm leaves on various forms of traditional healing at the Archives, Pirivena Libraries, Institute of Indigenous Medicine library and the Ayurveda Research Institute. Referring to and understanding what is written in original manuscripts was not an easy task as it was written in Pali or in old Sinhala language which was quite different to the language we currently use in Sri Lanka.

I postponed the field work in the North to the last stage of my field research because the Northern community is pre-dominantly Tamil speaking and their culture, traditions and healing systems are quite distinct from the rest of the country. I needed to depend on translators to communicate with most of the healers in the Northern Province.

Data Analysis

Grounded theory[154] is the theoretical approach used to understand and interpret findings of field research.[155] Grounded theory begins with observations.[156] Based on the observations, patterns, themes, or common categories are proposed.[157] The analysis in grounded theory is not set up to confirm or disconfirm specific hypobook, but to analyse and to interpret the grounded findings. In a grounded theory approach, researchers' preconceived

---

[154] Grounded theory was developed by Glaser and. Strauss (1965), (1967).

[155] Grounded theory as explained by Kathy Charmaz 'consists of systematic, yet flexible guidelines for collecting and analyzing qualitative data to construct theories 'grounded' in the data themselves.' Charmaz (2006), p 2.

[156] To develop theoretical analysis, Grounded theory collects data from the beginning of the project. Charmaz (2006), p 2. Sampling for data collection is not aimed at population representativeness but theory construction.

[157] To do so, analytical codes and categories are constructed from data and constant a comparative method is used to analyse in each stage while memo-writing is used to elaborate each category. Glaser and Strauss (1967); Glaser (1978); Strauss (1987).

ideas or expectations will shape the new search for generalities. The openness of the grounded theory approach allows increased analytical power[158] and a greater chance for discovering the unexpected.[159] Analysis in grounded theory uses inductive reasoning moving from the particular to the general, from a set of specific observations to the discovery of a pattern that represents some degree of order among all the given events.[160]

I used content and discourse analysis to analyse the evidence gathered from the archival and field studies. Using the content analysis technique,[161] the content message and meanings of historical, records and interview were analysed. The technique enabled me to understand and interpret the historical records and the interviews in light of social change and political will to protect and safeguard traditional knowledge.

Discourse analysis is analysing written, vocal or sign language use or any semiotic event beyond the sentence boundary to naturally occurring language use.[162] This aim is to reveal socio-psychological characteristics of a person/ group of people.[163] Discourse analysis was conducted on the reported projects implemented by various institutions on safeguarding traditional knowledge in healing and wellbeing, interview notes, participant observations in order to consciously, deliberately, systematically and objectively note and produce accounts of what their investigations have revealed.

To integrate the field work into the book, I have used a uniform, systematic method to refer to interviews. I have used the name of the healer and number of the interview (in brackets as footnotes) for each interview referred to in the book. [164] These numbers in full are provided in 'Annex– list of interviews completed.' The annex provides details of the interview including name of the healer, designation, organisation if applicable, contact details, subject of the interview, date of interview and the place of interview.

---

[158] Bigus, Hadden & Glaser (1994); Charmaz, (1983), (1990), (1995b), (2003), (2006); Glaser, (1992), (1994); Glaser & Strauss, (1967); Stern, (1994b); Strauss, (1987); Strauss & Corbin, (1990), (1994).

[159] Babbie (1998), p 283. Also see Atkinson, Coffey and Delamont (2003).

[160] Babbie (1998), p 35.

[161] It is a technique to analyse the content of the text. For general survey, Neuman (2000), p 292-294; Holsti (1968); Stone et al. (1966).

[162] Cutting (2002).

[163] Cutting (2002).

[164] Although I have adopted Australian Guide for Legal Citation (AGLC) for referencing, due to extensive number of interviews, I have adopted a slightly differenct format to cite the interviews. According to AGLC (2010) p. 114, interviews conducted by author is cited as 'Interview with (Name of the Interviewee), (Location and Form of Interview, Full Date)'

I have contextualized interviewees' comments only when it is relavent and necessary to provide the background for the argument. In many cases it was not necessary or possible to contextualize the interviewee considering the word limit of the book and relavence for the argument.

Ethical Considerations

The study strictly adhered to Griffith University's Code for the Responsible Conduct of Research.[165] Before implementing the study, in accordance with Griffith University policy, an ethical application was submitted for expedited ethical review to the Human Research Ethics Committee. Approval was obtained on 25 May 2012.[166]

An information sheet on the research containing detailed explanation of the research inquiries, including project aims, process of data collection, strategies to maintain confidentiality, possible intervention measures and ethical obligations of the researcher and consent form was developed in English, Sinhala and Tamil. All subjects of the research were given a copy of the information sheet in the preferred language, the research was explained and written consent was obtained before conducting an interview.

Consent

Consent was an essential part of this research. There were a number of steps to obtain this. I explained the research to all interviewees, gave them a copy of the information sheet in the language they were familiar with and requested them to sign the consent form before starting the interview. Some interviewees signed the forms before starting the interview, most said they would sign the forms after the interview, while others refused to sign a written document. It is interesting that the extent of consent I received from the interviewee was vastly different. Some interviewees did not want to give consent at all to conduct an interview. Some interviewees did not want the interviews to be audio or video recorded, while some interviewees did not want me to even take notes on the interview.

---

[165] Griffith University Code for Responsible Conduct of Research See- https://policies.griffith.edu.au/pdf/The%20Responsible%20Conduct%20of%20Research.pdf (last retrieved 19 February 2019).

[166] Griffith University Human Research Ethics – http://www.griffith.edu.au/research/research-services/research-ethics-integrity/human (last retrieved 19 February 2019).

Limitations of the Study

There were limitations and difficulties faced in conducting the field work; analysing a large number of interviews, translation of interviews, ownership of knowledge, and in adopting a multi-disciplinary approach for the research.

My field work of conducting interviews and participant observations had limitations. At first, interviewees were reluctant to talk to and at times refused to participate in the interviews. The reasons stated for nonparticipation included the knowledge not being owned by an individual, but a group, and the indigenous healers being only the custodians of the knowledge. As a result, they were reluctant to share their knowledge openly. I also came across many cases where traditional healers were willing to share information but were not willing to sign the consent form. Traditional healing is usually practiced in an informal atmosphere. They do not believe in formalizing their form of practice. Entering into a written consent even for an interview is a form of formalizing and a few healers rejected signing a written document. The officials attached to the government feared whether there will be a conflict between the official stance vs. private voice. There were many interviewees who were concerned that I was attached to a foreign university and whether their knowledge might be stolen. Figure 3.20 portrays a field experience on which difficulties were faced in obtaining consent from an indigenous cancer healer.

On 16 August 2013, I met a very popular traditional healer for cancer in Balangoda. It was quite difficult to find her address as she lived in a very remote area. A one-way trip alone took me five hours of driving. This lady was about 75 years old. She was very kind and gave me an interview for more than one and a half hours. Before the interview, I explained the research to her and gave her the informed consent form. She said she would sign the informed consent after the interview as she didn't have a pair of specks with her.

Just as I completed the interview and when she was about to sign the informed consent form, three of her daughters who lived in the neighbourhood came in with about six neighbours and started shouting at me. I tried to explain what I was doing to them, but they didn't want to listen. They scolded me using bad language and ordered me to leave immediately. They saw me as a thief trying to steal their mother's traditional knowledge.

'We are not interested in sharing our knowledge.'

'Our mother is innocent. But we won't let people like you take unwanted advantage'

'This is secret knowledge. We don't want to share with anybody. Definitely not with a stranger'

'We are doing this for charity and are not interested in safeguarding it…or continuing it… we don't want anyone's help…please let us survive alone…this is the way we would like it to be sustained...'

'Please go away without trying to put our mother into trouble. If you want to do research, please go to the Ayurveda hospital or the Ministry of Indigenous medicine, we are innocent people… and this is a secret private practice that we don't want to share with an outsider. We don't want publicity; we don't want authenticity… we do it for spirituality.'

Figure 1.29 - Obtaining Consent from the Indigenous Cancer healer

Conducting field research also involved inherent unexpected risk. Figure 3.21 relates a field experience in which this was experienced

In many of my visits to study healing and healers I encountered some of the most remarkable men and women… Not all of them were friendly but without exception they all had knowledge that was not available in the public domain. During such a memorable field visit I almost became possessed by the spirits that were being expelled from possessed people who had come to visit a very erudite monk. He had in fact initially declined an interview when I visited him. He said 'I do not wish to share the knowledge I have accumulated with a scholar writing a book for a foreign university'. It all started when the monk healer declined to give an interview and I decided to climb a hill in his temple. Without my knowledge, I was walking in the same path that he would drive the spirits out of the possessed in the air.

My research into traditional health involved interviewing men and women with super natural powers. During a visit to Mountain in Hindagala, a Buddhist monk was in the process of dispelling evil spirits from men and women who came from around Sri Lanka to see him. The spirits were expelled in the direction of a mountain top. Not knowing this I started to climb this mountain with my son when I was rudely stopped by the monk's assistant. I started to argue with him that this was a common mountain. When I resisted, he screamed at me, saying, to come down immediately. And he went inside… another man told me that this is where the man who come with spirits are dispelled… the spirits need a body to survive and as I was with a small child, the child could possess the spirit… from this moment onwards I was feeling bad and guilty for bringing little Anuk with me.

There is inherent risk of participation observation research of healers and healing.

Figure 1.30 - A Field Experience

The number of interviews was very large due to the study being exploratory research, depending on a snowball sampling method to identify the respondents and geographic coverage of the research included all 25 districts of Sri Lanka. Due to the extensive number of interviews, translating and analysing, the interviews were a very tedious process.

Being a multi-linguist country, although I needed to depend on translators for interviewing traditional healers speaking Tamil, Malayalam, Telagu and Vaddha creole; I had unprecedented access to Sinhala speaking indigenous and traditional healers being a Sinhalese and being accustomed to the culture, value and practices of the Sinhala community.

The study was not intended to be an anthropological study but as a result of the lack of information on various healing methods, I had to do field work to obtain basic information. This, therefore, is a multi-disciplinary study covering history, politics, culture, society and law. I have conducted field work in all the nine provinces in Sri Lanka.

One of the major limitations faced in analysing and writing the book was the fact that there were contested definitions of concepts such as traditional knowledge, traditional cultural expressions, indigenous identity, authentic culture and traditional culture. In Chapter 1, 1.5, I have tried to explain the contested definitions and the meaning I have adopted for the purpose of the book: emphasizing that the book is not a legal or doctrinal analysis.

Part 7: Overview of the Book

This book argues that all forms of healing practices in Sri Lanka are significant. These healing practices matter not only because of their value in the health and wellbeing of the community, but also because they strongly contribute towards the intangible cultural heritage of Sri Lanka going forward. Identifying the diverse forms of healing practices existing in the country and the role of the existing regulatory mechanisms broadens the potential of protecting the diversity of healing. The book answers the research question 'What role doed the recognition, support and regulation of the Government of Sri Lanka in healing and wellbeing practices play in determining, promoting, protecting or destroying the cultural aspect of healing?'

To understand the diversity of healing and wellbeing practices, interviews and observations were conducted with anyone who claimed to contribute to the health and wellbeing of people. They include shamans, exorcists, astrologers, palm readers, healing monks, spiritual healers, Ayurvedic doctors, Siddha doctors, Unani doctors, ritual dancers, indigenous

Vaddha healers and various forms of indigenous healers. A total of 117 interviews were conducted in all the nine provinces of Sri Lanka, contributing towards the rich body of knowledge of health and wellbeing practices in Sri Lanka. In addition, this book draws on archival sources located in Sri Lanka on diverse practices related to health and wellbeing and the role of regulatory mechanisms.

Despite Sri Lanka being historically rich in traditional knowledge and expression, very little, if anything, has been written on regulating traditional practices related to health and wellbeing in Sri Lanka.[167] This book is important because it illustrates the diverse forms of knowledge systems that exist in Sri Lanka, the identification of which is essential in order to find ways and means to protect these knowledge systems and cultural heritage.

Chapter 2 titled 'Recognising and regulating practices related to health and wellbeing,' aims to recognise the regulating practices related to health and wellbeing in Sri Lanka. First, the chapter provides an overview of some of the schemes dealing, at least in some way, with traditional practices related to health and wellbeing. Then, the chapter will provide a brief overview of the international negotiations of traditional knowledge and traditional cultural expressions, particularly as they relate to recognising the right of indigenous peoples to self-determination, access and benefit sharing and intellectual property. First, the chapter traces the development of the protection regime in traditional knowledge from the recognition of rights to self-determination of indigenous peoples to calls for the safeguarding and protection of traditional knowledge, expression and practice, as well as for sharing the benefits resulting from the exploitation of traditional knowledge, expression and practice. Second, Sri Lanka's attempts to recognise and regulate traditional practices related to health and wellbeing are discussed by examining Sri Lanka's role in international institutions, Sri Lanka's domestic laws related to health and wellbeing and how the

---

[167] Some notable exceptions include Sri Lanka being a contracting party to many international instruments protecting traditional knowledge, developing a legal framework for the protection of traditional knowledge in Sri Lanka, having intellectual property law and a regulation mechanism in place, (see: WIPO- Sri Lanka - http://www.wipo.int/wipolex/en/profile.jsp?code=LK last retrieved 19 February 2019) implementing few cultural heritage laws in Sri Lanka, (see: UNESCO – Sri Lanka – http://www.unesco.org/new/en/unesco/worldwide/Asia%20and%20the%20Pacific/sri%20lanka last retrieved 19 February 2019 and Department of Ayurveda documenting the Ayurveda Pharmacopeia. (Kumar: 2000).

regulation of health and wellbeing is affected by colonialism, globalisation and current revival efforts.

Chapter 3, 4 and 5 are based on the empirical data I collected from the field. Chapter 3 titled 'Diversity of Healing Practices in Sri Lanka' concerns what healing practices are considered and used in Sri Lanka. To answer this question, this chapter examines various kinds of traditional healing in Sri Lanka. It identifies the diversity of healing practices used which include inter-generational practices adopted from other countries, cosmically-oriented healing practices, Western healing practices, practices using mixed methods, and a variety of less recognised and uncategorisable kinds of healing practices. This chapter has three parts. The first part describes government recognized traditional healing practices in Sri Lanka, namely Ayurveda, Siddha, Unani, Homeopathy, Acupuncture, and Deshiya Chikithsa. In so doing, it discusses the diversity of engagements within and between the practices. The second part outlines and briefly discusses the diversity of healing practices in Sri Lanka. In this part, the diversity of healing practices will be presented by mapping the forms of healing practiced in Sri Lanka using the categories of inter-generational healing, cosmic healing, adopted traditional healing, Western healing and integrated healing. The third part of the chapter describes the typology of relations between different forms of healing knowledges. The chapter is important as it sets the stage for the book by presenting the diversity and complexities of the prevailing healing systems in Sri Lanka and by questing for the definition of 'traditional' in healing practices and also in arguing that only some systematic healing practices are recognised and regulated by the Government of Sri Lanka.

Sri Lanka's health and wellbeing is a complicated mix of traditional and 'Western' practices. Chapter 4 on 'The Sri Lankan Government Support for Traditional Health and Wellbeing Practices in Sri Lanka' looks at how the Sri Lankan government has dealt with traditional health and wellbeing practices. The chapter first traces the history of government support for traditional medicine in Sri Lanka. Then it portrays how the government is administrating these traditional health care practices. Thirdly the role in systematising education in traditional healing is discussed. Subsequently, the government initiatives in establishing and maintaining curative services of traditional medicine are presented and then how the traditional medicine is regulated by the government, and government involvement in promoting traditional healing research and herbal gardens. Finally, the role of the government in promoting traditional community health care is discussed.

Chapter 5 is 'Inter-Generational Healing and Loss of Culture' which examines inter-generational healing in Sri Lanka, and argues that inter-generational healing in Sri Lanka is facing the threat of losing its cultural heritage aspects due, in large part, to Government interventions in recognizing, supporting and regulating healing practices. More specifically, this chapter presents cases of diverse inter-generational healing practices of Sri Lanka which are partially recognized by the Sri Lankan government such as *Sarvanga* (physicians), *Kadum Bidum* (orthopaedic), *Akshi Roga* (eye disease), *Anshabaga* (stroke and paralysis), *Pilika* (cancer), *Visa* (toxicology), and *Adivasi Vedakama* (tribal medicine). In so doing, the chapter tries to understand and recognise different forms of inter-generational healing practices, the nature of the healing practices and the nature and impact of government recognition, support and regulation on the healing practice. The chapter has three parts. Part 1 argues inter-generational healing is diverse, unstructured, informal and part of cultural heritage of Sri Lanka, by presenting reflections. Part 2 argues that largely due to the diverse, unstructured and informal character of inter-generational healing, inter-generational healers are faced with many challenges. These challenges include, lack of employment opportunities, secretive knowledge, inappropriate treatment by the fovernment and formal education. Part 3 further argues that government intervention in inter-generational healing threatens the rich and diverse cultural heritage of healing, due to approaches followed in systematizing and mainstreaming the diverse healing system. The conclusion of the chapter analyses how inter-generational healing practice could be strengthened in the country in a way so that the healing system and the traditional cultural aspects are protected.

Chapter 6, presents my concluding remarks. This chapter has five parts. The first part summarises the findings. The second part discusses observations based on the findings in this book. The third part is on the main concerns related to knowledge and practices related to health and wellbeing in Sri Lanka. The fourth part of the conclusion points out the limitations of this research. Finally, the fifth part presents recommendations for future work.

CHAPTER 2

RECOGNISING AND REGULATING TRADITIONAL PRACTICES RELATED TO HEALTH AND WELLBEING

Introduction

Traditional practices related to health and wellbeing are socially, culturally and economically important to many communities and individuals.[1] While these traditional practices are entrenched within many societies, they have particular significance for indigenous and local communities, where practice related to health and wellbeing continues to play a vital role in everyday life, interaction with nature and development of spirituality.

This chapter aims to recognise the regulating of traditional practices related to health and wellbeing in Sri Lanka in a legal pluralism context. The chapter starts with Kalu mama's story that highlights the importance of traditional practices related to health and wellbeing to local communities and provides a brief overview of concerns related to protecting traditional practices related to health and wellbeing. Then the chapter is presented in four parts. In the first part of the chapter a brief overview of some of the schemes dealing, at least in some way, with traditional practices related to health and wellbeing at the international level is provided. A discussion of the international negotiations of traditional knowledge and traditional cultural expressions, particularly as they relate to recognising the right of indigenous peoples to self-determination, access and benefit sharing and intellectual property then follows. To do this, the chapter traces the development of the protection regime in traditional knowledge from the recognition of rights to self-determination of indigenous peoples to calls for the safeguarding and protection of traditional knowledge, expression and practice, as well as for sharing the benefits resulting from their exploitation. The second part of the chapter focuses on Sri Lanka's attempts to recognise

[1] See, for example, World Intellectual Property Organization General Assembly (2000), p 71; Bubela and Gold (eds) (2012); Wiessner, (2008), p 1141.

and regulate traditional practices related to health and wellbeing. This part examines Sri Lanka's role in international institutions and the domestic laws related to health and wellbeing. The third part of the chapter discusses how the regulation of health and wellbeing is affected by colonialism. Finally, the fourth part of the chapter is on revitalisation efforts of traditional knowledge and its impact on the traditional healing and wellbeing practices of Sri Lanka. This chapter revels, that traditional healing is often based on individual relationship between healer and the patient, and as a result protecting traditional practices using Western ideas of tangible or intangible property results in traditional cultural aspects of healing being threatened and indigenous healing methods being neglected.

Many indigenous and local communities in Sri Lanka have developed a holistic relationship with their surroundings and habitat, particularly related to food, medicine, building material and handicraft.[2] Furthermore, the habitat in which the indigenous and local communities live is very closely interrelated with culture, beliefs, spirituality, and identity which in turn contribute towards a sense of belonging and self-determination. Kalu mama's story is a good example.

Kalu mama,[3] a 68-year-old villager from Lankagama, Southern Province, Sri Lanka, bordering the Sinharaja forest reserve has been living near the jungle all his life. Although he has not received a formal school education, he has developed a strong understanding of natural healing methods, plants and animals by interacting with nature. During my time with him, Kalu mama guided me in the Sinharaja forest, introducing me to rare and endemic plants, animals and medical values. We walked almost 20 kilometres over two days. As we walked, he explained how the villagers depend on natural remedies for their health and wellbeing:

> the fresh food, fresh air and the fresh water we can access here keep us healthy. We are used to a simple and nutritious diet, plenty of exercise and an easy-going, simple lifestyle with minimum needs. Our habitat and lifestyle keep us healthy. Even when we are sick, nature protects us. We

---

[2] Vishwakeerthi Vanaspathi Uru Walige Wanniya Attho (# 18). Also see, Kipuri (2009), pp 51-78. In her chapter on Culture of the World's Indigenous Peoples Kipuri presents the holistic relationship of indigenous people with their surroundings. The Gene Campaign movement also argue the interdependent relationship of indigenous community with their surroundings. http://genecampaign.org/indigenous-knowledge/ (last retrieved 19 February 2019).

[3] Kalu mama (# 89).

> have simple remedies for the common ailments and diseases of our community which we make from herbs we get from our habitat. [4]

Kalu mama also inducted me to various *Manthra* (sacred verbal formula repeated in prayer, meditation, or incantation, such as an invocation of a god, a magic spell), *Bara* (vows) and *Kem Krama* (practices conducted based on faith, for protection) used by the forest dwellers, for sickness, wellbeing and to catch animals.[5]

By interacting with their surroundings and habitat, the members of indigenous and local communities, like Kalu mama, continue to identify natural remedies and medicine. The ancestors of Kalu mama's village of Lankagama[6] are leprosy patients. As there has been no treatment for leprosy, and as it was believed to be a deadly and infectious disease, the past practice was for the sick to be isolated in Lankagama.[7] Lankagama has also been a part of the forest without road access to human habitats, and thus access to medical facilities, groceries or household items. These leprosy patients had to depend only on food and water they can access in Sinharaja forest. Surprisingly most of the sick people have recovered by living close to the nature and using fresh Sinharaja forest water.[8]

There are many concerns over the survival of diverse forms of traditional practices related to health and wellbeing. Indeed, traditional practices related to health and wellbeing have been subject to numerous threats as a result of colonialism and, more recently, globalisation, More specifically traditional practices have been threatened by the loss of knowledge,[9] misappropriation,[10] inappropriate commercialisation,[11] and the

---

[4] Kalu mama (# 89).

[5] Based on interview and interaction with Kalu mama (# 89).

[6] A village in the Southern Province of Sri Lanka bordering the Shinharaja forest reserve.

[7] Segregation of leprosy patients was the main way of controlling leprosy in Sri Lanka based on *Lepers Ordinance (1902).* Although dapsone monotherapy was introduced in Sri Lanka in the 1940s and the anti-leprosy campaign developed since 1954, it was only by 1983that multi-drug therapy was available nationwide. See: Pathmeswaran, Nugegoda, and Post (2008).

[8] Kalu mama (# 89).

[9] Reyes-García et al. (2013).

[10] Dutfield introduces a misappropriation regime to protect traditional knowledge from misappropriation. According to him 'a misappropriation regime should incorporate (1) the concept of unfair competition; (2) moral rights; and (3) cultural rights' (2006), p xi. He argues a misappropriation regime is a promising approach to protect traditional knowledge based on customary law (2006), p x.

[11] See Robinson (2010).

publication of secret or sacred knowledge.[12] There are a number of well-known cases where the law, particularly intellectual property rights, have been used to allow those in the West to profit from indigenous traditional knowledge, expression and practice such as by obtaining patents for inventions based on traditional medicinal knowledge.[13] Some examples include: the use of turmeric for healing wounds, the anti-fungal properties of neem, and a diabetes medicine made from extract of jamun.[14] Other cases globally include involving the Maasai people[15] of Kenya and Tuareg (also Touareg), a tribe which inhabit parts of North Africa.[16] The word 'Maasai' is used in connection with a range of goods (from Land Rover cars, to running shoes, to Louis Vuitton towels, hats, scarves and bags) and also in tourism and hospitality services,[17] while Volkswagen manufactures the SUV Touareg.[18]

Traditional practices provide opportunities for indigenous and local people to obtain economic and non-economic benefits. One way in

---

[12] Restraining of the publication of a book entitled "Nomads of the Australian Desert" the interlocutory injunction obtained by the members of the Pitjantjatjara Council of Australia for the breach of confidence in the case Foster v. Mountford (1976) 29 FLR 233, Tilousi v. Arizona State University, Case No. CV2004-0115 (Ariz Sup Ct, 2004) is an example of court upholding community's right to prevent sacred or secret knowledge from publication.

[13] See Robinson (2010).

[14] WIPO background brief No 6, Intellectual property and traditional medical knowledge.
http://www.wipo.int/export/sites/www/tk/en/resources/pdf/tk_brief6.pdf
(last retrieved 19 February 2019) has stated these examples. The background brief further notes that all three patents were subsequently revoked.

[15]Maasai are a semi-nomadic community engaged in herding cattle. They wear intricate jewellery and famous for traditional dancing. More on Maasai people see: MAASAI Association http://www.maasai-association.org/maasai.html
(last retrieved 19 February 2019).

[16] The Tuareg people had once controlled the caravan trade routes across the Sahara. See Who are the Tuareg? http://africa.si.edu/exhibits/tuareg/who.html (last retrieved 19 February 2019).

[17] The Maasai People Take Back Their Brand (September 2013)
http://www.theatlantic.com/magazine/archive/2013/09/big-in-kenya/309425/
(last retrieved 19 February 2019) and Brand Maasai: Why nomads might trademark their name (28 May 2013) http://www.bbc.com/news/magazine-22617001 (19 February 2019).

[18] Volkswagen Touareg was first produced by German automaker Volkswagen in 2002. It is a mid-size luxury crossover SUV and the vehicle was named after the Tuareg people. See History of the Touareg-
http://www.kingstonvw.ca/HistoryoftheTouareg.aspx?lng=2 (19 February 2019).

which indigenous and local people benefit from their traditional practices is the sustainable use and management of nature and natural resources including plants, herbs and animals.[19] The sustainable resource management practices of Sri Lanka's Vedda community, for example, illustrate best practice in utilising the land and resources for economic and non-economic benefits. The Vedda community do not recognise individual ownership of land, but instead they believe that the forest of the Wanni (which they inhabit and protect) belongs to their ancestor-spirits as well as the Vedda community. In this way, the Vedda community identify and discuss their land from natural landmarks and boundaries, such as hills and rivers.[20] The Vedda community were self-sufficient in the habitat they lived in. The spiritual/ sacred relationship they had with the land and the constant interaction with their habitat promoted sustainable management of the resources, self-reliance and healthy life-style[21] and protected the natural resources from being destroyed by over utilisation for commercial purposes.

Traditional practices do not fit neatly into Western ideas of tangible or intangible property nor do they cater to a market-oriented commercial economy. Herbs used for traditional and indigenous treatment were not commercially grown but were hand-picked by the healers or their assistants, who could walk for hours and sometimes days to find the herbs.[22] Perhaps more importantly healers looked at the time they gathered the herbs,[23] and the place where the plant was growing (ie plants that grow near a cemetery, polluted water or land would not be used for medicine), as the healers believed the energies derived from the nearby trees, soil and the environment have a great influence on healing.[24] Many indigenous healers did not believe in the commercial growing of herbal plants as they assumed the use of chemicals or artificially growing the plant (rather than in its natural habitat) could hamper the healing powers of the plant.[25] Recognising the importance of practices related to health and wellbeing for communities and individuals, international schemes have been initiated in regulating and

---

[19] See for example, Brown, Mitchell, and Beresford, eds (2005); Rodriguez-Navarro, Guillermo (2000), p 455-458.

[20] Kotagama (2013).

[21] Vishwakeerthi Vanaspathi Uru Walige Wanniya Attha (# 18).

[22] Ariya Vedamahathaya (# 84).

[23] H. D. Karunawathie (# 53) and W. H. Anulawathie (# 56).

[24] S. M. H. Seneviratne (# 95) and S. M. K. Nimal Karunaratne (# 93).

[25] R. M. P. Rathnayake (# 13), Vishwakeerthi Vanaspathi Uru Walige Wanniya Attho (# 18), S. Shantha (# 25), B. V. Punchimenike (# 42), H. D. Karunawathie (# 53), W. M. Anulawathie (# 56).

protecting such practices. The following part of the chapter looks at such initiatives.

Part 1: International schemes dealing with traditional practices related to health and wellbeing

The protection of social and cultural traditional practices is an important and contentious site of legal development and debate at national, regional and international levels. To protect social and cultural traditional practices from being exploited by Western commodification of culture,[26] and to ensure good global governance,[27] it is necessary to consider the protection of health and wellness practices and the idea of legal pluralism.[28] Part 1 and 2 of this chapter surveys the legal pluralism measures relevant, accepted and adopted in Sri Lanka in relation to traditional practices related to healing.

The development of legal mechanisms has involved the contribution of a large number of entities and organisations, including but not limited to the Wold Health Organization (WHO),[29] the United Nations Economic Social Cultural Organization (UNESCO),[30] the Office of the High Commissioner on Human Rights (OHCHR),[31] the World Trade Organization (WTO)[32] and the World Intellectual Property Office

---

[26] Conway (2009), p 302.

[27] Tobin (2013), p 144.

[28] Legal pluralism refers to the presence of more than one legal order in a social field. Griffiths (1986), p.1.

[29] WHO plays a significant role in promoting traditional medicine. ie WHO Strategies for Traditional Medicine 2002-2005/ 2014-2023; Resolutions of the World Health Assembly (WHA); WHO South-East Asia Region (SEARO); HerbalNet; WHO Collaborating Centres for Traditional Medicine; WHO Expert Advisory Panel on Traditional Medicine.

[30] See UNESCO role in protecting local and indigenous knowledge http://portal.unesco.org/en/ev.php-URL_ID=5065&URL_DO=DO_TOPIC&URL_SECTION=201.html. UNESCO Local and Indigenous Knowledge Systems portal http://www.unesco.org/new/en/natural-sciences/priority-areas/links/ (last retrieved 4 September 2015)

[31] See OHCHR role in protecting the rights of the Indigenous Peoples. http://www.ohchr.org/EN/Issues/IPeoples/Pages/IndigenousPeoplesIndex.aspx (last retrieved 19 February 2019).

[32] WTO Agreement on Trade Related Aspects of Intellectual Property Rights (TRIPS). See http://www.wto.org/english/tratop_e/trips_e/t_agm0_e.htm (last retrieved 19 February 2019).

(WIPO).[33] Over the last fifty years a range of treaty based mechanisms dealing with indigenous peoples, their knowledge and traditional practices has developed. First there are a range of international legal treaties that recognise the rights of indigenous peoples, regulate the access and transfer of genetic resources, and create specially crafted property rights over traditional knowledge that can (theoretically) be enforced through state and possibly international legal forums. Second has been the application of existing legal schemes such as patents and plant variety rights to indigenous people. There is a growing body of scholarship discussing and analysing these treaties, as well as working papers and technical documents from organisations such as the World Intellectual Property Organization ('WIPO'), the Secretariat of the CBD, and other organisations working on this topic. [34] Rather than repeating the scholarship in analysing these treaties, the next part of this book provides an overview of the types of protection given in three key areas—(1) indigenous peoples and self-determination; (2) access and benefit sharing; and (3) intellectual property of the international law.

1.1 Indigenous Peoples, Self-determination

In the 1950's, an assimilation approach to mainstream culture was adopted internationally with regard to indigenous peoples. One of the earliest organisations to recognise the rights of indigenous people was the International Labour Organization (ILO). The *Indigenous and Tribal Populations Convention, 1957 (No. 107)* of the ILO is an early example of international legislation dealing with the protection and integration of indigenous and other tribal and semi-tribal populations.[35] More specifically

---

[33] For a discussion see the role of the WIPO Intergovernmental Committee on Intellectual Property and Genetic Resource, Traditional Knowledge and Folklore (IGC). IGC's new mandate:
http://www.wipo.int/export/sites/www/tk/en/igc/pdf/igc_mandate_1415.pdf; IGC meeting documents: http://www.wipo.int/meetings/en/topic.jsp?group_id=110 (last retrieved 20 February 2019).

[34] See Dutfield (2000); Dutfield (2006); Twarog and Kapoor (ed) (2004); Gupta (1999) pp119-129; Subramanian and Pisupati (eds) (2010); Twarog (2003); Twarog and Kapoor (eds) (2004); Biber-Klemm (1998) pp1-21; Cottier (1997); Downes and Laird (1999a); Downes and Laird (1999b); Downes D.R. and Laird S.A. (1999a); Nijar (1996); UNEP/WIPO (2000); Axt et al. (1993); Cox (1997); Four Directions Council (1996); Posey (ed.) (1996); Rural Advancement Foundation International (1994); Tobin (1997), p 17-18; WIPO (2001).

[35] The history of ILO activity leading to adoption of *ILO Convention No. 107* is recorded by Hannum, 'As early as 1921, the ILO carried out a series of studies on

the *Indigenous and Tribal Populations Convention, 1957* concentrates on integration of indigenous and other tribal populations in independent countries[36] in terms of rights related to land;[37] recruitment and conditions of employment;[38] vocational training, handicrafts and rural industries;[39] social security and health;[40] and education and means of communication.[41]

In 1989, the ILO revised the *Indigenous and Tribal Populations Convention, 1957* with the *Convention Concerning Indigenous and Tribal Peoples in Independent Countries* (*ILO Convention No. 169 of 1989*). This introduced new international standards, considering the developments taken place internationally.[42] More specifically the preamble of *ILO Convention No. 169 of 1989* recognised 'the aspirations of these peoples to exercise control over their own institutions, ways of life and economic development and to maintain and develop their identities, languages and religions, within the framework of the States in which they live.'[43] The preamble also recognizes the diminishing nature of indigenous and tribal culture due to the erosion of implementing traditional laws, values, customs and perspectives.

Despite the potential for self-determination of indigenous people by participating in decisions affecting their lives, according to *ILO Convention 169*, it has been the state that has used their authority in

---

indigenous workers. In 1926, it established a Committee of Experts on Native Labour, whose work led to the adoption of a number of conventions and recommendations concerning forced labour and recruitment practices of indigenous groups. A second committee of experts on indigenous Labour first met in 1951. It encouraged states to extend legislative provisions to all segments of their population, including indigenous communities, and called for improved education, vocational training, social security, and protection in the field of labour for indigenous peoples. Finally, in 1953, the ILO published a comprehensive reference book, entitled *Indigenous Peoples: Living and Working Conditions of Aboriginal Populations in Independent Countries,* which provided a survey of indigenous populations throughout the world and a summary of national and international action to aid these groups. Hannum (2011), pp 652-653. (Footnotes excluded).

36 *ILO Convention 107, Preamble.*

37 *ILO Convention 107, A 11-14.*

38 *ILO Convention 107, A 15.*

39 *ILO Convention 107, A 16-18.*

40 *ILO Convention 107, A 19-20.*

41 *ILO Convention 107, A 21-26.*

42 *ILO Convention on Indigenous and Tribal Peoples 1989 (No. 169)*: A manual helps to understand the new rights enshrined in the convention and how to use the Convention is gaining recognition in promotion and protection of indigenous and tribal peoples' rights.

43 *Convention 169, Preamble.*

regulating the traditional knowledge of the local communities. According to Drahos, *ILO Convention 169*:

> …with its integrated approach to land rights, natural resources, culture, customary law, consultation and participation, an approach that is tied to complaints procedures that can be started by non-state actors, is an approach that should have been built upon and strengthened. This has not happened. Instead…states have strengthened their regulatory power over indigenous knowledge assets.[44]

Another international treaty to recognise indigenous people is the *United Nations Declaration on the Rights of Indigenous Peoples* (UNDRIP);[45] which was adopted by the United Nations General Assembly in 2007, after more than two decades of negotiation.[46] As a declaration, UNDRIP does not bind states; although it must be read in conjunction with other international law such as human rights law. UNDRIP provides a common global framework for protecting the rights of the indigenous peoples,[47] to listen to and to address all of the concerns of indigenous peoples that reclaim the essential identity of the indigenous people all over the world as well as their role on the global stage of decision making. The declaration sets out the individual and collective rights of indigenous peoples, as well as their rights to culture, identity, language, employment, health, education and other issues. The UNDRIP recognises the 'indispensable' collective rights. The contribution of the indigenous people to the common heritage of mankind through maintaining diversity and richness of civilization and cultures is recognized in the preamble. UNDRIP is a dynamic development towards protecting human rights of the indigenous people internationally.

Following the adoption of the UN Declaration, there is now a general consensus among international policy makers that there must be a focus on implementation of indigenous peoples' rights at the country-level to ensure that international instruments bring the necessary changes for the millions of indigenous peoples around the world, who are still living in marginalised and disadvantaged situations. The right to self-determination is a key right to protect the identity of these indigenous people and to ensure the thriving of their knowledge systems. The shared vision of the United

---

[44] Drahos, Peter (2014) above n p 79.

[45] *United Nations Declaration on the Rights of Indigenous Peoples 2007.*

[46] For a discussion of these negotiations see http://undesadspd.org/indigenouspeoples/declarationontherightsofindigenouspeoples.aspx (last retrieved 20 February 2019).

[47] Lawrence (2002)

Nations Indigenous Peoples' Partnership (UNIPP)[48] taking the initiative to deliver as one[49] in protecting self-determination of the indigenous people does have a strong impact at the country level in promoting cultural diversity. The concern, however, is to what extent have the international frameworks been able to promote self-determination at the grassroots. Are the indigenous people able to introduce and maintain their own education system, legal system, their own medical practices and the life style without the regulation and intervention of respective governments or authorities, or what level of freedom does the indigenous people possess in self-determination? The level of self-determination indigenous people possess in maintaining their traditional lifestyle determines the level of protection of traditional knowledge.

One of the most important aspects of the UNDRIP is the recognition of the connection of knowledge and traditional practices to the land of indigenous people. As Siegfried Wiessner explains, 'being "indigenous" means to live within one's roots,'[50] that is living in the ancestral lands. "Distinctive spiritual relationship" with their lands emphasised in art 25 refers to the collective consciousness of indigenous peoples, to their location of physical existence often expressed in creation stories or sacred tales of their origin. Indigenous sovereignty claimed by indigenous people is primarily to preserve their inherited ways of life, to make their cultures flourish and change those traditions as they see necessary.[51] The traditional practices relating to health and wellbeing of indigenous community are closely linked to their way of life and to the spiritual beliefs and understanding of the land they live in. As a result, indigenous sovereignty and right to land of the indigenous people is significantly important in protecting the indigenous health and wellbeing practices.

---

[48] UNIPP is an initiative to deliver as one at the country level in partnership with the indigenous peoples and governments. UNIPP member organisations are International Labour Organization (ILO), United Nations Development Programme (UNDP), United Nations Development Group (UNDG), United Nations Children's fund (Unicef), UNFPA and United Nations Office of the High Commissioner of Human Rights (OHCHR).

[49] United Nations Indigenous Peoples' Partnership (UNIPP) Delivering as one UN at the country level in partnership with indigenous peoples and governments. – http://www.ilo.org/wcmsp5/groups/public/---ed_norm/---normes/documents/publication/wcms_186284.pdf (last retrieved 20 February 2019).

[50] Wiessner (2008).

[51] Wiessner (2008).

1.2 Access and benefit sharing

In addition to acknowledging the self determination of indigenous peoples, the issues of how to provide access and benefit sharing of traditional knowledge, expressions and practices has been considered in a number of fora. Perhaps the most relevant are the Convention on Biological Diversity (CBD)[52] and the International Treaty on Plant and Genetic Resources on Food and Agriculture (ITPGRFA).[53]

1.2.1 The Convention on Biological Diversity

Recognising the vital role of biodiversity in building civilizations, and the importance of the Earth's biological resources for humanity's economic and social development, and understanding the threats of loss of bio-diversity for our food supplies, opportunities for recreation and tourism, and sources of wood, medicines and energy, the UN bodies looked into the possibilities of conserving biological diversity internationally. In November 1988, the United Nations Environment Programme (UNEP) convened the Ad Hoc Working Group of Experts on Biological Diversity to explore the need for an international convention on biological diversity. [54] The Ad Hoc Working Group of Technical and Legal Experts was established in May 1989 to prepare an international legal instrument for the conservation and sustainable use of biological diversity.[55] This working group became known as the Intergovernmental Negotiating Committee in February 1991.[56] Work of the Intergovernmental Negotiating Committee was adopted as the *Convention on Biological Diversity* on 22 May 1992. At the Rio "Earth Summit" (the United Nations Conference on Environment and Development), the Convention was opened for signature on 5 June 1992.[57] By 4 June 1993, it had received 168 signatures. The Convention entered into force on 29

---

[52] *Convention on Biological Diversity.*

[53] *International Treaty on Plant Genetic Resources for Food and Agriculture,* http://www.planttreaty.org/sites/default/files/i0510e.pdf (last retrieved 20 February 2019).

[54]History of the Convention https://www.cbd.int/history/ (last retrieved 20 February 2019)

[55]History of the Convention https://www.cbd.int/history/ (last retrieved 20 February 2019)

[56]History of the Convention https://www.cbd.int/history/ (last retrieved 20 February 2019)

[57] UN Treaty Collection, *Convention on Biological Diversity.*

December 1993.[58] The first session of the Conference of the Parties was held in the Bahamas from 28 November to 9 December 1994.[59]

The CBD was introduced as a means of preserving biodiversity. The objectives of the conservation are: the conservation of biological diversity, the sustainable use of the components of biological diversity and the fair and equitable sharing of the benefits arising out of the utilisation of genetic resources. The Convention could be seen as a compromise between the interests of industrialised Western countries and those in the developing world. Those who represented the developing world wanted to secure technological and economic benefits in exchange for allowing access to their biological asserts.

Article 8(j) is the key provision relating to the knowledge and innovation of indigenous communities. In applying this article of the Convention at the National level, Governments implement legal and non-legal strategies, including respect for indigenous customary laws, where indigenous and local communities get involved in protecting traditional knowledge. More specifically art 8(j) states:

> Subject to its national legislation, respect, preserve and maintain knowledge, innovations and practices of indigenous and local communities embodying traditional lifestyles relevant for the conservation and sustainable use of biological diversity and promote their wider application with the approval and involvement of the holders of such knowledge, innovations and practices and encourage the equitable sharing of the benefits arising from the utilization of such knowledge, innovations and practices.[60]

For example, the Secretariat of the *Convention on Biological Diversity* (CBD) defines traditional knowledge safeguarded by the Convention as 'knowledge, innovation and practices of indigenous and local communities embodying traditional lifestyles relevant for the conservation and sustainable use of biological diversity.'[61]

One effect of the CBD has been to draw together a range of people and organisations; all to discuss and debate issues related to indigenous knowledge. These organisations have included: the United Nations Development Programme, the ILO, the WTO, the United Nations Environment

---

[58] *Convention on Biological Diversity*, Introduction. https://www.cbd.int/intro/default.shtml (last retrieved 20 February 2019)

[59]History of the Convention https://www.cbd.int/history/ (last retrieved 20 February 2019)

[60] *Article 8 (j), CBD.*

[61] *Article 8(j), CBD.*

Programme and the Working Group on Indigenous Populations of the Commission of Human Rights. In addition to these organisations, the state members, indigenous groups, NGO organisations and business organisations also contribute in implementing the Convention.

At the international level CBD is the major protection regime for traditional knowledge related to bio-diversity, for example: the CBD's principles of prior informed consent, fair and equitable benefit sharing, and the Bonn Guidelines and most recently, the *Nagoya Protocol on Access to Genetic Resources and the Fair and Equitable Sharing of Benefits Arising from their Utilization (the Nagoya Protocol*). The *Nagoya Protocol* is a global agreement that implements the access and benefit-sharing obligations of the *Convention on Biological Diversity* (CBD). The *Nayoga Protocol* also covers traditional knowledge associated with genetic resources that are covered by the CBD and the benefits arising from its utilisation. It was adopted in October 2010, after six years of negotiations. The *Nayoga Protocol*'s objective is the fair and equitable sharing of benefits arising from the use of genetic resources which contributes to the conservation and sustainable use of biodiversity, implementing the objectives of the CBD.[62] The Protocol establishes a legally-binding framework that assists researchers to access genetic resources in return for a fair share of any benefits from their use. The Protocol applies when genetic resources are accessed and 'used'. The *Nagoya Protocol* on access and benefit-sharing of genetic resources entered into force on 12 October 2014.

1.2.2 International Treaty on Plant and Genetic Resources on Food and Agriculture

The *International Treaty on Plant and Genetic Resources on Food and Agriculture* (ITPGRFA) was adopted on 3 November 2001 by the Thirty-First Session of the Conference of the Food and Agriculture Organization of the United Nations.[63] The Treaty is vital in the fight against hunger and poverty. It supports the achievement of Millennium Development Goals 1 and 7.

The aims of the treaty include: 'recognising the enormous contribution of farmers to the diversity of crops that feed the world; establishing a global system to provide farmers, plant breeders and scientists with access to plant genetic materials; and ensuring that recipients share benefits they derive from the use of these genetic materials with the

---

[62] *Nayoga Protocol, A 1.*

[63] *International Treaty on Plant Genetic Resources for Food and Agriculture,* (entered into force on 29 June 2004.)

countries in which they originated.'[64] This treaty and its Standard Material Transfer Agreement has been able to practically implement the fair sharing of plant and genetic resources at the international level.

The multilateral system is an innovative solution for access and benefit sharing.[65] The global pool of genetic resources that is maintained as a part of the multilateral system, holds 64 of the most important crops on the planet, crops that together account for 80 percent of the food we derive from plants.[66]

Genetic resources could be accessed by the treaty's ratifying nations for research, breeding and training for food and agriculture.[67] Intellectual property rights over these genetic resources cannot be claimed by the recipients. The treaty also ensures that access to genetic resources already protected by international property rights is consistent with international and national laws.[68] Those who access genetic materials through the Multilateral System agree to share any benefits from their use through four benefit-sharing mechanisms established by the treaty.[69] The treaty has made provisions for protecting the traditional knowledge of the farmers, who have enormously contributed towards the development of plant genetic resources.[70] The treaty calls for participation in national decision-making processes and to share the benefits from the use of genetic resources.[71] The treaty enables the maximisation of the use and breeding of all crops, including local crops and promotes development and maintenance of diverse farming systems.[72]

Both the CBD and The *International Treaty on Plant and Genetic Resources on Food and Agriculture* (ITPGRFA) contribute to protecting practices related to health and wellbeing. Most of the traditional healing practices subscribe to the holistic notion of healing process which caters not

---

[64] *ITPGRFA,* Text of the Treaty: Official Versions. http://www.planttreaty.org/content/texts-treaty-official-versions?&session-id=a0e8b0f846b1d0c4c487c2c21c94b349 (last retrieved 20 February 2019).

[65] *ITPGRFA, A 10.*

[66] *International Treaty on Plant Genetic Resources for Food and Agriculture* Website http://www.planttreaty.org/content/overview (last retrieved 20 February 2019).

[67] *ITPGRFA, A 12.*

[68] *ITPGRFA, A 12 (3).*

[69] The four benefit sharing mechanisms established by art 13.2 of the treaty are, 1. Exchange of information, 2. Access to and transfer of technology, 3. Capacity-building, and 4. Sharing of the benefits arising from commercialization.

[70] *ITPGRFA, A 9 (2) (a).*

[71] *ITPGRFA, A 9.*

[72] *ITPGRFA, A 6.*

only to curing the symptom but acknowledges that body, mind, spirt and environment play an important role in the healing process. Todd J. Pesek, Lonnie R. Helton and Murali Nair argue that the current disconnection of individuals from their natural habitat affects the existence of healthy ecosystems, creates spiritual imbalance and hampers the full understanding of crucial matters such as environmentally derived illness, and unsustainable and damaging food production strategies.[73] Many scholars have presented the negative impact of ecological disruptions and the destruction of habitats, such as the alteration of disease transmission patterns, the accumulation of toxic pollutants, and the invasion by alien species and pathogens.[74] Timothy Johns and Pablo B. Eyzaguirre argue that biodiversity is essential for dietary diversity and health. Todd J. Pesek, Lonnie R. Helton and Murali Nair state, 'A healthy environment powerfully enables healthy and harmonious lifeways and is a necessary component in holistic health and wellbeing'[75] They further claim that by a mutually beneficial exchange of wisdom and practice of the traditional healers, all global communities can benefit from holistic collaboration and innovation in healing, and the generation of economically viable, culturally appropriate outlets for cultural self-empowerment and ecological integrity.'[76]

Understanding how the negative global impacts on biological diversity and ecological processes have affected the wellbeing of all species including humans,[77] scholars have attempted to define a new discipline called conservation medicine that links human and animal health with ecosystem health and global environmental change.[78] This new discipline has perhaps always been part of the healing practice of traditional healers, as it is holistic and linked with the eco system[79]. CBD and ITPGRFA play a significant role in promoting the discipline of conservation medicine by considering access and benefit sharing of traditional knowledge, expressions and practices related to health and wellbeing.

[73] Pesek, Helton and Nair (2006), p 115.
[74] Pongsiri et al (2009), Keesing et al (2010).
[75] Pesek, Helton and Nair (2006), p 115.
[76] Pesek, Helton and Nair (2006), p 118.
[77] Aguirre et al (2012), p 3.
[78] Aguirre et al (2002).
[79] Vishwakeerth Vanaspathi Uru Waligе Wannia Attho (#18), Dambane Gunarardena (#17), Venerable Wellawatte Seelagawesi (#66), Daya Dissanayake (#87).

1.3 Intellectual Property

Law, particularly intellectual property law, has increasingly contributed towards safeguarding and exploiting the knowledge, expression and practice of indigenous peoples.[80] Protection of intellectual property relating to traditional knowledge is a contested and divisive topic. Many traditional knowledge holders feel traditional knowledge is inalienable and cannot be protected as a property.[81]

In 2000, the General Assembly of WIPO established the Intergovernmental Committee on Intellectual Property and Genetic Resources, Traditional Knowledge and Folklore (WIPO-IGC).[82] The Intergovernmental Committee on Intellectual Property and Genetic Resources, Traditional Knowledge and Folklore (IGC) of the World Intellectual Property Organization (WIPO) is currently working on an international treaty protecting traditional knowledge and cultural expressions.[83] It has dealt most comprehensively with the meaning of traditional knowledge and traditional cultural expressions. In 2012, the IGC provided a draft text outlining various provisions of an international treaty protecting traditional knowledge and cultural expression. Most recently IGC 28 took place from 7 to 9 July 2014 where the interconnection of genetic resources, traditional knowledge and traditional cultural expressions was discussed.[84]

One of the objectives of the WIPO-IGC is to produce one or several legal instruments to protect genetic resources, tradition knowledge and traditional culture expressions. So far, three separate draft texts have

---

[80] See, Mugabe (1999) http://www.wipo.int/edocs/mdocs/tk/en/wipo_unhchr_ip_pnl_98/wipo_unhchr_ip_pnl_98_4.doc (last retrieved 20 February 2019).

[81] Vishwakeerth Vanaspathi Uru Walige Wannia Attho (#18), Dambane Gunarardena (#17), R. M. Premachandra (# 1113), Je Jeyalan (#100), Kalu mama (#89), H. M. Nandasena Herath (#68).

[82] See Intergovernmental Committee on Intellectual Property and Genetic Resources (2001). For discussion see WIPO, Intellectual Property and Traditional Knowledge. (Booklet no 2) http://www.wipo.int/edocs/pubdocs/en/tk/920/wipo_pub_920.pdf (last retrieved 20 February 2019).

[83] See WIPO, Traditional Knowledge - http://www.wipo.int/tk/en/ (last retrieved 20 February 2019).

[84] See Decision on Agenda Item 6 in Decisions of the Twenty Eighth Session of the Committee, WIPO Intergovernmental Committee on Intellectual Property and Genetic Resources, Traditional Knowledge and Folklore. 28th Session, 7-9 July 2014. http://www.wipo.int/edocs/mdocs/tk/en/wipo_grtkf_ic_28/wipo_grtkf_ic_28_ref_decisions.pdf (last retrieved 20 February 2019).

been proposed on: traditional knowledge; traditional cultural expression; and genetic resources, including traditional knowledge associate with those genetic resources. The proposed definitions and complexities associated with this were discussed in Chapter 1.5.

While there are international attempts to protect the intellectual property of traditional knowledge and traditional cultural expressions, it has been argued that Western intellectual property rights are inappropriate for protecting traditional knowledge as they are focused on individuals, limited by time, and require work to exist in material form, whereas traditional knowledge is very often communally created, transmitted from one generation to the next and is often not recorded in material form.[85] Protecting traditional knowledge as intellectual property gives an economic value for traditional knowledge. In non-capitalist economies traditional knowledge thrived due to spirituality, belief systems and traditional social structures, such as caste systems that passed the knowledge from one generation to other. Although traditional knowledge played a crucial role in everyday life of the community, traditional knowledge was not given an economic value nor catered for market-oriented social systems.

In this part an overview of the international negotiations of traditional knowledge and traditional cultural expressions, particularly as they relate to recognising the right of indigenous peoples to self-determination, access and benefit sharing and intellectual property have been presented. In doing this, the chapter has traced the development of the protection regime in traditional knowledge from the recognition of rights to self-determination of indigenous peoples and discussed calls for the safeguarding and protection of traditional knowledge, expression and practice, as well as for sharing the benefits resulting from the exploitation of traditional knowledge, expression and practice. In the light of international schemes dealing with traditional practices related to health and wellbeing, it is clear that the most challenging aspect is defining and understanding the concept of traditional knowledge. When analysing this concept many different political, economic and even social considerations are taken into account, many of which can only be touched upon in this book. These different dimensions can be observed partly through a consideration of the different objectives of those seeking to 'protect' traditional knowledge. These objectives range from a desire to prevent its misappropriation and safeguarding it as a crucial cultural resource, to facilitating indigenous development in the market economy based upon it.

[85] Wiessner. (2011).

In turn, many of these objectives are informed by fundamentally different views of what is meant by development. These different views could include, pursuing economic growth based on liberal market relations and the centrality of property rights; or pursuing a more ecologically sustainable and culturally-differentiated approach to achieving well-being. Protection of traditional knowledge can be aimed at by ensuring the local communities, life-styles and culture that gave rise to traditional knowledge in the first place are supported, and that the traditional knowledge is handed down to following generations. Or additionally, it can be directed towards ensuring that rights over the production and use of traditional knowledge are given to those institutions that have the best chance of defending them against international misappropriation.

Part 2: How Traditional Practices Related to Health and Wellbeing are Regulated in Sri Lanka

In Sri Lanka, traditional practices related to health and wellbeing are recognised and regulated under a range of laws. Sri Lanka has used multi-cultural Legal pluralism.[86] The main laws applicable in Sri Lanka are the Roman Dutch Law and the English law, both of which are a legacy of colonialism.[87] Although customary laws such as Thesawalamai, Kandyan law and the Muslim law are also applicable in Sri Lanka, it is applicable only in a limited context[88] such as marriage and property. Importantly, however in Sri Lanka when there is a conflict between the statute law and customary law, it is the statute law that prevails. The remainder of this chapter discusses the regulation of health and wellbeing practices in two areas. First, Sri Lanka's role in the application of international laws related to health and wellbeing. It will be shown that Sri Lanka has taken measures to comply with international schemes in protecting traditional practices related to health and wellbeing, although it is not fully compliant. Second, Sri Lanka's domestic laws and mechanisms related to health and wellbeing will be outlined. It will be argued that Sri Lanka's domestic laws and mechanisms related to protecting traditional practices in health and wellbeing appear adequate on paper. However, in practical implementation,

---

[86] Multicultural legal pluralism is when state and customary laws co-exist in parallel (yet distinct worlds) within the same jurisdiction, often when customary law conflicts with the state law, there is a tendancy to subordinate customary law. Walsh (2009)

[87] Cooray (2015), p 295.

[88] Cooray (2015), p 295.

the domestic laws and mechanisms are not fully protecting traditional practices in health and wellbeing.

2.1 Sri Lanka's Role in Application of International Laws Related to Traditional Practices in Health and Wellbeing

Sri Lanka has been taking measures to adopt and apply international laws connected to traditional practices related to health and wellbeing. In the following section, Sri Lanka's role in adopting the international schemes discussed in part 1 of the chapter is explored.

Sri Lanka is one of the 144 countries that have voted in favour of the *United Nations Declaration on Rights of Indigenous Persons* (UNDRIP).[89] Yet, *ILO Convention Concerning Indigenous and Tribal Peoples in Independent Countries*[90] has not been ratified by Sri Lanka[91] although it is in the process of discussing ratification.[92]

Sri Lanka is a contracting party to many of the international intellectual property mechanisms administered by WIPO, UPOV, WTO and UN. These include, *Trademark Law Treaty,*[93] *Nairobi Treaty on the Protection of the Olympic Symbol,*[94] *Patent Cooperation Treaty,*[95] *Convention*

[89] Voted on 13 September 2007 for the Adoption of the proposal at the General Assembly.

[90] *ILO Convention No. 169 of 1989.*

[91] Up-to-date Conventions not ratified by Sri Lanka., ILO – http://www.ilo.org/dyn/normlex/en/f?p=NORMLEXPUB:11210:0::NO::P11210_COUNTRY_ID:103172 (last retrieved 20 February 2019).

[92] See MacKay, Fergus, *A Guide to Indigenous Peoples' Rights in the International Labour Organization. Forest Peoples Programme.* http://www.forestpeoples.org/sites/fpp/files/publication/2010/09/iloguideiprightsju l02eng.pdf (last retrieved 20 February 2019).

[93] Entry into force in Sri Lanka on August 1, 1996. See WIPO Treaties and Contracting Parties – Trademark Kaw Treaty- Sri Lanka. http://www.wipo.int/treaties/en/remarks.jsp?cnty_id=445C (last retrieved 20 February 2019).

[94] Entry into force in Sri Lanka on February 19, 1984. See WIPO Nairobi Notification No.18 Nairobi Treaty on the Protection of the Olympic Symbol. http://www.wipo.int/treaties/en/notifications/nairobi/treaty_nairobi_18.html (last retrieved 20 February 2019).

[95] Entry into force in Sri Lanka on February 26, 1982. See WIPO The PCT now has 148 Contracting States. http://www.wipo.int/pct/en/pct_contracting_states.html (last retrieved 20 February 2019).

Establishing the World Intellectual Property Organization,[96] *Mardid Agreement for the Repression of False or Deceptive Indications of Source on Goods,*[97] *Paris Convention for the Protection of Industrial Property*[98] and *Berne Convention for the Protection of Literary and Artistic Works.*[99]

Sri Lanka has also taken many initiatives to adopt the international legal framework in access and benefit sharing and conserving bio-diversity. These initiatives include: ratifying the *International Treaty on Plant and Genetic Resources for Food and Agriculture*;[100] *International Plant Protection Convention*[101]; *Convention on Bio-Diversity*[102]; implementing a Framework for Action, that outlines conservation of four priority systems, namely, forests, wetland, coastal and marine and agriculture,[103] in 1999; ratifying the *Cartagena Protocol on Biosafety to the Convention on*

---

96 Entry into force in Sri Lanka on September 20, 1978. See WIPO Notification No. 100 Convention establishing the World Intellectual Property Organization. http://www.wipo.int/treaties/en/notifications/convention/treaty_convention_100.html (last retrieved 20 February 2019).

97 Entry into force in Sri Lanka on December 29, 1952. See WIPO Sri Lanka http://www.wipo.int/wipolex/en/profile.jsp?code=LK (last retrieved 20 February 2019).

98 Entry into force in Sri Lanka on December 29, 1952. See WIPO Treaties and Contracting Parties- Paris Convention – Sri Lanka http://www.wipo.int/treaties/en/remarks.jsp?cnty_id=314C (last retrieved 20 February 2019).

99 Entry into force in Sri Lanka on February 4, 1948. See WIPO Treaties and Contracting Parties- Berne Convention – Sri Lanka http://www.wipo.int/treaties/en/remarks.jsp?cnty_id=1028C (last retrieved 20 February 2019).

100 Entry into force in Sri Lanka on December 16, 2013. See The International Treaty on Plant Genetic Resources for Food and Agriculture. Sri Lanka Joins the International Treaty on Plant Genetic Resources for Food and Agriculture. http://www.planttreaty.org/news/sri-lanka-joins-international-treaty-plant-genetic-resources-food-and-agriculture (last retrieved 20 February 2019)

101 Entry into force in Sri Lanka on October 2, 2005. See WIPO IP-related Multilateral Treaties- Contracting Parties/ Signatories. http://www.wipo.int/wipolex/en/other_treaties/parties.jsp?treaty_id=276&group_id=22 (last retrieved 20 February 2019)

102 Entry into force in Sri Lanka on June 21, 1994. See Convention on Biological Diversity. Sri Lanka – Overview. https://www.cbd.int/countries/?country=lk (last retrieved 20 February 2019)

103 See http://www.cbd.int/doc/world/lk/lk-nbsap-01-en.pdf. This document was updated with the publication of an Addendum in 2007. (last retrieved 20 February 2019).

Biological Diversity[104]; drafting a *National Policy on Bio-Safety* in 2011, to regulate bio-technology and genetically modified organisms (GMOs). Yet, article 8(j) of the *Convention on Bio-Diversity* which refers to traditional knowledge of the country has received limited attention in Sri Lanka's policy framework.[105]

2.2 Sri Lanka's Domestic Laws and Mechanisms Related to Traditional Practices in Health and Wellbeing

This section argues that Sri Lanka's domestic laws and mechanisms related to protecting traditional practices in health and wellbeing appear adequate on the books. However, in practical implementation, the domestic laws and mechanisms are not fully catering towards protecting traditional practices in health and wellbeing. The argument that the practical implementation of domestic laws and mechanisms is not effective in protecting traditional practices in health and well-being is explored by looking at (i) the intellectual property law in Sri Lanka with an emphasis on compliance with international laws; (ii) the role of patents; (iii) the legal framework to protect traditional knowledge in Sri Lanka and (iv) the national mechanism in place to protect traditional healing.

(i) Intellectual property law in Sri Lanka

The main intellectual property law enacted by the legislature in Sri Lanka is the *Intellectual Property Act, No. 36 of 2003.*[106] *Intellectual Property Regulations No.1 of 2006* and *Regulations on the Antiquities Ordinance, No. 9 of 1940.* The National Intellectual Property Office (NIPO) of Sri Lanka established under the *Intellectual Property Act No. 36 of 2003*[107], is the main institution responsible for protecting intellectual property in Sri Lanka.

---

[104] Entry into force in Sri Lanka on July 26, 2004. See Convention on Biological Diversity. Sri Lanka – Overview. https://www.cbd.int/countries/?country=lk (last retrieved 20 February 2019)

[105] Hirimuthugodage (21 May 2013) Biodiversity as a Cornerstone of Sustainable Development: A Sri Lankan Perspective. See: http://www.island.lk/index.php?page_cat=article-details&page=article-details&code_title=79554 (last retrieved 20 February 2019).

[106] National Intellectual Property Office of Sri Lanka http://www.nipo.gov.lk/act.htm (last retrieved 20 February 2019).

[107] National Intellectual Property Office of Sri Lanka. About us http://www.nipo.gov.lk/about.htm (last retrieved 20 February 2019).

Sri Lanka is non-compliant with TRIP at present. The reason for the non-compliance as argued by Asanka Perera is, 'there is still no intellectual property protection for plant varieties in Sri Lanka.'[108] In order to be compliant with TRIPS, Sri Lanka has introduced the *Intellectual Property Act No. 35 of 2003*. However, this Act excludes plants and animals from the scope of the application.[109] There has been international pressure, particularly from the United States, for Sri Lanka to be TRIPS compliant in protection of plants and animals.[110] In order to fully implement intellectual property law regimes the proposed draft *Plant Varieties Bill 2001* was introduced by the National Intellectual Property Organisation in Sri Lanka in order to fulfil TRIPS obligation in art 27.3(b). The draft *Plant Varieties Bill 2001* is based on the *International Union for the Protection of New Varieties of Plant Convention* (UPOV).[111] However, a major criticism is that this Bill has still not been implemented. .[112] Perera argues that the proposed Bill does not deal with the traditional varieties of plants because it aims to protect new plant varieties.[113] Perera further argues that it is necessary to protect these traditional plant varieties to increase food security, eliminate poverty and maintain the environment.[114] Not having a mechanism to do this effectively is a threat to the protection of the traditional medical systems in Sri Lanka that use traditional plant varieties for the production of medicine.

The International Union for the Protection of New Varieties of Plants Convention (UPOV) arguably has negative consequences for developing countries, like Sri Lanka including the monopoly in the seed industry created by the Convention, would lead to a price increase for the seeds, which would in turn adversely affect the agricultural industry;[115]and public sector breeding could be impeded by protection of plant varieties.[116]

In order to protect traditional varieties of plants in Sri Lanka, the best approach would be a misappropriation regime, which is a non-intellectual property mechanism to protect plant variety rights. [117] Correa discusses the positive impacts of introducing a misappropriation regime as:

---

108 Perera, (2011), p 301.
109 Kamardeen, (2013).
110 Talagala (2012), p 17; Ramanna and Udgaonkar (2005), p 192.
111 Perera (2011), p 301.
112 Kamardeen, (2013).
113 Perera (2011), p313.
114 Perera (2011), p311.
115 Swaminathan, p 6.
116 Swaminathan, p 6.
117 Correa (2000) p 32-3 and Perera (2011), p 322.

- it would recognize the informal, collective and cumulative systems of innovation of local and indigenous communities and farmers;
- no novelty, inventiveness or secrecy would be required; there would be no arbitrary time limits for protection; the conferred rights would be 'non-monopolistic' and would not hinder the non-commercial use and exchange of germplasm within and among communities;
- no registration and therefore administrative machinery would be necessary;
- it would not oblige farmers or community members to keep secrets or change their traditional practices;
- as no monopolies would be recognized, possession of the same knowledge in different communities would be perfectly legitimate; and
- the rights against infringement would arise when a variety has been acquired in a manner contrary to certain rules, such as national access legislation or other acceptable practices on the collection of germplasm.'[118]

(ii) Role of patents

A patent is when the State grants the inventor, by means of a patent, the right to exclude others from making, using and selling the qualified invention for a period of 20 years from the date of application for patent. The owner of the patent can use, sell or license the patented technology and derive financial benefits.'[119] *Patent Ordinance* (*1907*)[120] has been in effect in Sri Lanka since 1st January 1907 until the enactment of the *Code of Intellectual Property Act No. 52 of 1979*.[121] *Intellectual Property Regulation No. 1 of 2006*[122] has been made by the Minister of Trade, Commerce, Consumer Affairs and Marketing Development under Section 204 of the

---

[118] Correa (2000) pp 32-3, also quoted in Perera (2011) pp 322- 323.
[119] National Intellectual Property Office of Sri Lanka. Patents.
http://www.nipo.gov.lk/patent.htm (last retrieved 20 February 2019).
[120] For a discussion on *the Patent Ordinance 1907* see: Swaminathan, Patent Law in Sri Lanka
http://www.juliusandcreasy.com/inpages/publications/pdf/pantent_law_in_sri_lanka.pdf (last retrieved 20 February 2019).
[121] This Act was amended by *Act No 30 of 1980, No 2 of 1983, No 17 of 1990, No 13 of 1997, No 40 of 2000* and the most current version of the *Act is No. 36 of 2003.*
[122] *Intellectual Property Regulation No. 1 of 2006*

Intellectual Property Act No. 36 of 2003. Part III of the Regulation deals with patents.

The National Intellectual Property Office (NIPO) of Sri Lanka is responsible for granting patents.[123] Except for the protection of plants and animals, Sri Lankan patent law is fully compliant with provisions in the TRIPS Agreement.[124] Therefore, the issues that are relevant with regard to TRIPS would become equally applicable in relation to Sri Lankan law as well.[125]

A patent is usually valid only in the country where it is granted, but being a member of the *Paris Convention for the Protection of Industrial Property,*[126] Sri Lankans can obtain patents for their inventions in all member countries of the Paris Convention, under the respective country's national laws. [127] Alternatively, as Sri Lanka is a member of the *Patent Cooperation Treaty*, Sri Lankan nationals or residents can apply for patents in any or as many of the member countries of *Patent Cooperation Treaty*.[128] Plant varieties, however, are an area that is highly significant for local and indigenous health and wellbeing practices, but that is not comprehensively covered by Sri Lanka law implementing international agreements.

(iii) Legal Framework for the Protection of Traditional Knowledge in Sri Lanka

The scope of the *Legal Framework for the Protection of Traditional Knowledge in Sri Lanka*[129] has made provisions for registration of traditional knowledge, a database for traditional knowledge in the public domain, controlling access to traditional knowledge, prior informed consent, licence contracts, traditional knowledge fund, and enforcements in protecting traditional knowledge. According to the legal framework, the

---

[123] National Intellectual Property Office. Patents. http://www.nipo.gov.lk/patent.htm (last retrieved 20 February 2019).

[124] Ramanna and Udgaonkar (2005), p 192.

[125] Talagala (2012).

[126] *Paris Convention for the Protection of Industrial Property*, A 2.

[127] National Intellectual Property Office. Patents. http://www.nipo.gov.lk/patent.htm (last retrieved 20 February 2019).

[128] National Intellectual Property Office. Patents. http://www.nipo.gov.lk/patent.htm (last retrieved 20 February 2019).

[129] Working document, version 1 (January 2009) See: http://www.wipo.int/wipolex/en/text.jsp?file_id=191824 (last retrieved 20 February 2019).

Director General of Intellectual Property is responsible for implementation. This legal framework is still in a draft format.

(iv) National mechanism in place to protect traditional healing

Nationally there is a structure in place to promote and safeguard traditional healing. The government body responsible for traditional and indigenous medicine is the Ministry of Indigenous Medicine. The two main arms under the supervision of the Ministry are the Department of Ayurveda responsible for curative services, regulatory functions, research, and certain matters pertaining to Ayurvedic educationand the Ayurvedic Drugs Corporation engaged in the production and sale of Ayurveda drugs. In order to execute some of the functions of the Department of Ayurveda, three statutory bodies were set up under the *Ayurveda Act No. 31 of 196*1, namely, the Ayurvedic Medical Council, Ayurveda Education and Hospital Board and the Ayurveda Research Committee; and one non-statutory committee, namely, the Ayurveda Formulary Committee. The Bandaranaike Ayurveda Research Institute in Nawinna, is the research institute and the National Institute of Traditional Medicine, is the training institute administered under the Department of Ayurveda. Also the Department monitors the 62 Ayurvedic hospitals including teaching and research hospitals, 208 central dispensaries and herbal gardens.[130] Although there is a mechanism in place to protect indigenous medicine, the Government's narrow approach to healing practices, ayurvedisation of healing practices and efforts to safeguard traditional healing practices from being informed and influenced by a biomedical framework has hampered the protection of traditional practices in health and wellbeing. This study will examine these regulatory bodies and areas of conflict and contestation in detail in Chapter 4.

Part 2 of the chapter has portrayed the legal pluralism mechanisms in place to protect traditional healing practices. Part 3 elaborates the historical influences in development of muti-cultural legal pluralism. Part 3: How the Regulation of Traditional Practices Related to Health and Wellbeing has been Affected by Colonialism. To understand the regulation of health and wellbeing, it is important to understand the historical factors that have impacted that regulation, particularly the values and moral principles that have governed the development, utilization and transmission of knowledge and cultural expressions. The most significant historical factor that has impacted Sri Lanka's knowledge systems and cultural

[130] The Ministry of Indigenous Medicine.
http://www.indigenousmedimini.gov.lk/About_us.html (last retrieved 20 February 2019).

expressions is European colonisation. Sri Lanka was a European colony from 1505[131] to 1948.[132] This section discusses how colonial influences in the traditional legal system, and health care system have negatively impacted the regulation of health and wellbeing in traditional practices in Sri Lanka.

2.3 Changes in traditional legal systems

The foundation of the traditional Sri Lankan law in pre-colonial Sri Lanka was the customs and traditions of the Sri Lankan community, based on religious beliefs. The sources of traditional law are religious law and Buddhist traditions, the Hindu law and traditions, Shakya and Mourya traditions, previous customs, caste customs, village customs and South Indian Customs.[133] For instance, Sinhala Law as portrayed in the *Niti-Niganduva*[134] was influenced by Buddhist principles and the *Theseawalami Law*[135] which was applied to Hindus was influenced by Hindu principals. The pre-colonial legal system was the key mechanism to promote and safeguard the traditional knowledge and it was reflected in the values and beliefs of the community.

According to the *Niti Niganduva* the main forms of law are, the Dhamma law, King's law[136] and the customary law.[137] However, Malwathu Mahanayake Thero's[138] letter to the Steering Committee to the Dutch Governor, refers to traditional Sri Lankan law as having two major

---

[131] 1505 is the year the Portuguese, Sri Lanka's first European colonizers, arrived in Sri Lanka (Pieris and Naish (1920)).

[132] Sri Lanka was ruled by Portuguese, Dutch and the British. In 4 February 1948 Sri Lanka (known as Ceylon) was granted independence and self-rule by the British Empire.

[133] Jayasekera, p 81.

[134] LeMasurier and Panabokke (1880).

[135] Thesawalami law codified by the Dutch in the seventeenth century is based on the foundation of customs and traditions of Tamils since Arya Chakravarthi's regime in Jaffna (fourteenth century) (Gamage (2007), p 2.

[136] The King in ancient Sri Lanka had the sole authority. Selection of the king, his duties and responsibilities were based on established customs. Kings commands include command on issues that cannot be solved from any of the prevailing laws and command to change a law being practiced. The laws and system of control laid-down by the kings of Anuradhapura era was applied in all the kingdoms of Sri Lanka from ancient times. (Gamage (2007), p 7)

[137] LeMasurier and Panabokke (1880).

[138] Malwathu Mahanayake Thero is the chief Monk of one of the two Siam Nikaya monastic order, called Malwatta.

categories, namely, King's customs (King's law) and World customs (worldly law). According to the interpretation of Gamage, the reason to exclude 'Dhamma law' from the major categories of law could be that the worldly law would cover the Dhamma law as the meaning of Dhamma according to the ancient sources including Mahavamsha is 'customs.'[139]

The Dutch introduced and applied the Roman-Dutch law[140] together with customary laws, such as Kandyan law,[141] Tesavalamai law,[142] Islamic law.[143] Unfortunately the new Roman Dutch law did not have a relationship with the traditional spirituality and was alien to the Sri Lankan community. The new legal system thus had an effect in changing the values, customs and social practices of traditional Sri Lanka.

2.4 Changes in Health and Wellbeing

In the pre-colonial history Sri Lanka's concept and practice of health and wellbeing was influenced mostly by Buddhism and also Hinduism and Islam. Religion, particularly Buddhism, and its ideals play a key role in influencing the beliefs the healing systems are based on and the rituals.

The three major traditional healing practices in Sri Lanka that is still practiced today and is recognized by the Government of Sri Lanka are Ayurveda, Siddha and Unani healing practices. Originally Ayurveda[144] and

---

[139] Gamage (2007), p 13.

[140] Gamage (2007) argues the introduction of Roman Dutch law in the coastal area controlled by the Dutch during their time of colonization (1656-1796) had a negative impact on the ancient local legal system in the country.

[141] Kandyan law was applied as territorial law to all inhabitants in the Kandyan provinces who happened to be almost exclusively Sinhalese during the time of Sinhalese kings. Later Kandyan law came to be regarded as a personal law applicable only to Sinhalese who were domiciled in the Kandyan provinces. Cooray (2015), p. 213.

[142] Customs of the Tamils of Jaffna was codified for the first time during Dutch period as Thesavalami law. Gamage (2007).

[143] Laws of Muslims were safeguarded by applying Islamic law to the Muslim community.

[144] The history of Ayurveda in India is traced back to 5,000 BCE. (Mackenzie and Rakel (2006) 215) During the Medieval period, Ayurveda was used as a travel tool in which Indian traditional knowledge systems were spread. Various forms of folk medical systems in India were called Ayurveda. Ayurveda, is not, however, a single homogenous healing practice; instead, it is a multi-phased system. (Wujastyk, Smith, and ebrary, edited book *Modern and global ayurveda: Pluralism and paradigms* analyses the multi-dimensions of Ayurveda.) The types of Ayurveda first introduced to Sri Lanka included Ayur medicine, Vedic Medicine, Hindu medicine

Siddha were both influenced by Hinduism. Ayurveda was adopted and was practiced commonly among the Sinhalese Buddhist[145] while Siddha was adopted in Northern Sri Lanka and practiced mostly by the Hindu Tamils. Unani medicine that has Arab origins[146] is commonly practiced by the Muslims of Sri Lanka. Development of Ayurveda in Sri Lanka took place principally in a Buddhist matrix and the Sanga played a major role.[147] Buddhism is also closely associated with folk healing practices including spirit healing and inter-generational healing.

Traditional and indigenous healing flourished in Sri Lanka for many centuries until the colonial invasions introduced Western medicine into the Island. The neglect and oppression of traditional healing systems including Ayurveda by the colonisers in the early period of colonisation led to a steady decline of the practice of Ayurveda.[148]

As there had been no systematic process to promote or monitor traditional and indigenous healing since the beginning of colonial administration, quaks with little or no knowledge of Ayurveda appeared all over the country as Ayurveda practitioners. The practice of Ayurveda became a source of great danger to the community.[149] In the public interest it was clearly necessary for Ayurveda to be completely banned or restored and developed.[150] Due to the deep-rooted public faith and demand for traditional medicine, it was not possible to ban Ayurveda completely.[151] The

---

and Indian medicine. (Based on the lecture delivered by Dr. Danister Perera on 'Ayurvedization of Indigenous Medical Knowledge' on 30 December 2013 at the Royal Asiatic Society, Colombo 7.). Liyanaratne argues, Ayurveda in Sri Lanka is a mixture of traditions: *Ātreya* and *Dhanvantari*, *Pulasti* and *Agastya*, and the tradition of *rasa*. Although Ayurveda found in Sri Lanka is similar to the Ayurveda of India (particularly in respect of principles and doctrines), there are certain differences with regard to therapeutics, medicinal composition and the plants used. (See, for example, Jayasinghe (1968), Liyanaratne (1999), pp 25-26).

[145] Buddhists, adding new insights to Ayurveda have taken it along with religion to many lands, including Tibet, Sri Lanka, Burma and China. Frawley (2000), p 6.

[146] Based on Ministry of Indigenous Medicine website http://www.indigenousmedimini.gov.lk/ (last retrieved 20 February 2019)

[147] Liyanaratne (1999), p xi.

[148] Ministry of Health (1955), p.3.

[149] Ministry of Health (1955), p.3.

[150] Ministry of Health Proposals for the Revival and Development of Indigenous Medicine in Ceylon (1955) has clearly identified the threats faced by Ayurveda due to colonial influence and the reservations of the colonial administration in reviving Ayurveda in the country. p 3.

[151] For a detail discussion on public demand and the establishment of a Government controlled traditional medicine system in Sri Lanka, see Chapter 4 (Part 1).

Ceylonese Government in 1916 declared it would consider the possibilities of granting of assistance for the teaching of indigenous medicine.

Up to now part 3 has argued how colonialism has influenced the traditional legal system, and health care system of Sri Lanka and have threatened the existence traditional knowledge and practices related to health and wellbeing.

Part 4: Revitalisation Efforts of Traditional Knowledge and its Impact on Traditional Healing and Wellbeing Practices of Sri Lanka

This section argues that revivalist movements in the last years of colonial rule and in the post-colonial era have been influential in reviving some aspects of traditional knowledge systems, practices and culture. Traditional cultures, religions, arts and crafts, occupations, healing practices were interrelated. As discussed in the preceding section, the dominance achieved by Christianity as well as colonial influence in changing traditional laws, policies and social systems, threatened pre-colonial traditional knowledge systems. As a reaction to colonial influences, revivalist movements that contributed towards the independence of Sri Lanka on 4 February 1948, sprang up in the country in the second half of the nineteenth century.[152] It was through the 'cultural nationalism'[153] ideologies created through the revival movements, that the activists managed to create national consciousness[154] among the people and revive traditional knowledge. These revival movements significantly influenced religion, education, language and traditional health care systems that in turn contributed towards reviving some aspects of traditional knowledge systems, practices and culture.

4.1 Religious revival

The introduction of Christianity and the loss of state patronage had a drastic negative effect mainly on Buddhism, the dominant religion in Sri Lanka in the pre-colonial era and also on Hinduism and Islam. Buddhists, Hindus and

---

[152] Samaraweera (1997), p 293.

[153] A national identity shaped by cultural traditions and language contributed in constructing an alternative lifestyle that rejected Western values, rather than directly confronting the British Colonial Administration.

[154] 'National Consciousness,' an understanding that a group of people in a certain geographic area share a common ethnic or linguistic or cultural evolution is a first step of gaining colonial independence. Kannangara (2011), p xii.

Muslims who had acquired wealth sponsored and funded the revival of their faiths as well as the establishment of modern schools teaching in English, based on respective faiths.[155]

The Buddhist Revival Movement dating back at least to the eighteenth-century,[156] immensely contributed towards the growth of national consciousness and the recovery of national pride via the promotion of Buddhism. The movement witnessed various interpretations of Buddhism by the Buddhist laity.[157] The early Buddhist reformers started reacting by imitating protestant Christianity strategies of organising religious practice. These strategies include establishing Buddhist schools, establishing Buddhist organisations such as the Young Men's Buddhist Association and printing Buddhist advocacy material, and organising debates. These early Buddhist reformers were called the Protestant Buddhists[158]. The traditional or neo-traditional Buddhism resurged during the Buddha Jayanthi period. The V*ipassanā Bhāvanā* (insight meditation) Movement resumed and reinterpreted meditation among the laity. Sarvodaya Shramadana Movement[159] was established based on Buddhist interpretations of addressing issues in society. Reinterpretation and branching out of Buddhism contributed greatly towards the revival of Buddhism.

The Panadura debate of 1873 was the most notable Buddhist-Christian confrontation. The establishment of the Vidyodaya Pirivena in 1872 and the Vidyalankara Pirivena in 1876 as centres of Oriental learning were initiatives to revitalise the oriental culture. The initiation of the Buddhist education movement, establishment of an education fund and a Buddhist national fund, the celebration of Vesak, and the design and adoption of a Buddhist flag were contributions by Colonel Henry Steel Olcott[160] towards the revival of Buddhism, with the support of leading Bhikkhus and laymen.[161]

---

[155] Jayawardena (2012), p xxv.

[156] Bastian (2009), p 127.

[157] The four patterns of reinterpreting Buddhism is based on Bond's clustering (1988).

[158] Obeysekera (1970).

[159] Ministry of Education, p 2.

[160] Colonel Henry Steel Olcott (2 August 1832 – 17 February 1907), played an important role in revival of Buddhism in Sri Lanka. Being an American, Olcott viewed and interpreted Buddhism through a westernised lens. Hence he is considered as a Buddhist modernist. For more on Olcott see, Motwani (1955); Murphet (1972); Prothero (1996); Guruge (2007).

[161] De Silva (1981), p 342.

The Hindus were in a more advantageous position in relation to resistance to the intrusion of the Christian missions as it was possible to draw on the resources of Hinduism in India and the Tamil elite. In the nineteenth century, Hinduism as a religion and a culture was revived. The Hindu revival pre-dated that of Buddhism by a whole generation.[162]

The arrival of Ahmed Orabi Pasha[163] (1829-1911) and his key lieutenants to Sri Lanka in January 1883[164] aroused Muslim interest in reviving their identity and culture.[165] Pasha became a symbol around which the Muslims could gather. [166] Carol S. Anderson has characterised Muslim revival as 'increased lay devotion and increased use of religious texts'.[167] Education was the initial focus of this Muslim revivalism. Before the Muslim revival efforts in early 1880s, Muslim education was confined to a few madrasas and one or two irregular newssheets until the early 1880s.[168] Muslim revivalism should be seen as a heightening of the collective identity of Muslims as a community, a separated group.[169]

4.2 Educational revival

Sri Lanka's education system was revived in the late nineteenth and early twentieth century when Buddhist[170] and Hindu religious organisations established their own schools. These Buddhist and Hindu religious schools[171] were an outcome of the nationalist movements' efforts to promote national consciousness. Education, based on traditional religions practiced in the country for generations, was a means of promoting the traditional value systems, transmitting traditional knowledge and

---

162 De Silva (1981), p 351.

163 Orabi Pasha was an Egyptian army leader, and a nationalist who led a national revolt against injustice in 1879 against Turkish ruler Fewfik. See Udugama. That exile from Egypt who inspired many. Kandy Times. (March 2, 2008) http://www.sundaytimes.lk/080302/KandyTimes/kandytimes_0026.html (last retrieved 20 February 2019).

164 Orabi Pasha also referred as Arabi Pasha was exiled in Sri Lanka for nineteen years between 1883 and 1901. Wickremasinghe (2014).

165 Wickremasinghe (2014).

166Anderson (2003), p184.

167 Anderson (2003), p 184.

168 Wickremasinghe (2014).

169 Samaraweera (1997), p 308.

170 The Buddhist education movement was initiated by Olcott with the help of leading monks and laymen. De Silva (1981), p 342. By 1890 the Theosophical society had established forty Buddhist schools. De Silva (1981), p 347.

171 Ministry of Education, p 2.

safeguarding traditional identity. Yet, all the schools of the country followed the National Education Curriculum which was greatly influenced by Western thinking and Western forms of knowledge. However, the education received from a Christian school was different from that which was received from a Buddhist or Hindu school since the religions taught and languages of instruction were not the same.

4.3 Revival of language

The Official Language Act no. 33 of 1956 prescribed the Sinhala Language as the only official language of Ceylon and enabled transitory provisions to be made. The act is an example of Sri Lankan Government efforts to revive Sinhala, the language used by majority of Sri Lankans. The following statement by Phillip Gunaradena, illustrates the important role of the Sinhala Only Bill in the national revival:

> We are completing by this [Sinhala Only] Bill an important phase in our national struggle. The restoration of the Sinhala language to the position it occupied before the occupation of this country by foreign powers marks an important stage in the history of the development of this island.[172]

Munidassa Cumaratunga's (1897-1944) contribution to language revival is also noteworthy. As a scholar of Sinhala, he revived the cultural landscape of the country through his Sinhala writings. Cumaratunga's three books, *Sidat Sangara Vivaranaya* (1935) [173] which was a critical analysis of the *Sidat Sangarava, Kriya Vivaranaya* (1936) [174] a treatise on the Sinhala Verb and *Vyakarana Vivaranaya* (1938) [175] a comprehensive grammar of Sinhala have been seen as extremely important in reviving the structure and distinctiveness of Sinhala language.[176]

4.4 Health care revival

Although the colonial administration wanted to see the eradication of an Ayurvedic system of medicine and replace it with the Western medical system, due to the public agitation for revival and development of indigenous medicine, the need for a change of policy was becoming more

[172] Phillip Gunawardene, Sri Lankan Cabinet Minister, *Hansard* (14 June 1956).
[173] Dharmadasa (1991), p 271.
[174] Dharmadasa (1991), p 271.
[175] Dharmadasa (1991), p 271.
[176] Dissanayake (2005), p 41.

apparent.[177] Detailed analysis of the Sri Lankan Government revival efforts of traditional health care are presented in Chapter 4.

This part has argued how revival movements significantly influenced in reviving Buddhism, Hinduism and Islam; introducing education based on pre-colonial religions; reviving Sinhala language and traditional health care system. Influence of the revival movement in each of these areas had an impact in reviving some aspects of traditional knowledge systems, practices and culture.

Conclusion

This chapter has recognised the multi-cultural legally pluralistic nature of the regulation of traditional practices related to health and wellbeing in Sri Lanka. To do so, chapter has provided an overview of some of the international schemes dealing, at least in some way, with traditional practices related to health and wellbeing, focusing on the right of indigenous peoples to self-determination, access and benefit sharing and intellectual property.

The chapter has started with a focus on international schemes dealing with traditional practices related to health and wellbeing. In this part, an overview of the international negotiations of traditional knowledge and traditional cultural expressions, particularly as they relate to recognising the right of indigenous peoples to self-determination, access and benefit sharing and intellectual property have been presented. To do so, the chapter has traced the development of the protection regime in traditional knowledge from the recognition of rights to self-determination of indigenous peoples to calls for the safeguarding and protection of traditional knowledge, expression and practice, as well as for sharing the benefits resulting from the exploitation of traditional knowledge, expression and practice.

Keeping in mind the role of international schemes in dealing with traditional practices related to health and wellbeing, part 2 of the chapter has explored how Sri Lanka regulates traditional practices related to health and wellbeing under a range of laws. Looking at Sri Lanka's role in application of international laws related to health and wellbeing, it has been shown that Sri Lanka has taken measures to comply by international schemes in protecting traditional practices related to health and wellbeing, although not fully compliant. Then, looking at Sri Lanka's domestic laws and mechanisms related to health and wellbeing it is argued that Sri Lanka's domestic laws and mechanisms related to protecting traditional practices in

[177] Ministry of Health (1955), p 3.

health and wellbeing appear adequate on the books. However, in practical implementation, the domestic laws and mechanisms does not fully protect traditional practices in health and wellbeing. This argument has been explored by looking at (i) the intellectual property law in Sri Lanka with an emphasis on the compliance with international laws; (ii) the role of patents; (iii) the legal framework to protect traditional knowledge in Sri Lanka and (iv) the national mechanism in place to protect traditional healing.

To obtain a clearer understanding of the regulation of health and wellbeing in Sri Lanka, part 3 and part 4 of the chapter has looked into it the historical factors that have impacted regulation, particularly the values and moral principles that governed the development, utilization and transmission of knowledge and cultural expressions. Part 3 of the chapter focuses on the influence of European colonisation in the regulation of health and wellbeing. This part has argued that colonial influence in the traditional legal systemand health care system have had a significant negative impact on traditional practices in health and wellbeing and its regulation in Sri Lanka. Part 4 of the chapter portrays how traditional knowledge systems, practices and regulation in Sri Lanka were linked to traditional legal system, and as a result the colonial influence threatened the existence traditional knowledges and practices related to health and wellbeing.

As a reaction to colonial influence in Sri Lankan society, there were many efforts towards revitalisation of traditional knowledge. Part 4 of the Chapter has looked into how these revitalisation efforts impacted on traditional healing and wellbeing practices. This part has discussed how revival movements significantly influenced the revival of Buddhism, Hinduism and Islam, introducing education based on pre-colonial religions, reviving Sinhala language, and traditional health care system. The influence of the revival movement in each of these areas in turn had an impact on reviving some aspects of traditional knowledge systems, practices and culture.

This review of the historical background and current legislations has highlighted the need for a more comprehensive recognition of the diversity of Sri Lankan healing practices and an examination of how effectively these healing practices are being safeguarded as part of this country's cultural heritage. Arguments in this chapter has revealed, that traditional healing is based on individual relationship between healer and the patient, and as a result protecting traditional practices using Western ideas of tangible or intangible property results in the traditional cultural aspects of healing being threatened and indigenous healing methods being neglected. One way of introducing more effective legal protection of diverse healing practices could be through the adoption of an intercultural approach to legal pluralism;[178]' particularly as an interim measure until laws can be introduced to ensure consistency. This book therefore aims to contribute to and supplement this current body of knowledge. The following chapter presents the methodology used in this study.

---

[178] Intercultural approach to legal pluralism refers to a system that 'promotes respect for distinct legal jurisdictions while drawing upon a wide range of legal sources including state, customary and international law for the development of law in areas such as equity, criminal, land, family and constitutional law as well as human rights.' Tobin (2012), p 160.

CHAPTER 3

THE DIVERSITY OF HEALING PRACTICES IN SRI LANKA

Introduction

What healing practices are considered and used in Sri Lanka? To answer this question, this chapter examines various kinds of traditional healing in Sri Lanka. It identifies the diversity of healing practices used which include inter-generational practices adopted from other countries, cosmically-oriented healing practices, biomedical healing practices, practices using mixed methods,[1] and a variety of less recognised kinds of healing practices. Some examples of less recognised practices in Ayurveda include Siddhayurveda, Hybridayurveda and Keraminiya. There are also many less recognisedcategories of healing practices even within other traditions of healing. Each form of healing practice has its own associated cultural values, beliefs and traditions of practice which makes it distinct from other healing practices.

This chapter is organised into three parts. The first part describes government recognised traditional healing practices in Sri Lanka, namely Ayurveda, Siddha, Unani, Homeopathy, Acupuncture, and Deshiya Chikithsa. In so doing, it discusses the diversity of engagements within and between these practices. The second part outlines and briefly discusses the diversity of healing practices in Sri Lanka. This is presented by mapping the forms of healing practiced using the categories of inter-generational healing, cosmic healing, adopted traditional healing, biomedical healing and integrated healing. The classification is to better understand the role of the Government of Sri Lanka in recognising, supporting and regulating healing practices and the status of traditional cultural aspects of healing practices. The third part of the chapter describes the typology of relations between different forms of healing knowledge. The chapter is important as it sets the

[1] Examples for healing practices using mixed methods are inter-generational and Ayurveda; Ayurveda and western healing; cosmic healing and inter-generational healing.

stage for the book by presenting the diversity and complexities of the prevailing healing systems in Sri Lanka and arguing that only some systematic healing practices are recognised and regulated by the Government of Sri Lanka.

Part 1: Government Recognised Traditional Healing Practices in Sri Lanka

Only a few healing practices in Sri Lanka are recognised by the government as traditional healing practices, namely: Ayurveda, Siddha, Unani, Homeopathy, Acupuncture and Deshiya Chikithsa. An introduction to these healing practices is presented here as this description is necessary for this book to develop a sense of the approach of the government in characterising traditional healing.

The Sri Lankan Government generally uses the words ‘indigenous medicine’[2] and ‘traditional medicine’[3] interchangeably to refer to traditional healing systems. These terms, however, are not interchangeable: they do not mean the same thing nor does the Sri Lankan Government treat them in the same way.[4] One of the issues of the Sri Lankan Government using the terms indigenous medicine and traditional medicine terms is that, in the Sri Lankan context, the terms indigenous or traditional healing do not necessarily mean a healing system that originated in the country. For example, traditional healing systems currently covered under the scope of the Ministry of Indigenous Medicine are, Ayurveda (healing system adopted from North India),[5] Siddha (healing system adopted from South India), Unani (healing system adopted from Arabs) and Desheeya Chikitsa (indigenous system of medicine in Sri Lanka).[6] Only the last of these is usually claimed to have originated from Sri Lanka. In *Mahinda Chinthanaya*, (the election manifesto of the former President of Sri Lanka, Mahinda Rajapaksa from the 2005 Presidential elections) traditional Sinhala medicine,

---

[2] Indigenous medicine is used in the context of ‘Ministry of Indigenous Medicine’, ‘Institute of Indigenous Medicine.’

[3] Traditional medicine is used in the context of ‘National Institute of Traditional Medicine.’

[4] For a detail discussion on Government recognition, support and regulation of traditional healing see Chapter 6.

[5] This is how the Ministry of Indigenous Medicine has introduced Ayurveda. (See:http://www.indigenousmedimini.gov.lk/ (last retrieved 20 February 2019) In part 1 of this chapter I have analysed what Ayurveda really is in Sri Lanka.

[6] Ministry of Indigenous Medicine: Herbal Medicines in Sri Lanka. http://www.indigenousmedimini.gov.lk/index.html (last retrieved 20 February 2019).

Ayurveda, Siddha, Unani, Homeopathy and Acupuncture are referred to as indigenous health care.[7] In contrast to the Ministry of Indigenous Medicine, *Mahinda Chinthanaya* has additionally recognised Homeopathy and Acupuncture as part of the indigenous health care system. The definition of traditional Sinhala medicine in *Mahinda Chinthanaya* is not clear, however. Is it referring to inter-generational healing practices? Does it also cover cosmic healing practices? Are the healing practices covered under traditional Sinhala medicine limited to the healing practices of the Sinhala community? That the Ministry of Indigenous Medicine's definition of indigenous health care is different from *Mahinda Chinthanaya* illustrates that there is no consensus of the ambit of indigenous healing at the policy level.

In the next chapter, I analyse how the Sri Lankan Government supports and regulates these government recognised traditional healing practices. The following sections describe the government recognised traditional healing practices: Ayurveda, Siddha, Unani, Homeopathy, Acupuncture and Deshiya Chikithsa.

1.1 Ayurveda

Ayurveda is an Indian medical system,[8] popular in the context of India[9] as well as globally.[10] The guiding principle of Ayurveda is that the mind exerts a profound influence on the body[11] as the physical body reacts to the thoughts and experiences of the mind. More specifically, it is a system of healing that controls, directs, builds-up and finally prolongs life by warding off illness and ageing.

The history of Ayurveda in India is traced back to 5 000 BCE.[12] During 900-1300, Ayurveda was one of the Indian traditional knowledge systems that were spread to other countries of the world.[13] Ayurveda, is not, however, a single homogenous healing practice; instead, it is a multi-phased

---

[7] GOSL (2005), p.71.

[8] Ministry of Indigenous Medicine recognize 'Ayurveda' as an Indian medical system in its website. http://www.indigenousmedimini.gov.lk/ (last retrieved 20 February 2019)

[9] Lodha (2000).

[10] Patwardhan, Warude, Pushpangadan, and Bhatt (2005), p 465.

[11] Liyanaratne (1999), p xvi based on Patrick Drouot (1993) *Guersison spirituelle et immoralite: Les voies therapeutiques du futur*. Paris: Editions du Rocher, p 156.

[12] Mackenzie, and Rakel (2006), p 215.

[13] Ayurveda along with Indian culture has spread to many lands, including Tibet, Sri Lanka, Burma and China (Frawley (2000), p 6.

system.[14] The types of Ayurveda first introduced to Sri Lanka included Ayur medicine, Vedic Medicine, Hindu medicine and Indian medicine.[15] Liyanaratne argues that Ayurveda in Sri Lanka is a mixture of traditions: *Ātreya* and *Dhanvantari*, *Pulasti* and *Agastya*, and the tradition of *rasa*.[16] Although Ayurveda found in Sri Lanka is similar to the Ayurveda of India (particularly in respect of principles and doctrines), there are certain differences with regard to therapeutics, medicinal composition and the plants used.[17]

Although in Sri Lanka there existed various forms of indigenous, folk healing systems before the introduction of Ayurveda, the Ayurveda system of healing dominated culturally, historically, educationally and professionally primarily due to the colonial administrative interventions in the latter periods of British colonial rule including the laws starting from 1927.[18] More specifically, the Ceylonese government attempted to support and encourage the Ayurveda medical system considering the public demand for Ayurveda and lack of health care facilities, by implementing various legal, political and social measures.[19] Under the Sri Lankan colonial rule Ayurveda was recognised as a socio-medical system where it was considered to be very similar to western medical science.[20] One of the key differences between Ayurveda and the western medical system is the use of modern technology in western medicine.[21] Based on the Majority Report of 1927, the Ceylonese Government decided to establish training colleges, hospitals and other facilities for Ayurveda, to protect and promote the livelihoods of the indigenous healers.[22] The term 'Ayurveda' was used for all forms of traditional and indigenous healing practices; and all of the

---

[14] Wujastyk and Smith (2008) analyses the multi-dimensions of Ayurveda.

[15] Based on the lecture delivered by Dr. Danister Perera on '*Ayurvedization of Indigenous Medical Knowledge*' on 30 December 2013 at the Royal Asiatic Society, Colombo 7.

[16] Liyanaratne (1999), p. 25.

[17] See, for example, D. M. Jayasinghe (1968)" *Āryurveda in Wickremarachi Felicitation Volume*, Kelaniya, pp 71-96. Quoted in Liyanaratne (1999), p 25-26.

[18] The Indigenous Medical Board was established on 1927; *Ayurveda Medical Council Ordinance No. 46* was passed in 1935; *Indigenous Medical Ordinance No. 17* was passed in 1941.

[19] The process followed by the Indian Colonial Government to uplift the Ayurveda Medical System was replicated in Sri Lanka. (Based on Dr. Danister Perera's Lecture on "Ayurvedization of Indigenous Medical Knowledge," 30 December 2013, Organized by the Royal Asiatic Society of Sri Lanka).

[20] Dr. M. W. S. J. Kumari (#11).

[21] Mr. Palitha Weerakoon (#3).

[22] Report of the Committee on Indigenous System of Medicine. No. 1 of 1927.

structures established to promote traditional and indigenous healing during this time were referred to 'Ayurveda.' For instance, the Department of Ayurveda (responsible for protecting Ayurveda, Siddha, Unani and Indigenous Medicine), the Ayurveda Hospital, the Ayurveda Dispensary, Ayurveda Sanrakshana Sabha (to protect indigenous medicine), the Ayurveda Pharmacopeia, and Ayurveda Medical Practitioner (legally there is no one called indigenous medical practitioner), were all established at this time.

Indigenous methods of healing were assumed by the policy makers to be included in the legal definitions of Ayurveda. The *Ayurveda Act No 31 of 1961*, which is the primary law directed to the protection of indigenous medicine in Sri Lanka refers only to Ayurveda. That is all traditional and indigenous healing practitioners are referred to as 'Ayurveda practitioner', all traditional/ indigenous dispensers of medicine are referred to as 'Ayurveda Pharmacist,' and all nurses practicing in traditional healing are called 'Ayurveda Nurse.' It is unclear from the *Ayurveda Act* whether and what other indigenous medicine systems are covered. As per the Ministry of Indigenous Medicine website, indigenous medicine in Sri Lanka are, 'the Ayurveda system of medicine from North India, the Siddha system of medicine from South India, Unani system of medicine of Arabs enriched with the contributions from the traditional system of medicine called Desheeya Chikithsa.'[23] Even the main task of the Ministry is to 'provide Ayurveda services to the nation.'[24] The work of the Ministry however shows that its work is not limited to Ayurveda healing practice, but includes other indigenous medicine, and the word 'Ayurveda' is used to incorporate other indigenous and traditional healing practices.[25] It is not clear what indigenous and traditional healing methods are covered in legal documents. Indigenous medicine has been absorbed within the definition and is therefore recognised as a sub-type of Ayurveda. Not recognising the diverse forms of indigenous healing as different categories, has potentially a great negative impact in safeguarding such healing practices. Chapter 6 on Inter-Generational Healing and Loss of Culture discusses this issue further.

---

[23] Ministry of Indigenous Medicine Website See: http://www.indigenousmedimini.gov.lk/ (last retrieved 20 February 2019).

[24] M inistry of Indigenous Medicine Website See http://www.indigenousmedimini.gov.lk/ (last retreived 20 February 2019).

[25] For example, the Ministry provides educational programmes through National Institute of Traditional Medicine for Ayurveda, Siddha, Unani, Traditional medicine; Ayurveda Medical Council register Ayurveda, Siddha, Unani qualified Doctors, Traditional healing practitioners; hospitals and dispensaries under the Ministry provide Ayurveda, Siddha, Unani and traditional health care services.

Sri Lanka's state sponsored system of Ayurveda which is presented in Figure 3.1 can be summarised as based on education levels, government employment prospects, documentation of Ayurveda, form of research conducted, type of healing practices available, type of hospitals and the form of administration.

Education	PhD Post-Graduate Diplomas Bachelor's Degree Diploma in Ayurveda (Syllabus – Universal, Medium of Instruction – English)
Employment	Government Employment for persons with Bachelor's degree or above qualification from a Sri Lankan or foreign recognised University
Documentation	Mostly based on Indian Text books
Research	Using Western techniques
Practice	Imitating the Western Medical Practitioner OPD – Clinics In-House Patients
Hospitals	Western Hospital structure
Administration	Western structure of Administration. Western Medicine qualified Doctors in highest levels of Indigenous Medicine Administration

Figure 3.1 – The existing government system of Ayurveda in Sri Lanka

Based on my field research findings, despite the efforts of Sri Lankan Government in introducing a homogenous Ayruveda in Sri Lanka, the prevailing Ayurveda system in Sri Lanka can be divided into three areas, namely: Hybrid Ayurveda, Siddha Ayurveda and Keraminiya Ayurveda. Figure 3.2 summarises these three categories of Ayurveda:

Siddha Ayurveda	Hybrid Ayurveda	Keraminiya Ayurveda
Practice only Ayurveda without combining with modern practices	Ayurveda combined with Western systems of healing	Ayurveda practices mixed with inter-generational healing practices
Siddha Ayurveda Vidyalaya, Gampaha	College of Indigenous Medicine, Borella (now known as Indigenous Institute of Medicine, University of Colombo)	Traditional Ayurveda Medical College of Keraminiya, Mawanella
The Siddha Ayurveda system was championed by Pandith Wickramarachchi	The Hybrid Ayurveda system was championed by Dr. A. N. N. Panikkar and Dr. R. B. Lenora	The Keraminiya Ayurveda system was championed by Venerable Aluthnuwara Anomadassi

Figure 3.2 – Different types of Ayurveda practiced in Sri Lanka

Acknowledging the differences of Ayurveda is important as the Ayurveda teaching institutions as well as practitioners tend to distinguish themselves based on the form of Ayurveda healing practice they are disseminating or have acquired.

1.1.1 Siddha Ayurveda

The Siddha Ayurveda practiced in Gampaha refers to 'pure – Ayurveda.'[26] This tradition was first introduced in 1929 by Ayurveda Pandit G. P. Wickraramarachchi by establishing Gampaha Siddhayurveda Vidyalaya[27] in 1929. Pandit Wickramarachchi studied the Siddha Ayurveda tradition in Calcutta and introduced it to Sri Lanka.[28] Siri Vajiraghanodaya Pirivena,

[26] Dr. Saranadasa Devaraja (# 9), Dr. E. A. S. C.S. Edirisuriya (# 7) and Dr. M. Chithra Nalini (# 8) (Based on discussion of the meaning of Siddha Ayurveda).
[27] Since the institute was affiliated to the University of Kelaniya, it has been known as Gampaha Wickramarachchi Ayurveda Institute.
[28] Mr. W. A. D. Chithrananda (# 46).

Siddhayurveda Medical Institute still continues to teach the Siddha Ayurveda tradition.[29] The Gampaha Siddh Ayurveda tradition is different to the Siddha – Ayurveda healing tradition in Jaffna. As the healers interviewed for this work explained, the major difference between the two traditions are: Siddh Ayurveda in Gampaha is a form of purc Ayurveda while Siddha Ayurveda in Jaffna is a mix of the Siddha healing system and Ayurveda healing system.[30]

1.1.2 Hybrid Ayurveda

Hybrid Ayurveda refers to the Ayurveda practices that have integrated with modern diagnostic technology, medicine, surgery and western forms of research.[31] Hybrid Ayurveda tradition follows from the Indigenous Medical College (*Swadeshiya Vaidya Vidyalaya*) established on 10th June 1929.[32] The Indigenous Medical College was established on *Ayurveda Sammelana Sabha* recommendations of establishing an institute of indigenous medicine integrating with modern science and technology.[33] To achieve the objectives of introducing integrated indigenous medical system (a system of Hybrid Ayurveda), Dr. A. N. N. Panikkar from India who had western medical qualifications and a sound training in Ayurveda sciences was made the first Director of the College of Indigenous Medicine from 1929 to 1950[34] The next main advocate of Hybrid Ayurveda was Dr. R. B. Lenora, Director of the College of Indigenous Medicine from 1952 to 1965.[35] Dr. Lenora, a prominent physician in Colombo had earned a scholarship from the Oriental Medicine Society in Ceylon to attend the Jamini Bhushan Astanga Ayurveda College in Calcutta, where he has studied an integrated curriculum of

---

[29] Dr. Saranadasa Devaraja (# 9). The purpose of establishing Siri Vajiraghanodaya Pirivena, Siddhayurveda Medical Institute is to protect the pure- Ayurveda tradition.

[30] Dr. E. A. S. C.S. Edirisuriya (# 7); Dr. Saranadasa Devaraja (# 9), Je-Jeyalan (# 100).

[31] Dr. M. W. S. J. Kumari (# 11).

[32] Indigenous Medical College is now known as the Institute of Indigenous Medicine, University of Colombo. For a discussion of this institution see Chapter 5, 3.3.

[33] Ayurveda Sammelena Sabha is an Advisory Committee established by the State Council in 1928. The committee was chaired by Dr. K. Balasingham.

[34] Past Directors, Institute of Indigenous Medicine. https://iim.cmb.ac.lk/index.php/past-directors/ (last retrieved 20 February 2019).

[35] Past Directors, Institute of Indigenous Medicine. https://iim.cmb.ac.lk/index.php/past-directors/ (last retrieved 20 February 2019).

Ayurveda. Later he studied medicine in Edinburgh and Glasgow.[36] Charles Leslie introduces Dr. R. B. Lenora as,

> Dr. Lenora belonged to the generation of college-trained physicians who had imagined a national medical system inspired by indigenous tradition but incorporating modern science and technology.[37]

Dr. L. B. Lenora had wanted to 'add x-ray and laboratory facilities to the teaching hospital, to improve instruction in anatomy and surgery and to raise the standards of examinations' for which the then Minister of Local Administration and the Chairman of the Board of Indigenous Medicine, Bandaranaike did not agree.[38]

With the objective of introducing 'pure Ayurveda' in Sri Lanka, Bandaranaike invited Pandit Shiv Sharma, leading advocate of 'pure Ayurveda' in India and repeatedly elected President of the All India Ayurveda Congress since 1938[39] to advise on the integrated programme of indigenous and cosmopolitan medicine.[40] In Pandit Shiv Sharma's report he recommended 'that the teaching hospitals at indigenous medical colleges eliminate whatever uses they had made of modern diagnostic technology, chemotherapy, and surgery, and that the curriculum in the first years of training be limited entirely to concepts and practices from ancient and medieval texts.[41] These recommendations were opposed by the students of the College in Indigenous Medicine, Colombo who went on strike.[42] A

---

[36] Leslie (180), p180.

[37] Leslie (180), p 180.

[38] Minister Bandaranaike had held this post from 1937 to 1944. Leslie (1992) p 179-180.

[39] Pandit Shiv Sharma was invited by then the Minister of Health, Bandaranaike using the Colombo Plan for mutual aid between South Asian countries. Leslie (1992), p 180. Leslie also points out although Pandit Shiv Sharma was a leading advocate on pure Ayurveda publicly, he had been self-instructed in using modern diagnostic technology and for his patients, and he had ordered laboratory tests and x-rays. Pandit Shiv Sharma's only son had become an allopathic doctor. (1992), p 182.

[40] Earlier committee report by the *Ayurveda Sammelena Sabha* advised on an integrated programme of indigenous and cosmopolitan medicine. Ministry of Health Bandaranaike's invitation to Pandit Shiv Sharma was to present a report to revise the decision on an integrated programme of medicine made in the earlier report. Leslie (1992), p180.

[41] Leslie (1992), p182.

[42] Leslie (1992), p182.

hundred and fifiteen students were sent to integrated colleges in India to complete their education by Dr. Lenora.[43]

Since the College of Indigenous Medicine was affiliated to University of Colombo as the Institute of Indigenous Medicine,[44] and since Gampaha Siddha Ayurveda Vidyalaya was affiliated to the University of Kelaniya as Gampaha Wickremarachi Ayurveda Institute,[45] both institutions have incorporated hybrid Ayurveda into the curriculum where Ayurveda practice have integrated with modern diagnostic technology, medicine, surgery and western forms of research.[46]

1.1.3 Keraminiya Ayurveda

In many ways Keraminiya is an indigenised school of Ayurveda, that has been systematically developed in Sri Lanka, to treat all bodily disorders[47]. Kereminiya is based on the principles of Ayurveda and inter-generational healing.[48] In the process of developing Keraminiya as a systematic healing tradition, it has incorporated many components of Ayurvedic medicine. The Keraminiya system of medicine has been stabilised by establishing training institutions,[49] drug manufacturing centre,[50] and Keramiya Medical Centres that are spread in many parts of the island.

The system of Keraminiya Ayurveda has been given legal recognition by various legal schemes. For example, the *Palaka Sabhawa of Samastha Lanka Paranparika Ayurveda Vaidya Vidyalaya of Keraminiya, Mawanella (Incorporation) Act (No. 1 of 1986)* has given powers to:

- conduct, maintain and administer the Vidyalaya as a national institution providing instructions in the traditional Ayurveda system of medicine;[51]

---

[43] Leslie (1992), p182.

[44] In 1977 College of Indigenous Medicine was incorporated as Institute of Indigenous Medicine under *University Act no. 1 of 1972.*

[45] In 1982 Gampaha Siddha Ayurveda Vidyalaya was incorporated as Gampaha Wickramarachchi Ayurveda Institute under the Ministry of Indigenous Medicine by the *Parliamentary Act No 30, in 1982.*

[46] For a discussion on Institute of Indigenous Medicine and Gampaha Wickremarachchi Ayurveda Institute see Chapter 4, 3.3 and 3.4.

[47] Venerable. Dr. Kehalpannala Chandaloka (#83).

[48] Venerable. Dr. Kehalpannala Chandaloka (#83).

[49] The Keraminiya Indigenous Medical School is located in Mawanella.

[50] Keraminiya Drug Manufacturing Centre is located in Mawanella.

[51] *Palaka Sabhawa of Samastha Lanka Paranparika Ayurveda Vaidya Vidyalaya of Keraminiya, Mawanella (Incorporation) Act no. 1 of 1986* (Sri Lanka) s 3 *(a)*. The

- to establish an Ayurveda hospital to train medical students and provide free treatment to patients;[52]
- to conduct examinations to ascertain person who have acquired proficiency in the traditional Ayurveda system of medicine[53] (the examinations are to be conducted with the approval of the Commissioner of Ayurveda); and
- to construct, equip and maintain buildings that are necessary for the Vidyalaya.[54]

The Keraminiya Ayurveda Medical College is open to any person who meets the entrance educational requirement and is interested in being a Keraminiya healer.[55] As the training institute is not affiliated to a Sri Lankan University, it has a lower standard of entry. More specifically, the institute only requires that its students pass G. C. E. Advance Level[56] in any stream and is not limited to the Bio-Science stream[57]. Most of the students in the Keraminiya School are from traditional (inter-generational) healing backgrounds. The title of the school which in Sinhala is '*Samastha Lanka Paramparika Ayurveda Vidyalaya.*' is the 'All Island Inter-Generational Ayurveda Medical College.' Figure 3.3 is a photo of the entrance of the Keraminiya college, hospital, and drug manufacturing centre with the name board.

---

concern here is, what does the traditional system of Ayurveda refer to? Does it refer to inter-generational Ayurveda practice that is inclusive of indigenous methods of healing?

52 *Palaka Sabhawa of Samastha Lanka Paranparika Ayurveda Vaidya Vidyalaya of Keraminiya, Mawanella (Incorporation) Act no. 1 of 1986* (Sri Lanka) s 3 (b).

53 *Palaka Sabhawa of Samastha Lanka Paranparika Ayurveda Vaidya Vidyalaya of Keraminiya, Mawanella (Incorporation) Act no. 1 of 1986* (Sri Lanka) s 3 (c).

54 *Palaka Sabhawa of Samastha Lanka Paranparika Ayurveda Vaidya Vidyalaya of Keraminiya, Mawanella (Incorporation) Act no. 1 of 1986* (Sri Lanka) s 3 (d).

55 Venerable Dr. Kehalpannala Chandaloka (#83).

56 General Certificate of Education (G.C.E.) Advanced Level (A-level) is a qualification in Sri Lanka, taught in Year 12 and 13 (final two years) of schooling. It is regarded as the entrance exam for Sri Lankan State Universities. The examination is conducted by the Department of Examination of the Ministry of Education, in three languages, English, Sinhala and Tamil.

57 G.C.E. Advanced Level qualification diversifies over five major fields of study, 1. Physical Science stream, 2. Biological Science stream, 3. Commerce stream, 4. Arts stream and 5. Technical stream. Admission to Sri Lankan State University Medical College or for Ayurveda, Siddha and Unani programmes is limited to students qualifying and obtaining the Z-score (above the cut-off marks) in the Biological Science stream.

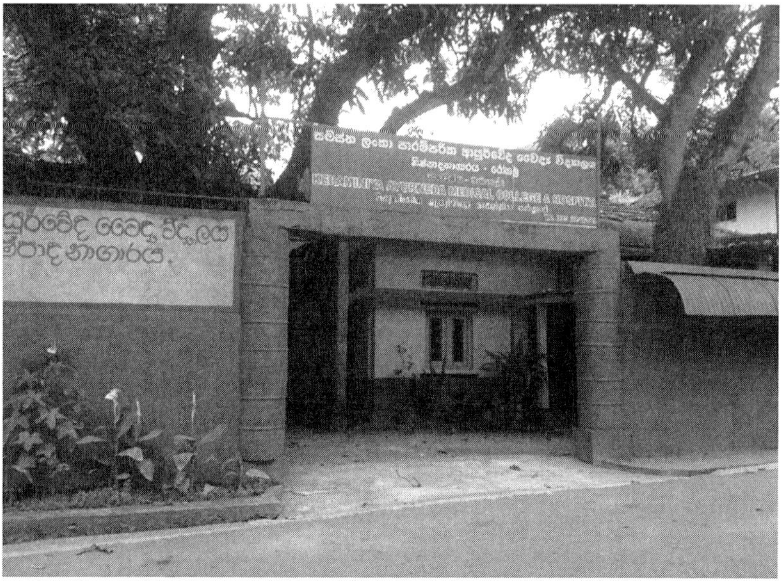

Figure 3.3- The Entrance View of Kereminiya Ayurveda Medical College and Hospital – Mawanella

1.2 Siddha (South Indian traditional medicine)

The Siddha treatment system, practiced mostly by Hindus, particularly in the north of Sri Lanka, is a tradition of medicine from South India.[58] This practice is systematically taught at the Department of Siddha medicine[59] in the University of Jaffna and Unit of Siddha Medicine, Trincomalee Campus, Eastern University at Bachelors degree and post-graduate diploma level. To enter the Siddha Department for the Bachelors degree at the university, the candidates have to possess the required Z-score[60] in G. C. E. Advanced Level. The candidates who complete a university degree qualification in Siddha are called 'Siddha Doctors' and those who possess the above degree

[58] Based on the Ministry of Indigenous Medicine website http://www.indigenousmedimini.gov.lk/ (last retrieved 20 February 2019).
[59] Department of Siddha Medicine, University of Jaffna – http://www.siddha.jfn.ac.lk/ (last retrieved 20 February 2019)
[60] Z-score is the quota system that admission of students to university is based on. (Warnapala and Silva, p 2)

qualifications in Siddha are called 'Siddha Specialists.'[61] Lanka Siddha – Ayurveda Medical College awards diplomas in Siddha medicine after five years of training.[62] Candidates who qualify through the Siddha-Ayurveda Diploma are called 'Siddha-Ayurveda' healers. People who acquire the inter-generational healing practice of Siddha without any academic qualifications are called 'traditional healers' or 'Siddha healers.'

The Siddha healing system is practiced in government hospitals including the Siddha Teaching Hospital in Jaffna District and Rural Siddha hospitals in the northern and eastern Provinces and in some Ayurveda hospitals in the other parts of the country. There are many Siddha doctors, Siddha-Ayurveda healers and traditional Siddha healers who conduct private practice. Most Siddha practitioners or Siddha-Ayurveda practitioners are located in north and the eastern provinces of Sri Lanka.

An inter-generational Siddha healer without a university degree will still fall under the scope of the government traditional healers. But they are not recognised as 'Siddha Doctors'.[63] Such healers belong to the category of 'Traditional Healers.'[64] A good example is the interviewee Paranasivamullai.[65] Paranasivamullai has learned the Siddha system of treatment from his ancestors and he also possess a Diploma in Ayurveda. He is registered as a traditional healer with the Ayurveda Medical Council. Paranasivamullai says the inter-generational healing system is very diverse. Although some inter-generational healers have called themselves 'Siddha', 'Ayurveda', 'Siddha-Ayurveda' practitioners, if they have learnt the practice from their family tradition, rather than following a systematic course, the practice is unique and diverse, as they practice with their own knowledge, family traditions and experience, rather than based on a systematic training. The indigenous Siddha healers have no connection with the Department of Siddha of University of Jaffna. Paranasivamullai's healing practice also illustrates the integration of healing practices. Paranasivamullai says, 'for some sicknesses I use either one of Siddha or Ayurveda treatments, some

---

[61] Dr. S. Sivashanmugarajah (# 99).

[62] Mr. S. Sivalingam (# 104).

[63] Such healers have to register as an inter-generational Ayurveda healer according to Ayurveda Medical Council Guidelines. Guidelines are available on http://www.ayurvedicmedicoun.gov.lk/web/images/download/guid01_sa_.pdf (last retrieved 20 February 2019)

[64] Traditional healer is a contested term. In Ayurveda Medical Council registration guidelines they are referred to as 'Hereditary Ayurveda Physicians' Ayurveda professional classification in the Ayurveda Medical Council refers to healers as 'Traditional (General)' and 'Traditional (Special)'

[65] Mr. S. Paranasivamullai (#102).

sicknesses require a mixture of both treatments, it depends on what I feel is best for that particular sickness.'[66] Paranasivamullai's specialised area of treatment is for rheumatic pains, asthma, and fever, yet he treats all forms of bodily disorders. Most of the medicines Paranasivamullai uses are prepared at home using natural herbs, based on Siddha and Ayurvedic medical recipes. He harvests some herbs required for the medicine and some are brought in by the patients themselves, after being directed as to where to find them.

Paranasivamullai has no fixed consultation fee for the patients. Only a nominal amount is charged to cover the expenses of preparing treatments. Paranasivamullai says, 'the money we receive by treating the patients is not too much, but it is sufficient to survive.'[67] Paranasivamullai believes 'it is the effectiveness of the treatment that will bring popularity to the healer and that would result in sustaining the healing system.'[68]

'There are some inter-generational practitioners who receive support from the government' says Paranasivamullai. He says 'If I want, I assume I too can receive support, but I am not sure of the process and eligibility criteria. I prefer to maintain my individuality and independence in the practice. I feel there is no need for governmental or other influence to obtain popularity.'[69]

The Government can support the inter-generational healers by enabling access to medicine ingredients. Current laws prohibit or have strictly regulated the usage of some herbal ingredients like '*Abing*.'[70] Paranasivamullai believes that these restrictions hamper the efficient practice of indigenous healers.

Paranasivamullai possesses some documentation about the traditional healing practices, which came from his ancestors, and he updates it according to the knowledge he has acquired from learning and experimenting. Paranasivamullai has an idea to publish this work in order to transfer the knowledge, but he has considered that right now is not the best time. Presently he is focusing on improving the practice and methods of treatment.

Paranasivamullai's case shows how inter-generational traditional healers in Siddha are different from the Siddha doctors with a formal university education in Siddha and who are given government appointments as Siddha doctors.

---

[66] Mr. S. Paranasivamullai (#102).
[67] Mr. S. Paranasivamullai (#102).
[68] Mr. S. Paranasivamullai (#102).
[69] Mr. S. Paranasivamullai (#102).
[70] Dr. Parakrama (#15).

1.3 Unani (medicine of Unan origin)

Unani is another traditional medical practice recognised, supported and regulated by the Sri Lankan Government.[71] The Unani medical practice has a Greek-Arab origin[72] and has developed a very good practice in Sri Lanka. Unani is widely known as a traditional medical system practiced mostly by the Muslims in the country; however, it is not limited to population group.[73] The formal academic courses are offered in Unani from the Institute of Indigenous Medicine, University of Colombo[74] and are mostly taken by Muslim students. Yet, a few Sinhala and Tamil students also study Unani. Most of the Unani medicine is still imported from India and the Middle East.[75] To understand the practice of Unani in a Sri Lankan context, a case of an Unani doctor practicing in Sri Lanka is considered.

Dr. Hameed A. Azeez J. P.[76] is a Unani qualified doctor practicing at the Azeez Medical Centre, Mawanella (see Figure 3.4) and a visiting lecturer at the Institute of Indigenous Medicine, University of Colombo for the past 25 years. Azeez's father had been a famous orthopaedic (*Kadum bindum*- fracture and dislocation) healer. Instead of carrying out the inter-generational healing practice based on learning from his father, Azeez has pursued academic qualifications in Unani. Being a Muslim, his cultural background has influenced him to select Unani instead of Ayurveda or Siddha. Azeez had been inducted to the practice when he was a child. Although Azeez is a doctor who has received a formal education in Unani, at his medical centre Azeez is practicing Unani together with homeopathy and the ancestral healing specialty Kadum Bindum. Azeez believes in an integrated form of medicine. He says, 'each treatment system has its

---

[71] The Ministry of Indigenous Medicine has recognised Unani as a traditional system of medicine in Sri Lanka. http://www.indigenousmedimini.gov.lk/ (last retrieved 20 February 2019).

[72] See Ministry of Indigenous Medicine http://www.indigenousmedimini.gov.lk/ (last retrieved 20 February 2019).

[73] Dr. M. U. N. Z. Farzana (#5).

[74] The Bachelor of Unani Medicine and Surgery is offered by the Institute of Indigenous Medicine. Annual intake for the programme is 50. The programme is conducted in English and Tamil. Based on the interviews with Dr. M.U.N.Z. Farzana (#5).

[75] Mr. L. H. Thilakaratne (# 4). Minister of Indigenous Medicine Salinda Dissanayake has said, 'steps should be taken to produce Unani medicine in Sri Lanka without depending on imports. Jamaldeen, Naalir (30 June 2013) Unani Medicine makes headway in Sri Lanka. http://www.sundayobserver.lk/2013/06/30/fea10.asp (last retrieved 20 February 2019).

[76] Dr. Hameed A. Azeez J. P. (# 38).

strengths and limitations. If we amalgamate the systems to treat the patients, we can achieve better results. I prescribe Unani, homeopathy and indigenous mixed medicines to my patients.'

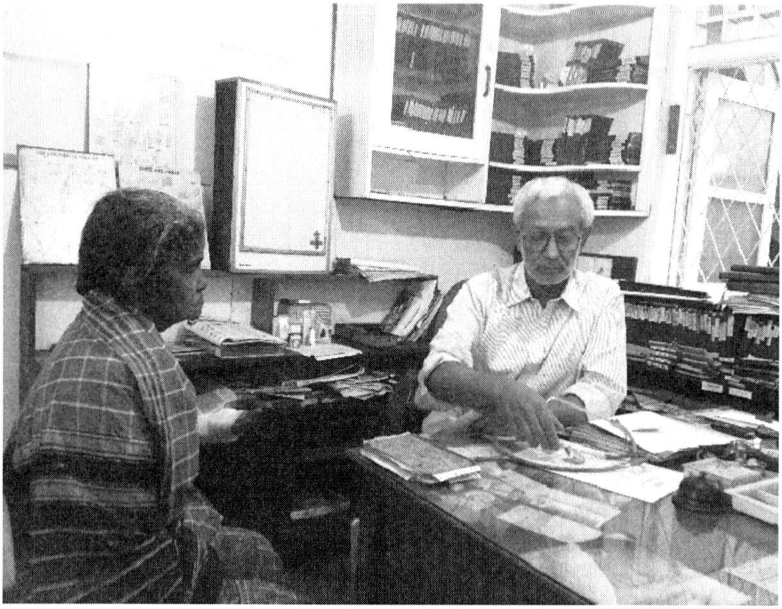

Figure 3.4 – Dr. Hameed A. Azeez consulting a patient at the Azeez Medical Centre

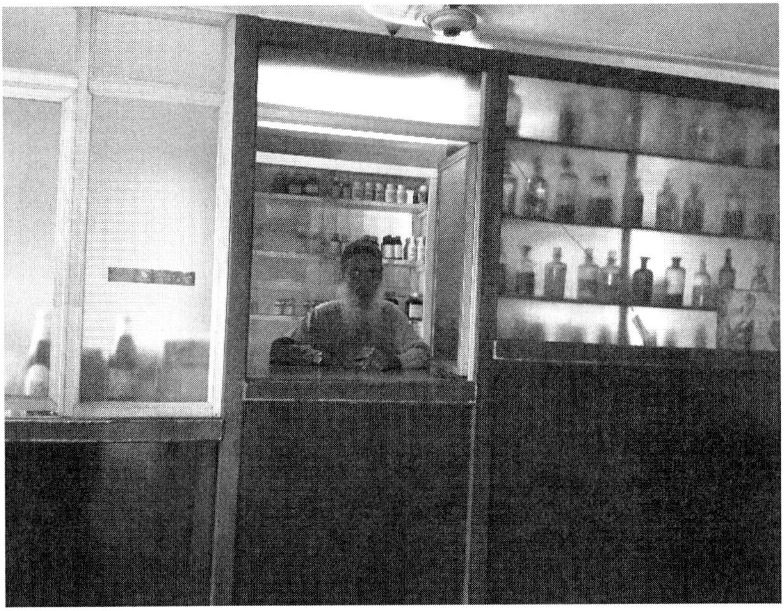

Figure 3.5– Pharmacy in the Azeez Medical Centre

Most of the drugs and oils used for treatments are prepared by his assistants at his home under his supervision and are distributed at the pharmacy (Figure 3.5) that is part of the Azeez Medical Centre. Some of the medicines he prepares are based on inter-generational recipes while others are Unani. Azeez says most of his patients are Muslims.

Azeez's case reveals the cultural divisions in the practice of traditional healing. Most students study Unani in Sri Lankan universities and most patients seeking Unani treatment are Muslims. It is also noteworthy that Unani education at university level is supported by the Government of Sri Lanka[77] and Unani qualified doctors are given government appointments.[78]

[77] Institute of Indigenous Medicine, University of Colombo is offering a degree programme leading to Bachelor of Unani Medicine and Surgery (BUMS). See message from the Head of the Unani Section. http://iim.cmb.ac.lk/unani (last retrieved 20 February 2019)

[78] By 2013, over 350 Unani Doctors were working in Government Institutions. Jamaldeen, Naalir (30 June 2013) Unani Medicine makes headway in Sri Lanka. http://www.sundayobserver.lk/2013/06/30/fea10.asp (last retrieved 20 February 2019)

1.4 Homeopathy

Homeopathy is another healing system that has received government recognition due to organised advocacy by Homeopathy Associations. However, Sri Lanka has been struggling to regulate the homeopathy due to irregularities in the performance of Homeopathy Council, illegal registration of homeopathic practitioners and sub-standard training in homeopathy.

The homoeopathy system of medicine was founded by Samuel Hahnemann[79], a German physician (1755- 1843).[80] The principle of homeopathy[81] is 'like cures like,'[82] that means 'diseases are treated with remedies that in a healthy person would produce symptoms similar to those of the disease. Rather than fighting the disease directly, medicines are intended to stimulate the body to fight the disease.'[83] The highest ideal cure is rapid, gentle and permanent restoration of the health, or removal and annihilation of the disease in its whole extent, in the shortest, most reliable and most harmless way.[84] Its remedies are manufactured in a manner that does not render them toxic. Homoeopathy is a safe and effective system of medicine used by millions of people worldwide for over 200 years. Today homoeopathy is practiced in many countries[85] and the efficacies of homoeopathic medicines are acknowledged worldwide.[86]

---

[79] The three major publications authored by Samuel Hahnemann that contributed towards development of Homeopathy are, *The Organon of the Healing Art* (1810) (revised by Hahnemann six times. Final revision in 1842), *Materia Medica Pura* (published in six volumes. Vol I in 1811 and Vol VI in 1827) and *The Chronic Diseases* (1828).

[80] For origins of Homeopathy see, Kayne (2006); Eschenbruch (2005); Rizza (1994); Meissner (1992); Dietrich. (1958); Dietrich (1958)

[81] 'Homoios' in Greek means similar, 'Pathos' means suffering.

[82] Although the laws of similar were previously discovered, it was Hahnemann who codified the law similar to a systematic medicine. See Ullman, Dana '*A Condensed History of Homeopathy*' https://www.homeopathic.com/Articles/Introduction_to_Homeopathy/A_Condensed_History_of_Homeopathy.html (last retrieved 20 February 2019).

[83] WHO (2001), p 3.

[84] Adopted from the definition given on Homeopathy by Buddhika Vittahchchi Hospitals (Pvt) Ltd http://www.srilankaayurvedicresorts.com/homeopathy.htm (last retrieved 20 February 2019).

[85] Homeopathy is practiced throughout Europe, Asia and North America. Some of the countries homeopathy has been integrated into the national health care system include India, Mexico, Pakistan, Sri Lanka and the United Kingdom. WHO (2001), p 3.

[86] Ullman (2007).

The history of homeopathy in Sri Lanka is traced back to 1906, when Cap. R. T. Samaraweera[87] practiced homeopathy informally among his friends and relatives. Historically, two homeopathic associations played a significant role in establishing homeopathy in Sri Lanka and advocating for state recognition for homeopathy. In 1951, a branch of the International Hahnemann Association USA was founded in Sri Lanka by Cap. R. T. Samaraweera.[88] In 1954, this association changed its name to the Ceylon Homeopathic Society. The Ceylon Institute of Homeopathy and the first private hospital[89] in homeopathy was established under the sponsorship of the Ceylon Homeopathic Society.[90] In 1951, Dr. C. V. S. Corea[91] also initiated a homeopathic association, mainly with homeopatheic patients as its members. In 1956, in response to persistent demands of the two homeopathic associations, the government appointed a committee of enquiry on homeopathy, with Dr. P. N. Banerjee of India as Chairman.[92] The Committee's recommendations led to state recognition of homeopathy.[93]

Homeopathy in Sri Lanka received state recognition, support and regulation with the passing of the *Homeopathy Act No. 7 of 1970.*[94] It is an act to provide for the establishment of a Homeopathic Council.[95] The Council is responsible for the regulation and control of the practice of

---

[87] Capt. R. T. Samaraweera was a cadet Master at Royal College, Colombo. He learnt homeopathy when he was studying medicine in Calcutta, India, from F.R. Augustus Muller, a lay practitioner of homeopathy and a Christian missionary from Germany, who was living in Manglore, India. See: Homeopathy from Inception – Sri Lanka. http://amcofh.org/sites/default/files/History%20of%20Homeopathy%20in%20Sri%20Lanka.pdf (last retrieved 20 February 2019)

[88] Homeopathy from Inception – Sri Lanka. http://amcofh.org/sites/default/files/History%20of%20Homeopathy%20in%20Sri%20Lanka.pdf (last retrieved 20 February 2019)

[89] Private Homeopathic Hospital has been established in Bambalapitiya, Colombo 4, with 10 beds.

[90] Das (2005), p. 230.

[91] Dr. C. V. S. Corea has been elected President of the association and first Government appointed Homeopathic Council and later appointed as an Advisor to the Government on Homeopathy. Das (2005), p 230.

[92] Das (2005), p 230.

[93] Effects of Government appointed Homeopathy Committee Recommendations includes passing of *Homeopathy Act No 7 of 1970* (Sri Lanka).

[94] *Homeopathy Act No. 7 of 1970* was passed in Parliament on 12 February 1970. The Act can be retrieved at http://www.commonlii.org/lk/legis/num_act/ha7o1970197/ (last retrieved 20 February 2019)

[95] *Homeopathy Act No. 7 of 1970* (Sri Lanka), *ss 2-24* deals with establishment and functioning of the Homeopathic Council

medicine according to homeopathy;[96] promotion and encouragement of the homeopathic system of medicine,[97] the registration of homoeopathic practitioners,[98] the establishment,[99] regulation and control of homoeopathic institutions,[100] the regulation and control of the manufacture, importation, sale and dispensing of homoeopathic medicines, drugs and other preparations.[101] There have been many controversies regarding the implementation of *Homeopathy Act No. 7 of 1970.* These controversies include, dissolving the Homeopathy Council by the Minister of Indigenous Medicine overnight in 2009;[102] illegal registration of homeopathic practitioners[103] and sub-standard training.[104]

---

[96] *Homeopathy Act No. 7 of 1970,* (Sri Lanka) *s 22 (a).*

[97] This includes the practice of medicine and study and research of Homeopathy. *Homeopathy Act (No. 7 of 1970), s 22 (b-c).*

[98] *Homeopathy Act No. 7 of 1970,* (Sri Lanka) *ss 25-37* deals with the registration of Homeopathy Medical Practitioners, including the process of registration (ss 25- 26*),* qualifications *(*s27*),* registration fees *(*s 31*),* certificates of registration *(*art 32*),* privileges of registered practitioners *(*s 35*),* disabilities of unregistered practitioners *(*art 36)

[99] *Homeopathy Act No. 7 of 1970,* (Sri Lanka) *s 22 (d)* states the establishment and maintenance of the Homeopathic Medical College as an Object of the Council.

[100] *Homeopathy Act No. 7 of 1970,* (Sri Lanka) *s 22 (e).* The first Government Homeopathic Hospital was established on January 4, 2013 in Welisara, Western Province of Sri Lanka. This Hospital is regulated from the *Homeopathy Act.*

[101] *Homeopathy Act No. 7 of 1970,* (Sri Lanka) *d 22 (g)*

[102] According to then Minister Tissa Karaliyadda, the reason for dissolving the Homeopathy Council is the Council has been taking many decisions, without consulting the Minister. Fazlulhaq, Nadia (January 4, 2009) Homeopathy Act to be overhauled. Sunday Times. http://www.sundaytimes.lk/090104/News/sundaytimesnews_10.html (last retrieved 20 February 2019) February 8, 2015 facebook post in 'In defence of Homeopathy and Homeopaths in Sri Lanka' states Ministry of Indigenous Medicine has discussed with the former Council Members on re-establishing the Council and appointing a committee to probe into all the irregularities of implementing the Homeopathy Act since dissolving the Council in 2009. https://www.facebook.com/pages/In-defence-of-Homoeopathy-Homoeopaths-in-Srilanka/284696298336616 (last retrieved 20 February 2019)

[103] In December 2008, half hour exam has been convened by the Homeopathic Council to register personnel as Homeopathy doctors for persons who haven't obtained formal four year Homeopathy qualification, but who have managed to obtain a letter from an official such as Grama Niladari (the Government representative at the village level) stating they have experience in practicing Homeopathy for more than ten years.

[104] Hahnemann Institute of Homeopathy Colombo in association with AIHMS academy, Kerala has been offering a Diploma in Homeopathy after a 27 day training

The preceding discussion explains how homeopathy has received government recognition in Sri Lanka as a result of the organised advocacy by homeopathy associations. Despite this Sri Lanka has been struggling in regularising homeopathy due to irregularities of the performance of the Homeopathy Council, illegal registration of homeopathic practitioners and sub-standard training in homeopathy.

1.5 Acupuncture

Acupuncture[105] literally stands for needle piercing, and involves the practice of slowly pushing very fine needles into the skin. Sri Lanka has many forms of acupuncture. These include the most popular government recognised form of acupuncture based on Chinese practice and the Korean practice; and the Sri Lankan inter-generational form of Acupuncture known as Nila *Wedakama* (healing).

Professor Anton Jayasuriya, a medical officer attached to the Health Department of Sri Lanka and former President of Medicina Atlernative, managed to obtain government support and recognition for acupuncture. Under the directorship of the late Professor Jayasuriya the Chinese practice of acupuncture was taught and practiced in the Colombo South Teaching Hospital for nearly three decades. Since his passing in April 2005, Professor Jayasuriya's contribution and legacy of re-introducing acupuncture has been kept alive by the Medicina Alternativa Organisation and its team of experienced physicians and practitioners in Colombo, by opening the Anton Jayasuriya Memorial Clinic.[106]

---

programme and these diploma holders have been registered as Homeopathy practitioner. Facebook page on 'In defence of Homeopathy and Homeopaths in Sri Lanka' has constantly questioned the legality of registering Diploma holders who qualify from the above mentioned progamme and how substandard qualification affect the quality of Homeopathy practice in Sri Lanka. See https://www.facebook.com/pages/In-defence-of-Homoeopathy-Homoeopaths-in-Srilanka/284696298336616 (last retrieved 20 February 2019).

[105] There is Archaeological evidence to suggest acupuncture has originated in Sri Lanka. See Prof. Lakshman Madurasinghe http://madure.multiply.com/journal/item/191?&item_id=191&view:replies=reverse (Last Retrieved on 28 February 2013).

[106]Anton Jayasuriya Memorial Clinic is in no. 8, International Buddhist Centre Road, Colombo 6. The clinic provides acupuncture, homeopathy, laser therapy, rheumatology and massage. All treatments and medicines are provided free of charge. This initiative is funded by the Anton Jayasuriya Foundation. As many as 300 patients are treated per day free of charge at the Anton Jayasuriya Memorial Clinic, providing students with limitless opportunity to gain hands on experience in

Korean acupuncture treatments were introduced in the National Ayurveda Teaching Hospital in 2003 with the funding of the Korean International Cooperation Agency (KOICA). As part of the project the Korean Clinic was established and Dr. Han, Gyu-Eco, a Korean Oriental medical doctor was appointed as the head of the clinic under KOICA's World Friends Advisory Programme.[107] Initially the Korean Clinic was solely managed by Dr. Han, Guy-Eco but since 2009, Ayurvedic doctors trained in Korean acupuncture support Dr. Guy-Eco to manage the clinic.[108] One hundred and fifty to one hundred and sixty patients are treated in the clinic on a daily basis.[109] Since 2004, Sri Lankan Ayurveda doctors have been trained in Korean acupuncture treatment[110] with the support of KONICA.

Professor Jayasuriya argued that archaeological evidence proved acupuncture originated in pre-historic Sri Lanka over 30,000 years ago,[111] based on Dr. Siran Deraniyagala's archaeological research.[112] R. M. Premachandra, inter-generational practitioner of the Nila system of healing says the Nila healing system practiced by his ancestors for many generations is a local version of acupuncture.[113] Nila healers are recognised as traditional healers in Sri Lanka.[114] Yet there is no government programme to recognise and support the Nila system of healing.[115]

---

acupuncture while helping others. Daily News (30 May 2005) Anton Jayasuriya Memorial Clinic Opened. http://archives.dailynews.lk/2005/05/30/news28.htm (last retrieved 20 February 2019).

[107] KOICA helps promote acupuncture treatment. 7 November 2013. Daily Mirror (Colombo, Sri Lanka)

[108] 'Korean Clinic,' a combination of traditional healing methods. (Posted on 8 April 2013) http://www.koica.go.kr/english/board/news_events/1303942_3532.html (last retrieved 4 September 2015)

[109] 'Korean Clinic,' a combination of traditional healing methods. (Posted on 8 April 2013) http://www.koica.go.kr/english/board/news_events/1303942_3532.html (last retrieved 4 September 2015)

[110] 14 month Certificate programme on Korean Acupuncture. Up to 2013, six batches of Ayurveda doctors (totaling up to 133 doctors) have been trained in Korean acupuncture
http://www.koica.go.kr/english/board/news_events/1303942_3532.html
(last retrieved 20 February 2019)

[111] At the 39th World Congress of Alternative Medicines (November 27-30, 2001), B.M.I.C.H.

[112] Medicina Alternativa – Sri Lanka. Epicenter of Alternative Medicine.
http://www.medalta.8m.net/ (last retrieved 20 February 2019).

[113] R. M. Premachandra (#113).

[114] R. M. Premachandra (#113) is registered as a traditional healer in Ayurveda Medical Council.

[115] R. M. Premachandra (#113).

It is interesting to note that the Chinese practice of acupuncture received government support to be established and treated in the Colombo South Teaching Hospital, which is a hospital that caters for Western forms of medicine as acupuncture was introduced by a physician qualified in Western medicine, and professionally highly regarded internationally. The Korean form of acupuncture received government support to be established in the National Ayurveda Teaching Hospital as the project was funded by KOICA.

1.6 Deshiya Chikithsa

'Deshiya' refers to local and 'Chikithsa' refers to medicine.[116] There is no clear definition on what comes in the ambit of Deshiya Chikitsa. The Department of Ayurveda refers to Desheeya Chikitsa as the Indigenous System of Medicine in Sri Lanka.[117] According to the Ayurveda Medical Council[118] the practitioners of Deshiya Chikitsa are the hereditary physicians. Different types of hereditary physicians include general physicians and physicians with a special hereditary knowledge of healing.[119] The list of Ayurveda hereditary healers registered under the Ayurveda Medical Council section 55 (2)(b) include the following categories –

- eye disease,
- balaroga (paediatrics),
- snake bites,
- boils and ulcers,
- haemorrhoids,
- animal diseases,
- fractures and dislocation,
- goitre diseases,
- dysentery,
- cut and burns,
- fever,
- mental diseases,
- suthikaroga,
- arthritis,
- diabetes,
- hydrophobia,
- wheeze,
- elephant diseases,
- nervous diseases,
- falling sickness,

[116] Dr. M. W. S. J. Kumari (# 11).

[117] Department of Ayurveda. http://www.ayurveda.gov.lk/index.html (last retrieved 20 February 2019).

[118] Ayurveda Medical Council. http://www.ayurvedicmedicoun.gov.lk/web/ (last retrieved 20 February 2019).

[119] Type of registration under Ayurveda Medical Council include hereditary physicians (55(1)E- General Physicians and 55(2) Special Physicians http://www.ayurvedicmedicoun.gov.lk/web/index.php?option=com_content&view=article&id=89&Itemid=54&lang=en (last retrieved 20 February 2019).

- blood pressure,
- sthriroga (women's health),
- catarrh,
- shawasankajwara.
- skin diseases,
- palsy diseases (paralysis),
- typhoid,

At the Institute of Indigenous Medicine of the University of Colombo, course curriculum for the Bachelor of Ayurveda Medicine and Surgery (2011) covers the following subjects for Deshiya Chikitsa:[120]

- *Akshi Roga* (eye disease),
- *Devum Pilissum* (traditional treatment for burns),
- *Gedi Vana Pilika* (wound management),
- *Peenasa* (sinusitis),
- *Vata Roga,*
- *Kedum Bidum* (orthopedic),
- *Sarpa Visa* (snake bites),
- *Vidum Pilissum* (burning and penetrating skin with special tools),
- Unmada (mental sickness).

The Centre for Traditional Knowledge of University of Kelaniya has listed the following healing practices as Sri Lanka's indigenous or traditional medicine:[121]

- *Sarvanga Chikitsa* (general medicine),
- *Kedum Bidum Chikitsa* (Orthopedic practices),
- *Manasika Roga Chikitsa* (Psychiatric medicine),
- *Visha Chikitsa* (Toxicology),
- *Gedi Vana Pilika Chikitsa* (Wound management),
- *Akshi Chikitsa* (Traditional Ophthalmology),
- *Devum Pilissum Chikitsa* (Traditional treatment for burns),
- *Nila Chikitsa* (Accu Pressure treatment),
- *Buthavidya Chikitsa* (Demonology),
- *Adivasi Vedakama* (Tribal Medicine),

---

[120] IIM (2011) Bachelor of Ayurveda Medicine and Surgery (BAMS) Course Unit System – Rules and Regulations – Course Curriculum. p 76. See http://iim.cmb.ac.lk/wp-content/uploads/2010/08/BAMS-CURRICULUM-2011.pdf (last retrieved 20 February 2019).

[121] Centre for Traditional Knowledge. University of Kelaniya. http://www.kln.ac.lk/institutes/wickramarachchi/ayurex2014/ (last retrieved 20 February 2019).

- *Pashu Chikitsa* (Traditional Veterinary medicine),
- *Vrukshayurveda* (Traditional treatments for trees and plants.)

All the healing practices listed under Deshiya Chikitsa in the above lists are inter-generational healing practices. The lists illustrates that there is no consensus on what is called Deshiya Chikitsa practice or terminology used for different forms of practice. Using different terminology also suggests the informal nature of Deshiya Chikitsa where the government has not been able to fully recognise the practice. Without full recognition of the practice by the government, it is not possible to fully formalise and regulate the practice.

Part 2: Diversity of Healing Practices in Sri Lanka

The preceding section highlighted the traditional healing practices recognised by the Government of Sri Lanka. In this part I reveal the diversity of the healing practices in the country, which is far more extensive and richer than those practices only recognised by the government. As shown in Figure 3.6 below, I have clustered the diverse forms of healing in Sri Lanka into 5 categories, namely: inter-generational healing, cosmic healing, adopted traditional healing, biomedical healing and integrated healing. This attempt to classify practices is based on the need to obtain a broader understanding of all the healing practices, without limiting discussions to just government classifications. Only through a broader understanding of the healing systems currently practiced, the cultural values, and beliefs associated with each form of practice and social recognition received due to acceptance by the government as well as communities, can the cultural aspect of healing be protected and promoted.

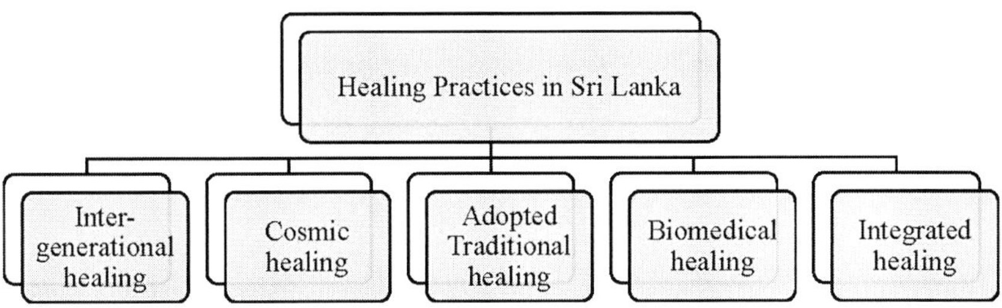

Figure 3.6 – Healing practices in Sri Lanka (Author's Classification)

The diverse healing practices of Sri Lanka as presented in Figure 4.6 include practices that have evolved in Sri Lanka and practices that have been adopted from other countries. As many indigenous healing practices have adopted healing components of healing practices of other countries it is difficult to distinguish authentic Sri Lankan healing practices. I have explained each type of healing belowin the way I have interpreted them for the purposes of this book.

2.1 Inter-Generational Healing

Here I have referred to inter-generational healing practices as beliefs, knowledge and practices of local and indigenous community in Sri Lanka that have been used in healing through medical practices and have been passed down from generation to generation.[122] Inter-generational practices are diverse, vivid and informal. Some of the inter-generational healing practices[123] include:

- *Sarvanga* (are physicians. The treatments cover arthritis, diabetes, blood pressure, dysentery, fever, typhoid, haemorrhoids, goitre diseases, stokes and paralysis. Some Sarvanga physicians specialise in treating one or few forms of these diseases);[124]
- *Kadum Bidum* (orthopaedic);[125]
- *Akshi Roga* (eye disease);[126]
- *Devum Pilissum* (traditional treatment for burns); [127]

---

[122] Knowledge passed down from generation to generation is considered traditional knowledge practices for protection in the draft international legal instrument of WIPO Intergovernmental Committee on Intellectual Property and Genetic Resources, Traditional Knowledge and Folklore. See: (c) art 1, Subject Matter of [Protection]/[this Instrument] is art 1, Subject Matter of [Protection]/[Instrument] in The Protection of Traditional Knowledge: Draft arts Rev. 2 (March 28, 2014), WIPO/GRTKF/IC/27/REF/FACILITATORS DOCUMENT REV.2

[123] This is not an attempt to list all inter-generational healing practices in Sri Lanka.

[124] H. D. Karunawathie (#53) practices general *Sarvanga*. R. M. D. J. Gunasekera (# 58) is specialised in Diabetics, Cholesterol and Pressure. Wanasinghe Mudianselage Sudu Banda (#59) is specialised in stroke and paralysis.

[125] *Kadum Bidum* inter-generational healers interviewed include Sunil Shantha (#25); W. M. Anulawathie (#56), R.V. Piyadasa (#55), Ariya (#84), S. M. K. Nimal Karunarathne (#93), R.A. Sudath Priyantha (#94), Sandan (#106).

[126] Healing system practiced by S. K. Liyanarachchige (# 27) and P. Weerasinghe (# 52).

[127] Based on the Deshiya Chikitsa subjects covered for the Course Curriculum for Bachelor of Ayurveda Medicine and Surgery (2011) at the Institute of Indigenous

- *Visa* (toxicology);[128]
- *Peenasa* (sinusitis);[129]
- *Vata Roga* (is one of the three doshas in Ayurveda, condensed from the elements air and space. It is the principle of kinetic energy in the body, is concerned with the nervous system and with circulation, movement and pathology, and is eliminated from the body through defecation);[130]
- *Gedi Vana Pilika Chikitsa* (wound management);[131]
- *Vidum Pilissum* (burning and penetrating skin with special tools);[132]
- *Nila Chikitsa* (Acupressure treatment);[133]
- *Adivasi Vedakama* (Tribal Medicine);[134]
- *Pashu Chikitsa* (Traditional Veterinary medicine);[135]

Medicine of the University of Colombo, p.76 See http://iim.cmb.ac.lk/wp-content/uploads/2010/08/BAMS-CURRICULUM-2011.pdf (last retrieved 20 February 2019)

128 *Visa* healers interviewed include Rathnawathie (#29); W. A. Kusuma Wijesekera (#32); S.D.M. Mahipala (#51); Ven. Kapugama Somalankara (#54).

129 Based on the Deshiya Chikitsa subjects covered for the Course Curriculum for Bachelor of Ayurveda Medicine and Surgery (2011) at the Institute of Indigenous Medicine of the University of Colombo, p 76 See http://iim.cmb.ac.lk/wp-content/uploads/2010/08/BAMS-CURRICULUM-2011.pdf (last retrieved 20 February 2019)

130 Explained by Dr. E. A.S.C.S. Edirisuriya (#7) and Dr. M. Chithra Nalini (#8) *Vata Roga* is also a Deshiya Chikitsa subject covered for the Course Curriculum for Bachelor of Ayurveda Medicine and Surgery (2011) at the Institute of Indigenous Medicine of the University of Colombo, p 76. See http://iim.cmb.ac.lk/wp-content/uploads/2010/08/BAMS-CURRICULUM-2011.pdf (last retrieved 20 February 2019)

131 The Centre for Traditional Knowledge of University of Kelaniya list of Sir Lanka's indigenous or traditional medicine: See http://www.kln.ac.lk/institutes/wickramarachchi/ayurex2014/ (last retrieved 20 February 2019)

132 The Centre for Traditional Knowledge of University of Kelaniya list of Sir Lanka's indigenous or traditional medicine: See http://www.kln.ac.lk/institutes/wickramarachchi/ayurex2014/ (last retrieved 20 February 2019)

133 Healing system practiced by R. M. Premachandra (#113).

134 Healing system practiced by the Vaddha Community of Sri Lanka comes under this category. VishwakeerthiVanaspathi UruWalige Wanniya Attho (#18).

135 Ajith Liyanage (#96) practice healing for elephants. The Centre for Traditional Knowledge of University of Kelaniya also list *Pashu Chikitsa* in the list of Sir Lanka's indigenous or traditional medicine: See

- *Vrukshayurveda* (Traditional treatments for trees and plants);[136]

Many inter-generational healing practices adopt cosmic healing practices as well. The main distinction I am making between cosmic healing and inter-generational healing is that while cosmic relationship is primarily based on cosmic beliefs and related rituals, inter-generational healing includes the application of medicine. The other significant difference is, while inter-generational healing is passed down from one generation to the next, cosmic healing practices are learnt in different ways, including developing the mind, through dreams, or through an inter-mediator spirit. It is noteworthy that there are some cosmic healing practices such as astrology, or the performance of rituals that are passed down from generation to generation. For a detailed discussion on inter-generational healing, see: Chapter 4.[137]

2.2 Cosmic Healing

In this work I refer to cosmic healing as healing from the power of spirituality, spirts, cosmic energy, faith, beliefs, rituals and astral connections.[138] The various kinds of cosmic healing practices that this work reflects upon are in Figure 3.7 below.

---

http://www.kln.ac.lk/institutes/wickramarachchi/ayurex2014/ (last retrieved 20 February 2019)

[136] The Centre for Traditional Knowledge of University of Kelaniya list of Sir Lanka's indigenous or traditional medicine: See http://www.kln.ac.lk/institutes/wickramarachchi/ayurex2014/ (last retrieved 20 February 2019).

[137] Analysis of intergenerational healing practice is limited due to the semi-formal, semi-regulated nature of the practice. As all the inter-generational healers are not registered under the Ayurveda Medical Council due to the criteria for registration (discussed in Chapter 5), and as there has not been a survey conducted to identify all inter-generational healing practitioners in Sri Lanka, it is not possible to determine the number of inter-generational healing practitioners. Due to inter-generational healers practice in informal settings, it is not possible to make any statements about the volume or popularity of practice. Also due to lack of scientific research conducted on the effectiveness of the treatment practices it is not possible to consider effectiveness of treatment.

[138] All cosmic healing practices discussed are informal and unregulated healing practices. Due to the nature and status of healing practices, it is not possible to determine the number of practitioners, popularity of practice or the effectiveness of the practice.

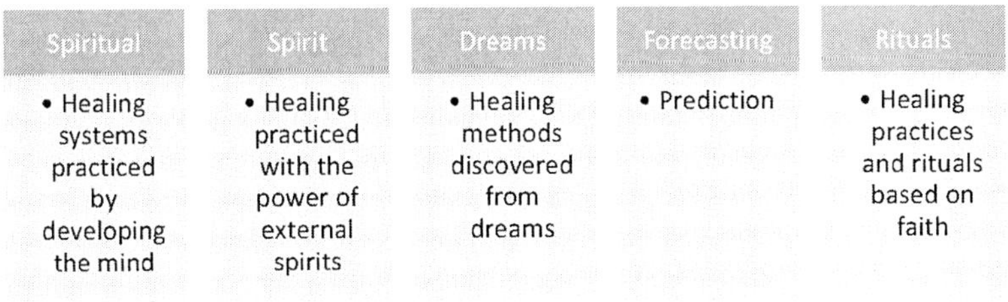

Figure 3.7 – Types of cosmic healing practices in Sri Lanka

Spirit healing is healing using the power of the spirit. This includes the exorcist who channels the power of spirits, and *kattadiyas* or *Aduras*[139] who perform rituals to take away the spirits out of human bodies or protect land and houses from the impact of negative spirits or to gain the protection of gods and positive spirits in healing and well-being. Charms[140] and amulets[141] are commonly used in spirit healing for protection. Although rituals, charms and amulets are a common practice in spirit healing, they are also practiced when prescribed by spiritual healer, religious dignitary, astrologer, or when felt by an individual.[142]

Spiritual healing and wellbeing refer to when individuals practice mind training methods for their own healing and wellbeing and when individuals who have developed their minds spiritually use their

[139] Kattadiya and Adura are Sinhalese names used to refer to a spirit healer who acts as an intermediator and performs rituals on behalf of the believer to the spirit or god. (Interview with R. P. Udayapala # 28).

[140] Charms are used for luck, for blessing or to cast a spell (Interview with P. M. Punchibanda # 67).

[141] The Amulets (*yanthra*) are divided into two categories: namely, astrological yanthra and Buddhist yanthra. The astrological yantra are tailor made, considering the astrological chart of the person concerned. Buddhist yanthra are not tailor made. They are general amulets that could be used by anyone based on their need for protection. The amulets are created using hand drawings according to what is mentioned in ola leaf books. The amulets are usually worn in a neckless, around the stomach, around the arm. Some amulets are kept in the entrance or worshipping place in the house, inside the pillow case, inside the vehicle or inside the purse. (Interview with Venerable Mihindupora Mahindawansa Nayaka # 72).

[142] For example charms and amulets are prescribed by astrologer P. D. Premachandra (# 64); astrologer Tennison Perera (# 109) religious dignitary Venerable Mihindupura Mahindawansa Nayaka (# 72).

understanding to heal other people.[143] Commonly-used spiritual healing methods in Sri Lanka are meditation, pirith and yoga. Some spiritual practitioners use unique methods for healing. An example is Venerable Wellawatte Seelagawesi[144] who uses techniques such as telepathic healing, neuro-psycho immunity, behavioural therapy and endocrine therapy for healing his patients. Ven. Seelagawesi's case is discussed in Chapter 1.

Forecasting methods can also be considered as a part of cosmic healing. Forecasting methods are used to make statements about events where the actual outcome has not yet been observed. Forecasting was quite often used as a planning tool.[145] Based on the forecast, people are advised to practice various forms of rituals to ensure mental and physical wellbeing.[146] Most often, the forecasters (Astrologers,[147] Palm Readers, [148] and Spirit Healers [149]) were also skilled in guiding ritual practices or performing the ritual on behalf of the devotee to ensure healing and wellbeing.

---

[143] Based on Venerable Wellawatte Seelagawesi's definition of the healing system practiced by him. (# 66).

[144] Venerable Wellawatte Seelagawesi (# 66).

[145] Tennisson Perera (# 109).

[146] Rituals performed are diverse and vary from situation to situation and forecaster to forecaster and based on religion of the devotee. Some examples of prescribed popular rituals can be *Bodhi pooja* (veneration of the Bodhi tree), *pahan pooja* (lighting of coconut-oil lamps as an offering), *Ass Vaha Kata Vaha Mathirima (*also known as *Dehi Kepima)* is a protection from evil looks and evil words, *Shanthi Karma* (practiced for health, protection and wellbeing of individuals as well as society at large). *Seth kavi* (is a composed poem tailor made for each individual based on their problems or concerns. It is a form of healing the sick or granting the wishes of a person by using the power of sound), performing pooja for a particular god.

[147] Astrologers P. D. Premachandra (# 64), Nandasena Herath (# 68) and Tennisson Perera (# 109) perform rituals based on their astrological forecast.

[148] Leelawathie (# 75) conduct Malayalam Palm Readings and predict the future by reading the lines of the palm; suggesting rituals and deeds to overcome or lessen the effects bad *karma*. (Bad deeds performed in this birth or previous births.)

[149] Spirit healers are also called Exorcists. A problem a person is facing currently or the future of a person could be predicted by the power of spirits. It is a common practice of the Sri Lankans, particularly the villages to consult an exorcist to understand the cause for a problem and how to overcome it. Ghana Manio (# 60), and W. S. Pushpakumara (#61) are spirit healers who forecast based on the power of spirits and perform rituals for healing.

2.3 Adopted Traditional Healing

The adopted traditional healing practices are the traditional healing practices in other countries that have been adopted and practiced in Sri Lanka and are recognised by the government as traditional healing practices. As discussed earlier in the chapter, government recognised and adopted traditional healing practices are Ayurveda[150], Siddha[151], Unani[152], Homeopathy[153] and Acupuncture.[154] In addition to those traditional healing practices there are many other adopted traditional healing systems in Sri Lanka. These include, traditional Chinese herbal medicine, Vedic Alchemy,[155] Shiatsu.[156]One example of traditional healing, that has been adopted in Sri Lanka but is not recognised by the government as a separate form of healing is *Rasa Shastra* (Vedic Alchemy).

Practitioners of *Rasa Shastra*[157] claim to be able to cure all health problems in the twenty first century.'[158] It is considered a highly effective way of treating illnesses using alchemical fusion between mineral and organic compounds including such diverse materials as mercury, gold, silver, tin, lead, zinc, sulphur, copper and diamond.[159] The *Rasa* medical system can treat HIIV/ AIDs, all types of cancer, diabetes, leukaemia, all types of skin diseases, neuro and spinal disorders, cardiac problems, hypertension, urinary disorders, kidney problems and sexual disabilities and

---

[150] Chapter 3, Part 1 (1).

[151] Chapter 3, Part 1 (2).

[152] Chapter 3, Part 1 (3).

[153] Chapter 3, Part 1 (4).

[154] Chapter 3, Part 1 (5).

[155] Also known as Rasa Shastra. Based on interviews with R. L. Kularatne (#110) and C. Kularatne (#111).

[156] Shiatsu is a Japanese healing system to improve the nervous system functioning, the endocrine glands, and stimulate the circulation of blood and lympy. This healing system is offered at Thusare-Talking Hands in Colombo 7. Based on interviews with Ishikawa Naohito (# 76) and Thusare (# 77).

[157] Based on series of interviews with R. L. Kularatne (#110) and C. Kularatne (#111), Rasa Medical Practitioners at Sri Mangala Rasa Osu Hala (Pvt) ltd in Moratuwa and four patients cured by the above Doctors from November 2012-January 2013. The *rasa* tradition referred to here is the system of medicine attributed to Siddha Nāgārjuna. Jayasinghe (1968), p 74.

[158] R. L. Kularatne (#110) and C. Kularatne (#111).

[159] The raw metals and organic compounds used in *Rasa Shastra* are subjected to various purification processes called "*Shodhana,*" "*Marana,*" "*Bhashma*" says R. L. Kularatne (#110).

impotency. All forms of surgical operations too can be avoided and treated through this system.

Interviewees have learnt the Rasa healing tradition from Mr. Kularatne's father. Mr. Kularathe's father has learnt the Rasa healing tradition from an Indian Guru, whom he has sponsored to live in Sri Lanka for several years to teach him the practice of Rasa healing. Mr. Kularatne claims himself to be a self-made scientist. He says, 'I don't only rely on the knowledge passed down from my father, but constantly work on experimentation. It is I who discovered treatment for cures for HIV/AIDS, cancer and hepatitis using the knowledge of Rasa medicine.' He relies on lab reports to prove his findings but hasn't obtained a patent for the treatments he has discovered.

Mr Kularatne introduced me to two of the patients he has cured. One was a father of a 9 year old girl from Diyatalawa; the girl had been completely cured within 4 months while she was on the death bed for kidney related problems. The other person was the mother of a totally blind girl and son who was suffering from deafness, blindness, epilepsy and autism. Now, after 6 months of treatments, the girl has regained partial vision and the boy's conditions have significantly improved.

Mr and Mrs. Kularatne are looking forward to establishing a hospital and research centre in Rasa medicine. Most of his efforts to promote Rasa medicine has been blocked through the prevailing administrative system in Sri Lanka.

2.4 Biomedical Healing

The biomedical care system,[160] which can also be called orthodox medicine[161] was first introduced to Sri Lanka by the Portuguese colonisers of Sri Lanka.[162] During the period of Dutch colonisation a few hospitals were established in the Maritime Provinces.[163] Afterwards the British colonisers played a significant role in continuing the expansion of the biomedical care system in Sri Lanka.[164] The contribution of the British

---

[160] For history of the hospital system and health care based on biomedicine see, Jones (2009).
[161] Orthodox medicine is based on bio-medicine which is primarily centered on the use of drugs and surgery. Saks, Mike (2008) 29.
[162] Fernando (1999), p 14.
[163] Fernando (1999), p 14.
[164] The impact of colonial influence in the regulation of traditional healing practices has been discussed in Chapter 2, part 3.

colonisers include establishing military and estate health services;[165] establishing the Civil Medical Department in 1859; in 1915 the sanitary branch of the Civil Medical Department was established with the accountability of environmental sanitation and prevention of communicable diseases;[166] the first health unit was established in 1926 in Kalutara for the provision of preventive health care services at the community level and was replicated in other parts of the country during the colonial administration.[167]

In contemporary Sri Lanka, the biomedical (allopathic) health care system includes preventive, curative and rehabilitative care. The health care is provided both by the public and private sectors. In the public sector, the primary responsibility of the biomedical health care system lies with the Ministry of Health. At the provincial level, the provincial councils are responsible in the delivery of health care services for the respective provinces. The private sector mostly contributes to out-patient services through general practitioners. Fernando argues as the private sector is not regulated; it is difficult to assess the exact contribution of the private sector.[168]

2.5 Integrated Healing

Integrative healing systems are practiced by many healers in the country, where they mix and practice two or more forms of healing at once. In the following paragraphs I describe two case studies outlining the idea of integrated healing practices used in Sri Lanka.

Jeyalan,[169] who is the Siddha- Ayurveda healer in Jaffna (Figure 3.8), has an ancestry that has practiced Siddha healing since the Anuradhapura era. Jeyalan is the 25th person in his family taking this traditional healing system forward. Jeyalan has many ola leaf inscriptions of Siddha medicine in Tamil and Sinhala. He has been treating patients in Jaffna for the past 9 years.[170] Although, the inter-generational healing practice is Siddha, Jeyalan has acquired knowledge in many other forms of healing by self-study and by reading for a 5 year diploma at Lanka Siddha-Ayurvedic Medical College.[171]

---

[165] Fernando (1999), p 14.
[166] Uragoda (1987).
[167] Fernando (1999), p 14.
[168] (1999), p 15.
[169] Jeyalan (# 100).
[170] Jeyalan (# 100).
[171] Jeyalan (# 100).

Jeyalan treats for a diverse range of sicknesses: asthma, gastritis, kidney stones, skin diseases, fibroids, spirit influences and infertility.[172] He has made a name in the community for treating infertility issues. He has learnt about the treatment system by studying the ola leaf manuscripts (Figure 3.10). Now many patients come to Jeyalan for infertility treatment. 'Rasa Mani,' a treatment system using mercury is also practiced by Jeyalan.[173] For a Rasa Mani treatment, Jeyalan requests the patients to wear a neckless with mercury (Figure 3.11). 'The radiation of mercury heals the bodily impact of '*hunuyam*' (charms and spells) and effects of evil spirits,' says Jeyalan.[174]

When diagnosing patients, sometimes he requests the patients to bring lab reports (scans, blood tests, hormone levels, etc) while he also uses traditional forms of diagnosis.[175] For some sicknesses, Jeyalan prepares special medication by looking at patients' horoscopes for times to prepare medicine, while for common symptoms he prescribes medicine he has prepared or purchased from traditional medicine shops or exported from India (Himalaya range products).[176] The medicines prescribed by him are Ayurveda, Siddha or sometimes unique combinations that Jeylan himself has developed (see Figure 3.9).

[172] Jeyalan (# 100).
[173] Jeyalan (# 100).
[174] Jeyalan (# 100).
[175] Jeyalan (# 100).
[176] Jeyalan (# 100).

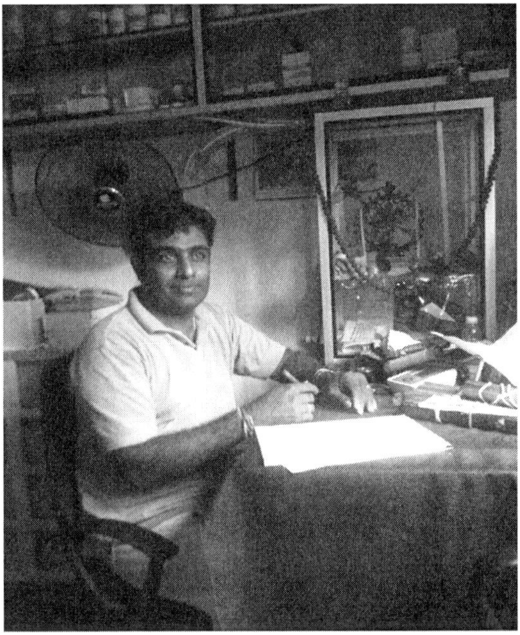

Figure 3.8 – Je Jeyalan, Siddha-Ayrveda healer at his desk in Sujjeevaah Clinic, Jaffna

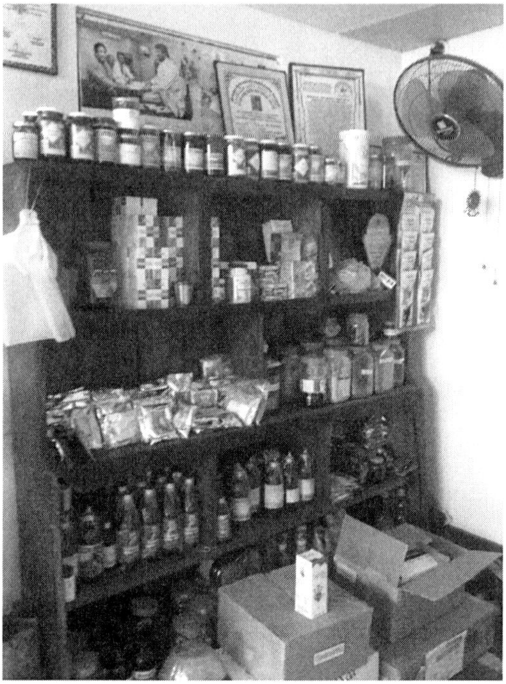

Figure 3.9 – Medicines that Je Jeyalan prescribes. Some of the medicines are prepared by him, while some are purchased from Ayurveda or Siddha traditional medicine shops in Sri Lanka and others (Himalayan products) exported from India

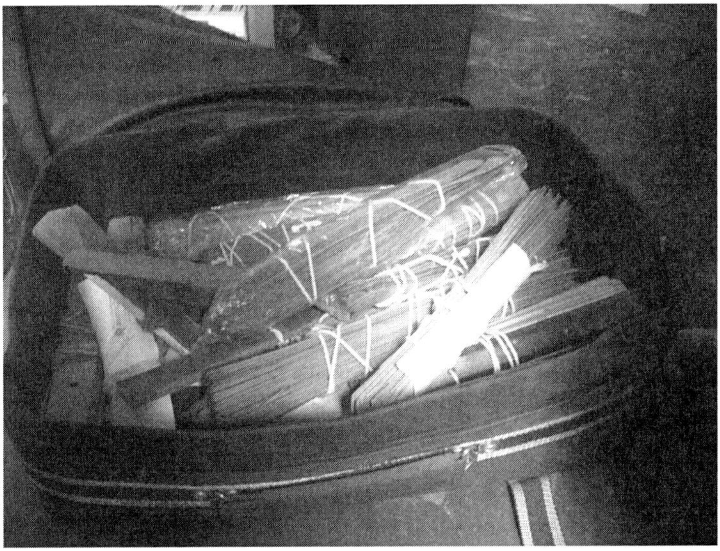

Figure 3.10 - Palm leaf manuscripts on healing, written in Tamil

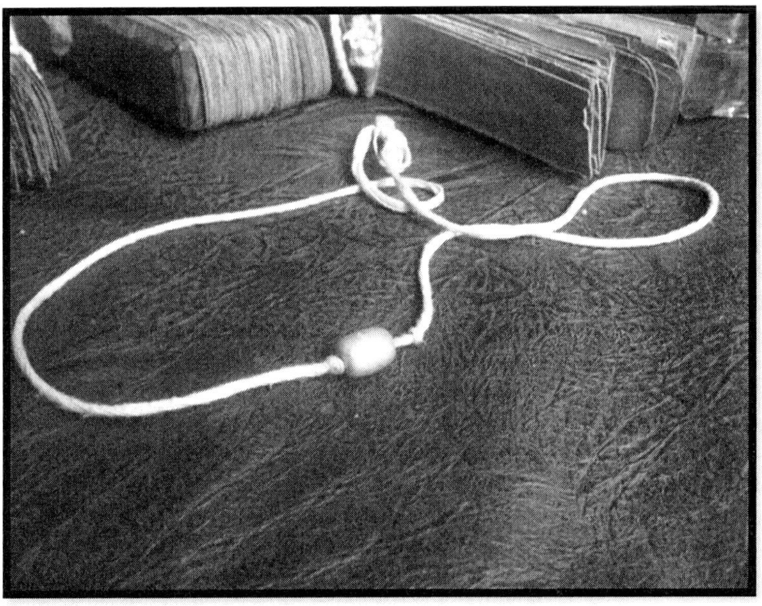

Figure 3.11 - 'Rasa Mani', healing and protection neckless

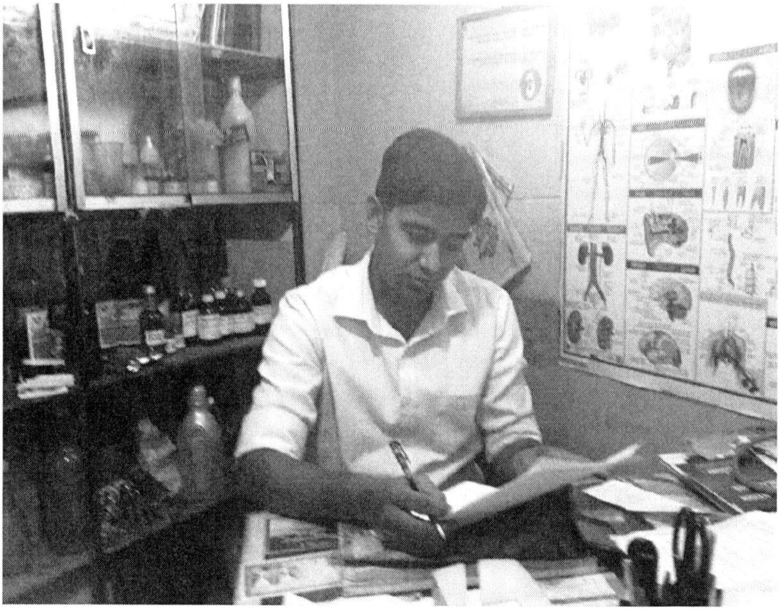

Figure 3.12 – Healer Chaminda Rajapakse at his healing centre

Another case that highlights the dilemma of classification is the healer Chaminda Rajapakse[177] (Figure 3.12) practicing in Bandarawela. Chaminda practices Sarvanga treatment based on Ayurveda and *Kadum Bidum, Sarpa Visa* and cancer treatments based on indigenous family practices. Chaminda is an indigenous healer, specialising in treatments for *Sarpa Visa* (serpent bites), *Kadum Bidum* (fractures, dislocation) and cancers.[178] He has acquired the inter-generational knowledge of the healing practices from his father, by observing and helping him since childhood.[179] Chaminda has also studied Ayurveda at the Uduwana Pirivena for three years and possesses a Diploma in Ayurveda. Ayurveda training has given him knowledge to treat any physical disorder (*Sarvanga).*[180] Chaminda is facing the dilemma of what to call himself. As he says:

> As I do not possess a Degree in Ayurveda, I cannot call myself an Ayurveda doctor. According to the government classification, I am a

[177] Chaminda Rajapakse (# 19).
[178] Chaminda Rajapakse (# 19).
[179] Chaminda Rajapakse (# 19).
[180] Chaminda Rajapakse (# 19).

> 'Traditional Healer.' But I feel I am both: Traditional/ Inter-generational healer cum Ayurveda Doctor.[181]

Chaminda explains how challenging it is to practice as a healer in Sri Lanka:

> The number of people who seek indigenous treatment for serpent bites and cancers at present have significantly reduced. When my father was practicing there were many such patients. Now people prefer the western medical option, as it is freely available and is sponsored by the Government. As a result of the competition with the western medical system in the country, it is difficult to practice as a traditional healer.[182]

Chaminda says he is still surviving as a healer because he has the traditional family background to healing, indigenous healing knowledge and academic qualification in Ayurveda.[183] In order to continue practice, he says he needs to adopt current trends. This includes charging a consultation fee from the patients, which his father or the ancestors did not practice.[184] At that time, a traditional healer was considered as an honorary service and they used to accept only what was given to them. Chaminda's friends who studied for the Diploma in Ayurveda with him have pursued other careers as it is not easy to survive as an Ayurveda practitioner without any form of formal support mechanism.[185]

In order to keep the indigenous forms of healing or to protect the profession of Ayurveda healers who have qualified with the Diploma in Ayurveda, he says it is necessary to systematically organise these two groups.[186]

In part 2 I have categorised the diverse forms of healing practices and complexities when trying to distinguish a practice into a certain category. The analysis in part 2 makes it clear that government recognised traditional healing practices are not the only forms of healing practices that exist in Sri Lanka. The Government has not recognised, regulated and supported all forms of healing practices due to various reasons, including the informal nature of some forms of healing practices and typology of relations between different forms of knowledge.

[181] Chaminda Rajapakse (#19).
[182] Chaminda Rajapakse (#19).
[183] Chaminda Rajapakse (#19).
[184] Chaminda Rajapakse (#19).
[185] Chaminda Rajapakse (#19).
[186] Chaminda Rajapakse (#19).

Part 3: Dynamics and Complexities of Diverse Healing Practices

Various factors, such as the characteristics of healing practices, socio-cultural and political dynamics have come into play in determining the status of knowledge systems, government recognition and traditional cultural aspects of healing and wellbeing in Sri Lanka. To protect and promote healing practices in a country, it is necessary to obtain a more nuanced understanding of the prevailing healing practices. This involves understanding the socio-cultural and political dynamics of healing practices along with the characteristics of practices recognised by the government. This part of the chapter tries to understand the dynamics and complexities between different forms of healing.

Differences between healing methods practiced in Sri Lanka can be understood based on the characteristics of healing practices, such as organisation of the practice, scientific testing, diagnosis, religious influence, documentation of healing practices, availability in public domain, accessibility of knowledge, nomenclature used to address the healer, fees charged, code of ethics, academic qualifications, method of treatment, use of rituals and use of forecasting methods. In Figure below (3.18) I summarise the differences between biomedical (allopathic) healing, government recognised traditional healing, inter-generational and cosmic healing in order to understand the dynamics and politics of healing and struggle for survival.

#		**Biomedical (Allopathic) Healing**	**Government Recognised Traditional Healing**	**Inter-generational Healing**	**Cosmic Healing**
1	Scientific approach	Scientifically tested using bio-medical methods. Treatments are designed after vigorous scientific research and testing.	Some aspects are tested using bio-medical methods while some aspects cannot be tested. Treatments are designed by the Rishis or the inventors of the traditional healing system based on their understanding of nature, causes of sickness and methods to overcome it	Most aspects are not scientifically tested. Treatments are designed based on dreams, inspirations, experimentation with nature	Most aspects are not scientifically tested. Treatments are designed based on dreams, inspirations, experimentation with nature
2	Recognition by the Government	Fully recognised by the Government	Recognised by the Government	Partialy recognised by the Government	Not recognized by the Government
3	Types of healing methods	Treats the symptoms. Does not use rituals for treatment. Does not use forecasting methods for diagnosis or treatment	Treats the cause. Sometimes use rituals for treatment. Sometimes use forecasting methods for diagnosis and treatment.	Treats the cause. Often use rituals for treatment. Often use forecasting methods for diagnosis and treatment.	Treats the cause. Treatment is mostly based on rituals. Often use forecasting methods for diagnosis and treatment.

4	Role of religion	Not based on a religious framework	Mostly based on a religious framework	Based on a religious framework	Based on a religious framework
	Practices/ Practitioners	Bio-medical practices Known as Western medical doctors	Ayurveda, Siddha, Unani, Homeopathy, Acupuncture Known as Ayurveda doctors, Siddha doctors, Unani doctors, Homeopathy doctors, Acupuncture doctors, etc.	See Chapter 3, 2.1 Known as healer, traditional healer, Intergenerational healer, Indigenous healer, Special doctor	See Chapter 3, 2.2 Known as exorcist, spirit healer, ritual performer, palm reader, astrologer, healing monk, heling priest (some individuals who practice cosmic healing are not referred to from a specific name)
5	Organized in terms of professional regulations; registration	Organised	Organised	Semi-organised	Semi-organised or Unorganised
6	Formal/ Informal Education	Taught in public domain. Knowledge is accessible for anyone	Used to be taught in private domain, now is available in public domain. Knowledge used to be passed down from generation to generation but now is accessible for anyone	Taught in private domains. Knowledge is passed down from generation to generation	Acquired by experimentation or taught in private domains. Knowledge is acquired by individuals by self exploration or acquired by generation to generation

7	Professional Fees	Professional fees are applicable when practiced privately. As Government Medical practitioners receive a monthly salary, services are provided free for the public.	Professional fees are applicable most of the time when practiced privately. Some traditional healers still practice without a set fee. As Government Medical practitioners receive a monthly salary, services are provided free for the public.	No set fee most of the time	No set fee most of the time
8	Transmission of knowledge or documentation	Systematically documented	Knowledge used to be passed down by word of mouth but now it is systematically documented	Knowledge is passed down by observation; word of mouth; or in hand written notes	Knowledge is acquired by self-exploration, or passed down by observation, word of mouth or notes of a healer

Figure 3.13 – Differences between biomedical allopathic healing, government recognised traditional healing, inter-generational healing and cosmic healing

The figure above is a general categorisation of healing practices based on characteristics of Western allopathic healing, government-recognised traditional healing, inter-generational healing and cosmic healing. Due to the diverse nature and over-lapping traits of healing practices, it is not possible to make absolute distinctions between healing practices. What is apparent from Figure 3.18 is that the distinction between diverse healing systems is based on two axes. The first (criteria 1-8 in Figure 3.13) concerns whether the healing systems knowledge base is in science or in religion and rituals. The second (criteria 9-17 in Figure 3.13) concerns whether the healing system is formalised in the public domain or informal, private domain.

Healing knowledge of Sri Lanka discussed above as Western allopathic healing, government-recognised traditional healing, inter-generational healing and cosmic healing can be further analysed based on the form of existence. These healing knowledge systems can exist as parallel systems of knowledge, as complementary systems of knowledge, as selective inclusion of knowledge and sometimes not openly.[187] Parallel knowledge of healing is different ways that knowledge coexists together without open interaction. Some examples of existence of parallel knowledge in Sri Lanka include allopathic, Ayurveda, Siddha, Unani, homeopathy, acupuncture, inter-generational healing (*Kadum Bidum, Ass, Pilika, Ansha Baga, Visa, Sarvanga*), meditation and yoga that exist in Sri Lanka as parallel systems of healing practices. Complementary systems of knowledge are when there are two or many different ways of knowing using mechanisms of exchange and mutual learning aiming at complementing each other. Examples in Sri Lanka include using astral charts, palm reading, telepathy, biological indicators and power of spirits for forecasting. Selective inclusion of elements of local knowledge in healing is when scientifically understood or validated knowledge in healing is accepted for enhancing the stock of scientific knowledge; this may imply assessment of local knowledge by outside scientists and lead to *ex situ* conservation of local knowledge. Some examples include *Kothala Hibatu* and some aspects of inter-generational healing (i.e, *Kadum Bidum, Visa, Pilika*) as part of Ayurveda. Politically suppressed knowledge continues to exist but not openly. For example, shamanism (which is also called spirit healers), *Yantra mantra, Bali, Shanthi karma*, indigenous healing of *Veddha*, *Dehi kepima*, protection, *thovil, kem karma* and sound therapy continue to exist not openly but underground.

[187] Based on Haverkort and Reijntjes (2010), p 12- 30.

It is important to note all the differences and distinctions of healing practices identified in this chapter are drawn from the diversities identified during interviews and during analysis of healing practices in Sri Lanka. As this chapter is discussing living healing systems, the characteristics of healing practices, the differences between healing practices, and their dynamics and complexities are not static but evolve and change with cultural, social, political, economic influences. This attempt to understand the diversity of healing practices is made because to recognise, support, and regulate healing practices by government to safeguard the cultural aspect of healing, it is necessary to understand the current status of these practices.

Conclusion

This chapter has presented the diversity of healing practices in Sri Lanka by categorising healing practices based on interviews and researcher's own analysis of characteristics of healing practices. In this chapter it is argued that only some healing practices are recognised by the Government of Sri Lanka. In making this argument, the chapter has first examined the government-recognised traditional healing practices of Sri Lanka namely, Ayurveda, Siddha, Unani, homeopathy, acupuncture, and Deshiya Chikithsa. The second part of the chapter established the wider scope of healing practices in Sri Lanka, recognising that the currently existing healing practices in the country are far more extensive and richer than the practices recognised by the Government of Sri Lanka. To obtain a broader understanding of the healing practices in Sri Lanka, the diverse forms of healing in Sri Lanka were clustered into 5 categories, namely: inter-generational healing, cosmic healing, adopted traditional healing, western healing and integrated healing. This classification was made to facilitate the analysis of how government has recognised, supported and regulated healing practices in Sri Lanka and the impact of government involvement or non-involvement in culture and practices of healing. The third part of the chapter is devoted to obtaining a better understanding of diverse healing practices of Sri Lanka. In this part, the complexities and dynamics of different forms of healing practices were analysed by trying to distinguish between Western allopathic healing, government-recognised traditional healing, inter-generational and cosmic healing according to characteristics of healing practices. The analysis of diverse healing systems has exemplified the distinctions of diverse healing systems being mainly based on: (1) how the healing system has been influenced by science compared with religion and rituals; and (2) whether the healing system is being practiced formally in public domain or informally in a private or secret setting.

This chapter plays an important role in understanding the diversity of existing healing practices, dynamics and complexities. Holistic understanding of prevailing healing practices is a pre-requisite for a government to recognise, support and regulate healing practices and ultimately, to safeguard the cultural aspect of healing. Government recognition, support and regulation play an important role in determining what healing practices including what aspects of healing practices will be protected and promoted. The next chapter focuses on the government role in recognition, support and regulation of traditional practices related to healing in Sri Lanka.

CHAPTER 4

THE ROLE OF SRI LANKAN GOVERNMENT IN RECOGNISING, SUPPORTING AND REGULATING 'TRADITIONAL' HEALING PRACTICES AND THE IMPACT ON CULTURE

Introduction

Having set out some of the types of healing practices in Sri Lanka in Chapter 4, this chapter examines the history and nature of the recognition, support and regulation of traditional healing practices in Sri Lanka and draws attention to the incommensurate ways in which the Sri Lankan Government recognises, supports and regulates these different healing practices. In this chapter 'traditional healing practices' refers to government recognised traditional healing practices. Healing practices such as Ayurveda, Siddha and Unani have the most government recognition and support; other healing practices such as inter-generational healing are partially recognised, while cosmic healing practices are not recognised and supported at all by the Sri Lankan Government.

This chapter argues that government recognition, support and regulation towards healing practices determine what healing practices and cultural aspect of it will be protected and promoted or diminished. This argument is presented in seven parts. In the first part the chapter argues that public demand for traditional and indigenous healing practices, particularly those associated with Ayurveda, was vital in the Sri Lankan Government's approach to healing practices. Indeed, from the early 1900s, the Sri Lankan public demanded more health care services and facilities that were not provided by Western (allopathic) doctors and medical administrators, and as a consequence the Sri Lankan Government established various departments and organisations to promote traditional healing. In this way the government became involved in research; education and training on traditional healing, the formalisation of traditional healing systems, the establishment, organisation and support of healing centres, herbal gardens and drug manufacturing centres, and the promotion of community healthcare based on Ayurveda. In effect this meant that, from the mid-1930s, many of the traditional healing structures were under government supervision.

From part two through to seven, the chapter discusses some of the most important steps that the Sri Lankan Government undertook to recognise, support and regulate traditional healing practices; particularly those associated with the Ayurvedic traditions. While there are numerous regulations and laws that indirectly affect healing practices, the focus of this chapter is on those healing practices that are recognised as traditional by the government and that come under direct government support, recognition and regulation.[1] These government interventions have an effect on education, training, research, hospitals, medicine and community healthcare. In the second part the chapter argues how the government administration of traditional health care system has contributed towards adopting a biomedical framework for traditional healing and Ayurvedisation of traditional healing. In the third part the chapter argues the government role in regulating, standardising and formalising education has had a negative impact on protecting culture and practices of healing systems. The fourth part of the chapter argues how hospitals and curative services for traditional healing that are sponsored by the Government have contributed to adopting Western styled places of treatment for traditional healing. This part also argues how the focus of traditional healing curative services has been mainly on Ayurveda and to a lesser extent on Siddha and Unani. Part five of this chapter argues that Ayurveda medicines and drugs receive attention from the Government of Sri Lanka in terms of standardising, sponsoring the production of and distribution to Government hospitals and dispensaries under the purview of Ministry of Indigenous Medicine. Part six of the chapter argues that the government focuses on Ayurveda in both research and gardens, and the government sponsored research has adopted a Western research framework to support the Western concepts of universalisation and standardisation of knowledge. The seventh part of the argument focuses on the programmes implemented by the Ministry of Indigenous Medicine to

---

[1] For example: the *Intellectual Property Act no 36 of 2003* that replaced the *Code of Intellectual Property Act no. 53 of 1979* covers a variety of Intellectual Property rights including copyright, related rights, expressions of folklore, industrial designs, marks, patents, unfair competition, geographical indications and lay-out designs of integrated circuits that has an impact on traditional knowledge in healing. The Act also provides for the management and enforcement of intellectual property rights. The National Intellectual Property Office of Sri Lanka is mandated under this act for the administration of the intellectual property system in Sri Lanka

develop community healthcare and inter-generational healing. The argument made in this part is that none of the community healthcare programmes and inter-generational healing programmes are well established and that in fact some of them are failures.

The chapter concludes by arguing that the Sri Lankan Government has adopted a rather narrow approach to traditional healing practices, where more formal practices are protected in a 'Western-like' framework and where there is a tendency towards the 'Ayurvedisation' of traditional healing practices. Throughout the chapter a significant trend in loss of cultural value in the process of standardisation and formalisation is illustrated. Another important aspect is the very limited support, recognition and regulation for inter-generational healing by the government and for cosmic healing practices this is non-existent due to the diversity and informal nature of the inter-generational and cosmic healing systems in the country. The chapter highlights that the real 'traditional knowledge' of healing in Sri Lanka - the inter-generational healing practices and cosmic healing practices - has therefore been overlooked.

Part 1: Public Demand and the Establishment of a Government Controlled Traditional Medicine System in Sri Lanka

This part argues that public demand for non-Western healing practices, particularly those associated with Ayurveda, was vital in the Sri Lankan Government's approach to healing practices. To present the argument, historical milestones that led to public demand and government initiations in the development of traditional medicine systems in Sri Lanka are discussed.

In the late nineteenth and early twentieth centuries non-Western healing practices in Sri Lanka were under threat.[2] This was in large part because of a complex mix of colonial influence, state neglect of traditional healing systems, changes in the traditional social and value systems[3] and the introduction of a Western medical system.[4] Due to the state sponsorship of Western medical system in the country, Western medical practices started to thrive. In the meantime, healing practices that existed in Sri Lanka prior

---

[2] Ministry of Health (1955), p.3. Also see Coperahewa (2009), De Silva (1981) for change in political consciousness and activities in Sri Lanka in this period.

[3] Coomaraswamy (1909) discusses how colonial influence has impacted in changes in traditional and social value systems in India.

[4] Wanninayaka (1982).

to colonisation faced the threat of extinction due to the introduction of Western social and administrative systems that suppressed the caste based social system.[5]

In the early twentieth century, however, public interest in traditional health methods grew. This interest was heightened by the fact that the Ceylonese Government—due to high costs and insufficient personnel—was not able to fulfil the health needs of all Sri Lankans through Western medicine.[6] As a consequence of the public demand for traditional healing and the limitations of resources available to roll out Western healthcare island-wide, in 1916, the Government declared it would consider favourably a scheme for granting of assistance for the teaching of indigenous medicine. Despite coming into focus in 1916, it was not until 1926 that a scheme to promote teaching of indigenous medicine was embedded in policy decisions.[7] In response to the public agitation about the lack of access and availability of traditional health care facilities, a committee, chaired by K. Balasingham, was appointed.[8] The committee was asked to report on the need for, and benefits of, granting financial and research assistance for indigenous medicine: most notably the committee was asked to evaluate the teaching, practicability and value of indigenous drugs.[9] To carry out the investigation, the committee held ten meetings, questioned many witnesses, and studied the report of the Indian Madras Committee on the Indigenous Systems of Medicine issued in 1923.[10] In the *Sessional Paper 1 of 1927* the committee recommended the constitution of a Board of Indigenous Medicine to deal with the teaching of indigenous medicine; the establishment of a college, a hospital, a dispensary and a research institute; the registration of qualified practitioners, and the award of scholarships for study in India.[11]

The Sri Lankan Government implemented some of the committee's recommendations. In 1928, the Legislative Council approved the committee's recommendation of establishing a Board of Indigenous Medicine that would develop and regulate indigenous medicine and research related to indigenous medicine.[12] In order to establish a Board of Indigenous Medicine, the Government allocated fifty thousand Sri Lankan rupees per

---

[5] For discussion see Chapter 2, Part 4.
[6] Ministry of Health (1955), p 4.
[7] Ministry of Health (1955), p 4.
[8] Ministry of Health (1955), p 4.
[9] Wickramasinghe, (2006), p 100; Ministry of Health (1955), p 4.
[10]*Sessional paper No. 1 of 1927*(Sri Lanka), c III.
[11] *Sessional paper No. 1 of 1927* (Sri Lanka).
[12] Ministry of Health (1955), p 5.

year for ten years.[13] The Board of Indigenous Medicine was responsible for executing the recommendations. Accordingly, the Board of Indigenous Medicine established a College of Indigenous Medicine in 1929, an indigenous pharmacy in 1932 and an indigenous hospital in 1933.[14]

Another important step in the recognition, support and regulation of traditional healing practices in Sri Lanka was implementing policies for the government's active involvement in the process of policy making related to traditional healing. In part this was achieved by government playing an active role in supporting and regulating the government-recognised traditional healing systems, where the power and control of these traditional healing systems, such as Ayurveda, Siddha and Unani, was transferred from healers to government control. This meant that many of the decisions related to traditional health care, such as training, practicing and medicine came under government control. In 1935, for instance, the policy review of the Indigenous Medical System was entrusted to a subcommittee of the Executive Committee of Health, where the committee observed, that:

> If the Government intends to satisfy the public demand for competent indigenous medical practitioners it should abandon the policy of non-interference and actively cooperate in making the present institution an efficient one.[15]

Based on the observation, the subcommittee of the Executive Committee of Health recommended the transfer of the college and its ancillary institutions to government control. This recommendation was approved by the Executive Committee of Health and was accepted by the State Council. *The Ordinance No. 17 of 1941* adopted the recommendations by the incorporation of the board, the continuance of the college, the hospital, the pharmacy, the dispensary and the herbarium as government institutions, and for the registration of practitioners of indigenous medicine.

Even though the Sri Lankan Government assumed control of traditional healing systems there were problems with spreading and systematically developing the traditional health care system in Sri Lanka. In 1945, for example, the State Council requested the appointment of a commission to examine the reasons for poor progress in the development of indigenous medicine. Accordingly, the Commission consisting of a well-

---

[13] Ministry of Health (1955), p 5.
[14] Ministry of Health (1955), p 5.
[15] Subcommittee of the Executive Committee of Health, *Report of the Subcommittee of the Executive Committee of Health on the Board of Indigenous Medicine and the Decisions on the Report by the Executive Committee.* Sessional Paper (1935), no. 94, class no. GP (27).

known Ayurveda physician from India and two Ceylon men who were not traditional healers, clergy or holding religious office were appointed in 1946. The Commission's report issued in 1947[16] disclosed the inadequacies of the state sponsored measures so far adopted and presented recommendations to revive and develop indigenous medicine. As per the report, despite state neglect in recognition or aiding indigenous medicine since 1929, over 70 percent of the population resorted to indigenous medicine in times of illness.[17]

In 1961, *the Ayurveda Act No. 31 of 1961*[18] ('the *Ayurveda Act'*) was enacted by repealing the *Indigenous Medical Ordinance No. 17 of 1941*. Based on the provisions of the *Ayurveda Act*,[19] four statutory boards were created: the Ayurveda Medical Council; the Ayurveda College and Hospital Board; the Ayurveda Research Committee; and the Ayurveda Drug Formulary Committee.[20] Broadly speaking these boards were established to implement the Government's plans for recognising, supporting and regulating traditional healing in Sri Lanka. In the *Ayurveda (Amendment) Act (no 9 of 1969*), the *Ayurveda Act, no. 31 of 1961* was amended by the insertion of sections 21A, 21B, 21C and 21D, of that Act. These sections deal with keeping accounts of the Council…;[21] auditing the Council Accounts by the Auditor General[22] (21 B); producing a report by the Auditor General;[23]and transmitting the Annual accounts… and the annual activities of the Council to the Minister.[24] There were a number of administrative, procedural and substantive changes made by the new laws.

One of the key areas in which the Government regulated traditional healing was the education and training of practitioners. In order to produce qualified medical practitioners of the Ayurveda, Unani and Siddha medical systems, the College of Indigenous Medicine was affiliated with the University of Colombo after renaming as the Institute of Indigenous Medicine by the *Institute of Ayurveda Statute No. 1 of 1977*.[25] The Siddha

---

[16] *Sessional Paper No. XXIV of 1947* (Sri Lanka).
[17] *Sessional paper No. XXIV of 1947*(Sri Lanka) *s17.*
[18] *Ayurveda Act No. 31 of 1961* (Sri Lanka).
[19] *Ayurveda Act No. 31 of 1961*(Sri Lanka).
[20] Also discussed in Chapter 2, Part 2. 2 (iv) National mechanism in place to protect traditional healing.
[21] *Ayurveda Amendment Act No. 9 of 1969* (Sri Lanka) s 21A.
[22] *Ayurveda Amendment Act No. 9 of 1969* (Sri Lanka) s 21B.
[23] *Ayurveda Amendment Act No. 9 of 1969* (Sri Lanka) s 21C.
[24] *Ayurveda Amendment Act No. 9 of 1969* (Sri Lanka) s 21D.
[25] Published in the Government Gazette Extraordinary bearing number 257 of March 30, 1977

section of the Institute of Indigenous Medicine, University of Colombo was transferred to Jaffna University on 2 July 1984 as a result of the civil conflict in the country.[26] The Gampaha Wickramarachchi Ayurveda Vidyalaya established in 1928 was incorporated under the Ministry of Indigenous Medicine by the *Parliamentary Act No 30 in 1982*. It was upgraded to a university institute in 1995.[27] To fast track the revival of the Ayurveda Medical Practice,[28] the Ministry of Indigenous Medicine was established on 14 February 1980.[29] The Ministry was granted cabinet status in 1994.

As a result of continued Government attention and support in systematically protecting and promoting traditional healing with the focus on Ayurveda, Siddha and Unani, currently (as at July 2015) there are 62 Ayurveda hospitals that offer residential curative services and 208 central dispensaries.[30] The services provided at these hospitals include consultation, residential facilities and treatment in these hospitals and dispensaries are offered free of charge. There are 1 424 physicians employed in the government Ayurveda hospitals.[31] In order to enhance community health work and to implement disease prevention programs of Ministry of Indigenous Medicine 325 community health officers and 325 assistant Ayurveda medical officers were were deployed from all over the island in 2009.[32] In addition, there are about 20,000 registered as traditional medical

[26] History, Department of Siddha Medicine, University of Jaffna. http://www.siddha.jfn.ac.lk/?page_id=33 (last retrieved 20 February 2019).

[27] History, Gampaha Wickramarachchi Ayurveda Institute, University of Kelaniya. http://www.kln.ac.lk/institutes/wickramarachchi/index.php/department/history.htm l (last retrieved 20 February 2019).

[28] As mentioned in the introduction given in the Ministry of Indigenous Medicine website -http://www.indigenousmedimini.gov.lk/About_us.html (last retrieved 20 February 2019).

[29] The Ministry of Indigenous Medicine, About Us – http://www.indigenousmedimini.gov.lk/About_us.html?&session-id=bf4e6b1982ea3f0348ebc843f9083fae (last retrieved 20 February 2019).

[30] Given statistics are based on the Ministry of Indigenous Medicine website – http://www.indigenousmedimini.gov.lk/About_us.html (last retrieved 20 February 2019).

[31] Given statistics are based on the Ministry of Indigenous Medicine website – http://www.indigenousmedimini.gov.lk/About_us.html (last retrieved 20 February 2019).

[32] Ministry of Indigenous Medicine – http://www.indigenousmedimini.gov.lk/About_us.html (last retrieved 20 February 2019).

practitioners in the Ayurveda Medical Council of the Ministry of Indigenous Medicine.[33]

Part 2: Administration of Traditional Health Care

This part argues how the government administration of traditional health care system has contributed to adopting a biomedical framework for traditional healing and the Ayurvedisation of traditional healing. To develop the argument, this section looks at the current government structure in administrating health care practices in Sri Lanka, with the aim of presenting a general overview of the nature and scope of the government's administration of healing practices. Or, to put it another way: what types of healing practices does the Sri Lankan Government support and regulate, and what types of healing practices does it not support and regulate? In order to do so the role of the Ministry of Indigenous Medicine, Department of Ayurveda, Provincial Administration of Indigenous Medicine and the Ayurveda Medical Council are discussed.

2.1 The Ministry of Indigenous Medicine

One of the ways in which the Government sought to control traditional health practices was through the establishment of the Ministry of Indigenous Medicine. The Ministry of Indigenous Medicine was established on 14 February 1980.[34] Significantly this was the first separate Ministry for Indigenous Medicine established anywhere in the world.[35] The first Minister of Indigenous Medicine, Hon. Dharmasenna Attygalle is a famous traditional Ayurvedic physician.[36]

The object of the Ministry has been the revival of traditional medical practice. The vision of the Ministry of Indigenous Medicine is to deliver healthcare facilities to all citizens through the system of indigenous medicine. It seeks to achieve its purposes by supervising and executing policy in respect of institutions, subjects and functions categorised under Ayurvedic medical services. In fulfilling the Ministry's vision, it has to compete with already established Western medical structures (allopathic

---

[33] Ministry of Indigenous Medicine http://www.indigenousmedimini.gov.lk/About_us.html (last retrieved 20 February 2019).
[34] Ministry of Indigenous Medicine www.indigenousmedimini.gov.lk/About_us.html(last retrieved 20 February 2019)
[35] Wanninayaka (1982), p 13.
[36] Wanninayaka (1982), p 13.

medicine), under the Ministry of Health in Sri Lanka for recognition and relevance. The institutions established under the Ministry of Indigenous Medicine, including the framework, administrative structure, bureaucracy, architecture, and services offered is an imitation of the system established by Ministry of Health for Western medicine.

Broadly speaking the Ministry provides government supported Ayurveda services to the nation for curative and preventive diseases.[37] More specifically the Ministry's two main objectives are: (1) to promote traditional medical practice locally and globally, contributing to the development of national economy; and (2) to create a healthy nation by optimum utilisation of the nationally available resources.[38]

To achieve their aims the Ministry is involved with a range of functions according to the Ministry of Indigenous Medicine website:

- policy planning and program implementation regarding indigenous medicine;
- developing the Ayurveda, Siddha, Unani medical systems;
- importing, marketing and distribution of raw and finished medicine required for Ayurveda, Siddha, Unani and Homeopathy;
- regulating the import of medicinal herbs and prepared medicine for Ayurveda, Siddha and Unani medicine;
- promoting the cultivation of herbs and extension activities associated with it;
- maintaining and promoting the Ayurveda research institute, the training institute and the research herbal gardens;
- registering and regulating the professional standards of Ayurveda medical practitioners and Ayurveda para-medical personnel;
- monitoring activities of Ayurveda Medical Council, Ayurveda colleges and hospital boards;
- regulating the activities of the Ayurveda medicine producers; developing and regulating the use of Homeopathy; and
- establishing Ayurveda Hospitals and administering them.[39]

---

[37] Home page, Ministry of Indigenous Medicine http://www.indigenousmedimini.gov.lk/index.html (last retrieved 20 February 2019).

[38] About Us, Ministry of Indigenous Medicine http://www.indigenousmedimini.gov.lk/About_us.html (last retrieved 20 February 2019)

[39] About Us, Ministry of Indigenous Medicine website http://www.indigenousmedimini.gov.lk/About_us.html (last retrieved 20 February 2019).

The two main arms under the supervision of the Ministry are the Department of Ayurveda (which is responsible for curative services, regulatory functions, research, and certain matters pertaining to Ayurvedic education) and the Ayurveda Drugs Corporation (which is engaged in the production and sale of Ayurvedic drugs).[40]

2.2 Department of Ayurveda

The Department of Ayurveda[41] of the Ministry of Indigenous Medicine plays a crucial role in controlling the traditional healing system of Sri Lanka. The Department of Ayurveda was established under the *Ayurveda Act, no. 31 of 1961*.[42] According to the Act the functions previously handled by the Commissioner for Development of Indigenous Medicine was transferred to the Commissioner for Ayurveda.[43] The role of the Department of Ayurveda according to Ministry of Indigenous Medicine website is:

- to recognise, support and regulate traditional healing practices by providing curative services on the basis of indigenous methods of treatment, through a network of hospitals and dispensaries;
- to provide for the establishment and services necessary for treatment of diseases; to preserve and promote of health according to indigenous methods of treatment;
- to provide for and standardise educational and professional levels in Ayurveda; and
- to encourage research in Ayurveda; and to provide ancillary services to facilitate treatment, study and research in Ayurveda.[44]

---

[40] Mr. Lalith Kannangara (# 1).

[41] Department of Ayurveda is located in Old Kottawa Road, Navinna, Maharagama, Tel 094-011-02896911, E-mail:- ita@ayurveda.gov.lk. See- www.ayurveda.gov.lk/dept.html (last retrieved 20 February 2019).

[42] *Ayurveda Act No. 31 of 1961* (Sri Lanka). Also see Department of Ayurveda and Statutory Bodies, Ministry of Indigenous Medicine http://www.indigenousmedimini.gov.lk/Deparment.html (last retrieved 20 February 2019).

[43] Commissioner for Ayurveda was appointed under *Ayurveda Act No. 31 of 1961* (Sri Lanka) 3.

[44] Department of Ayurveda and Statutory Bodies, Ministry of Indigenous Medicine http://www.indigenousmedimini.gov.lk/Deparment.html (last retrieved 20 February 2019).

In the process of fulfilling the role, the Department of Ayurveda is engaged in 'establishing and maintaining hospitals and dispensary services; conducting examinations at diploma level in Ayurveda for external students; registration of practitioners; conducting clinical, pharmacological and literary research; propagation of herb cultivation; and assisting projects to facilitate Ayurveda research.'[45]

In order to execute some of the functions of the Department of Ayurveda, three statutory bodies were set up under the *Ayurveda Act*, namely, the Ayurvedic Medical Council, Ayurveda Education and Hospital Board and the Ayurveda Research Committee; and one non-statutory committee, namely, the Ayurveda Formulary Committee.[46] The role of each of these statutory bodies and committees and their contribution towards traditional healing is discussed in this chapter[47]. The Bandaranaike Ayurveda Research Institute in Nawinna is the research institute and the National Institute of Traditional Medicine, is the training institute administered under the Department of Ayurveda. Also, the Department monitors the 62 Ayurvedic hospitals including teaching and research hospitals, 230 central dispensaries and herbal gardens.[48]

The institution name 'Department of Ayurveda' and the names of the sub-institutions under the Department of Ayurveda are misleading as the services provided by the Department of Ayurveda and the related institutions are not limited to Ayurveda but all traditional and indigenous healing practices. The institution name, 'Department of Ayurveda' also suggest government efforts in 'Ayurvedaisation'[49] of all traditional and indigenous healing practices.

---

[45] Department of Ayurveda Website- www.ayurveda.gov.lk/dept.html (Last retrieved 20 February 2019) and Department of Ayurveda and Statutory Bodies, Ministry of Indigenous Medicine http://www.indigenousmedimini.gov.lk/Deparment.html (last retrieved 20 February 2019).

[46] *Ayurveda Act No. 31 of 1961*(Sri Lanka).

[47] Parts of this chapter in which each of the bodies and committees are discussed are as follows -the Ayurvedic Medical Council – s 2.1, the Ayurveda Education and Hospital Board- s 3.1, the Ayurveda Research Committee – s 6.1, the Ayurveda Formulary Committee –s 5.1.

[48] Mr. Palitha Weerakoon (#3).

[49] Multi-faces of Sri Lanka Ayurveda where indigenous healing methods and cultural aspects are mixed is discussed by Nordstorm (1988) (1989).

2.3 Provincial Administration of Indigenous Medicine

The Provincial Councils governing system introduced to the eight Provinces in Sri Lanka through the 13th amendment of the Constitution of the country in November 1987,[50] created major reforms 'as it led to the devolution of the provision of health care to the Provincial Councils.'[51] The Provincial Council now possess 'the final responsibility for providing health care in the provinces.'[52] The President of Sri Lanka appointed a Governor for each province and a Provincial Government was established in each province by an election to assist the Governor.[53] The Provincial Government includes a Chief Minister and four other ministers.[54] The Provincial Council Ministry system is responsible for administering the services of preventive and curative indigenous medicine at the provincial level. This includes administering district Ayurvedic hospitals, rural Ayurvedic hospitals, central Ayurvedic hospitals and mobile units in the respective province.[55] The name of the responsible institution to administer indigenous health services differ from province to province. For example –

- The Ministry of Health and Indigenous Medicine[56](Northern Province);
- The Provincial Department of Ayurveda under the Ministry of Health, Indigenous Medicine, Social Welfare and Women Affairs, Probation and Child Care and Council Affairs[57] (Western Province);
- Medicine, Social Welfare and Probation and Child Care Services (Central Province).

---

[50] *The Constitution of the Democratic Socialist Republic of Sri Lanka 1978* (Sri Lanka), *13th Amendment* (1987).
[51] Fernando (1999), p15.
[52] Fernando (1999), p15. Also see Department of Ayurveda, www.ayurveda.gov.lk/dept.html (Last retrieved 20 February 2019).
[53] *Constitution of Democratic Socialist Republic of Sri Lanka* 1978 (Sri Lanka) *13th Amendment* (1987), s 154 (b)
[54] *Constitution of Democratic Socialist Republic of Sri Lanka* 1978 (Sri Lanka) *13th Amendment* (1987), s 154 (e)
[55] Mr. Palitha Weerakoon (# 3).
[56] Ministry of Health and Indigenous Medicine, Northern Province. http://www.np.gov.lk/index.php?option=com_content&view=article&id=179&Itemid=16 (last retrieved 20 February 2019).
[57] Ministry of Health, Indigenous Medicine, Probation and Child Care and Council Affairs (Western Province) http://www.healthmin.wpc.gov.lk/en/?page_id=215 (last retrieved 20 February 2019).

There are Provincial Indigenous Secretaries and Provincial Ayurveda Commissioners in each province to administer Ayurveda/ indigenous medical services.[58]

The national level Ayurveda Department and the Ayurveda Drug Corporation coordinate with the provincial Ayurveda Departments in providing services. Yet as the provincial Ayurveda Departments are managed by nine different administrative structures it is difficult to administratively coordinate, monitor the services and maintain standards. Since the delivery of traditional healing is administrated by different administrative structures it has been difficult to maintain the uniformity of traditional health care facilities within different provinces, but the Sri Lankan Government has managed to regulate traditional healing practices systematically to a great extent by creating a central structure to provide guidelines and support.

2.4 Sri Lanka Ayurveda Medical Council

The Indigenous Medical Board is the first legally authorised body in the field of Ayurveda in Sri Lanka.[59] It was established in 1928 on the recommendation made by a sub-committee of the State Council of 1927to recognise, support and regulate traditional healing practices in Sri Lanka.[60] Subsequently the Ayurvedic Medical Council was established by virtue of the *Ceylon Ayurveda Medical Council Ordinance No. 46 of 1935* which was re-established under the provision of the *Indigenous Medical Council Ordinance No. 17 of 1941* (amended by *No. 49 of 1945 and No. 49 of 1949*).[61] The currently functioning Ayurveda Medical Council is an organisation established under the *Ayurveda Act no.31 of 1961*.

The Ayurvedic Medical Council is intended to serve as the apex body of Ayurveda in Sri Lanka equipped with all required facilities.[62] The

[58] Department of Ayurveda. http://www.ayurveda.gov.lk/dept.html (Last retrieved 20 February 2019).

[59] Department of Ayurveda (2014), p 73.

[60] Department of Ayurveda (2014), p 73, and Ayurveda Medical Council, Ministry of Indigenous Medicine – http://www.indigenousmedimini.gov.lk/MEDICA_%20COUNCIL.html?&session-id=bf4e6b1982ea3f0348ebc843f9083fae (last retrieved 20 February 2019)

[61] Ayurveda Medical Council, Ministry of Indigenous Medicine – http://www.indigenousmedimini.gov.lk/MEDICA_%20COUNCIL.html?&session-id=bf4e6b1982ea3f0348ebc843f9083fae (last retrieved 20 February 2019)

[62] Vision of Ayurveda Medical Council, Ministry of Indigenous Medicine –

Council strives to protect the legal foundation necessary for the qualitative development of the Ayurvedic field, providing maximum service to the public through Ayurveda under professional ethics,[63] by conferring the legal authority on professionals who have the knowledge, attitudes, skills and experience necessary to provide qualitative services in the field of Ayurveda in accordance with provisions of the *Ayurveda Act no.31 of 1961*.'[64]

In terms of *section 2(i)* of the *Ayurveda Act no. 31 of 1961* the Ayurveda Medical Council is empowered:

- to make recommendations to the Minister as to whether any institute teaching Ayurveda should be approved by the Minister for the purposes of the Act;
- to register names of persons as Ayurveda practitioners, Ayurveda dispensers, Ayurveda nurses;
- to cancel or suspend such registrations aid; to make regulations for regularisation and control of professional behavior of Ayurveda physicians Ayurveda dispensers and Ayurveda nurses; and
- to make regulations required for any matter referred to from (a) to (f) in this section.[65]

The most important of all the functions assigned to the Council is the registration of Ayurvedic practitioners. Only a registered Ayurvedic practitioner is entitled to use the title "*Vaidyacharya*" (physician) and only such a practitioner is legally or duly qualified to practice Ayurvedic medicine.[66] It is an offense to practice Ayurvedic medicine without being

http://www.indigenousmedimini.gov.lk/MEDICA_%20COUNCIL.html?&session-id=bf4e6b1982ea3f0348ebc843f9083fae (last retrieved 20 February 2019)

[63] Mission of Ayurveda Medical Council, Ministry of Indigenous Medicine – http://www.indigenousmedimini.gov.lk/MEDICA_%20COUNCIL.html?&session-id=bf4e6b1982ea3f0348ebc843f9083fae (last retrieved 20 February 2019)

[64] Purpose of Ayurveda Medical Council, Ministry of Indigenous Medicine – http://www.indigenousmedimini.gov.lk/MEDICA_%20COUNCIL.html?&session-id=bf4e6b1982ea3f0348ebc843f9083fae (last retrieved 20 February 2019). Also see Ayurvedic Medical Council website – www.ayurvedicmedicoun.gov.lk/web/index.php?option=com_content&view=article&id=85&Itemid=55&lang=en (last retrieved 20 February 2019).

[65] *Ayurveda Act no. 31 of 1961* (Sri Lanka) *s 2 (i)*. Also see, Ayurveda Medical Council, Ministry of Indigenous Medicine – http://www.indigenousmedimini.gov.lk/MEDICA_%20COUNCIL.html?&session-id=bf4e6b1982ea3f0348ebc843f9083fae (last retrieved 20 February 2019).

[66] *Ayurveda Act No. 31 of 1961* (Sri Lanka) s 64 (1).

registered as an Ayurvedic practitioner.[67] The two categories Ayurvedic physicians that can be registered include:

(1) Physicians who possess medical qualifications laid down in the Act or recognised by the Ayurvedic Medical Council; and
(2) Paramparika (traditional) physicians.[68]

The registration system started in 1956 to give an opportunity to physicians who had had no institutional training. The original intention had been to restrict this facility for a limited period but the facility is still available.[69]

The above discussion of the administration of traditional health care has summarised the vision and objectives of the Ministry of Indigenous Medicine and the process of its administration. In the discussion it is apparent that the Ministry's priority has been in promoting Ayurveda and introducing a similar framework to that used in the administration of Western medicine in Sri Lanka. This approach, however, raises a number of questions and concerns. For example: what does the Ministry refer to as 'traditional' medical practice? In abstract the term 'traditional' suggests the know-how, skills, innovations, practices, teachings and learnings on healing of indigenous peoples and local communities of Sri Lanka that are dynamic and evolving, and that are intergenerational and which may subsist in codified, oral or other forms.[70] It appears, however, that the Ministry of Indigenous Medicine's reference to traditional healing is limited to formal healing practices such as Ayurveda, Siddha, Unani, Homeopathy and Acupuncture adopted in Sri Lanka from other foreign countries. This chapter argues that the government focus has mainly been on Ayurveda practice resulting in the colonisation of traditional healing practices by Ayurveda. This phenomenon is referred to as 'Ayurvedisation of traditional healing.'[71]This limited approach to traditional healing has threatened the existence of the traditional knowledge of healing of Sri Lanka, such as the inter-generational healing systems that are the focus of Chapters 6.

---

[67] *Ayurveda Act No. 31 of 1961* (Sri Lanka) s 64 (2).

[68] Wanninayaka (1982), p 16 and Overview, Department of Ayurveda http://www.ayurveda.gov.lk/Overview.html (last retrieved 20 February 2019)

[69] Overview, Department of Ayurveda http://www.ayurveda.gov.lk/Overview.html (last retrieved 20 February 2019)

[70] Based on IGC definition on traditional knowledge. See: WIPO/GRTKF/IC/27/4, Annex, p10 (January 23, 2014).

[71] Chapter 6, part 2.3 discusses inter-generational healers' perspective on Ayurvedisation of traditional healing.

Furthermore, and with reference to the second objective of the Ministry (to create a healthy nation) the focus is on curative aspects of health care, at the expense of preventative health. It is also necessary to introduce a healthy lifestyle and value system to the society. Currently the Ministry's focus is mostly the curative aspect of healing. The Ministry is also not sufficiently supporting the enhancement of the Sri Lankan heritage – the indigenous healing system as much as they are supporting the adopted knowledge systems as Ayurveda, Siddha and Unani.

Part 3: Education

This part of the chapter argues that the Government's role in regulating, standardising and formalising education has had a negative impact on protecting culture and practices of healing systems. In doing so, this part presents government efforts in promoting education in traditional healing and the impact of systematic regulation and constant efforts in standardisation of knowledge towards the culture and practices of healing systems. Government efforts discussed in this part include: Ayurveda Education and Hospital Board, National Institute of Traditional Medicine, Institute of Indigenous Medicine, University of Colombo, Gampaha Wickramarachchi Ayurveda Institute, and the Diploma in Ayurveda programme. In addition to the administration of the traditional health care system, the Ministry of Indigenous Medicine of the Sri Lankan Government plays a role in the education of traditional healing. Importantly, education in healing practices determines how the knowledge of healing is passed on to the next generation, and how the culture and practices related to healing should evolve and develop. As we will see the Government has focused its attention on some health practices, and traditional healing knowledge (such as Ayurveda, Siddha, Unani and Homeopathy) have received Government recognition, support and regulation. This means that these adopted traditional healing methods have been able to establish formal systems of education to pass down the knowledge, skills and practices.

3.1 Ayurveda Education and Hospital Board

The Ayurveda Education and Hospital Board was established according to section 22 of the *Ayurveda (revised) Act no 31 of 1961*. The focus of this Board, as the name suggests, is on supporting Ayurveda practice. It consists of 16 members made up of:

- the Commissioner;[72]
- the Principal of the College of Ayurveda Medicine;
- the Medical Superintendent of the Central Hospital of Ayurveda;
- Officer of the Department of Education appointed by the Minister on the recommendation of the Minister of Education;
- one member appointed by the Minister from the teachers of the College of Ayurvedic Medicine;
- two members elected by the teachers of the College of Ayurvedic Medicine from themselves;
- one member appointed by the Minister from the teachers of approved Ayurvedic teaching institutions;
- two members elected by the holders of diplomas granted or recognised by the Board of Indigenous Medicine, or by the Ayurvedic College and Hospital Board;
- not more than four members appointed by the Minister from the registered ayurvedic practitioners of whom not more than two shall be so appointed from a panel of six nominated by the AllCeylon Ayurvedic Practitioners Congress; and
- two members appointed by the Minister from persons who are not registered Ayurvedic practitioners.[73]

The roles of the Board include assessing the course curriculum of Ayurveda institutes, assessing the research conducted in the field of Ayurveda, conducting exams, issuing certificates for educational recognition, issuing scholarship and aid for students, and providing recommendations to the minister on administrating the Ayurveda hospitals and dispensaries.

The objectives of the Ayurveda Education and Hospital Board includes: 'to mobilise indigenous doctors with educational recognition in order to protect and enhance the traditional healing system, to encourage children of traditional healers to follow the path of traditional healing; to develop standards and maintain quality of Ayurveda hospitals and central dispensaries in satisfactory level and to develop guidelines and laws related to Ayurveda education and hospitals.'[74]

---

[72] The Ayurveda Commissioner is the Chair. *Ayurveda (revised) Act no 31 of 1961* (Sri Lanka) s 26.
[73] *Ayurveda (revised) Act no 31 of 1961*(Sri Lanka) s 22.
[74] Department of Ayurveda (2013), p 40.

3.2 National Institute of Traditional Medicine

In addition to the formal education on traditional healing in universities, the National Institute of Traditional Medicine (NITM) was established as an educational and training institute under the Department of Ayurveda, recognising the need for regular training, educating and updating knowledge of the traditional healing practitioners as part of the process of Government recognition, support and regulation. The main objectives of the NITM include:

- the development of traditional medicine and human resources for improvement of the health of the community through the systematic establishment of traditional health-care systems; and
- promotion of health care through the development of human resources which need to upgrade the systems of Indigenous medicine in the National Health Conservation structure. [75]

The NITM was established in Boralla Ayurveda hospital in 1984, with the funding of the United Nations Development Programme and the World Health Organisation.[76] The institution was shifted to its current location in the Navinna Ayurveda complex on 3 October 1996, after the ceremonial opening by the late Prime Minister, Sirimavo Bandaranayake.[77]

The NITM plays a vital role in regulating traditional medicine in Sri Lanka but its intervention often threatens the survival and livelihood of the inter-generational healers. The NITM does this through a range of activities including training programs for traditional physicians, medical officers, other staff and communities. Yet the administration of the NITM believes the training provided by the institute helps preserve inter-generational healing systems. They are dedicated to finding ways in which they can preserve and hand down this valuable knowledge to the younger generation and share the secret traditional knowledge of inter-generational healers with all other traditional doctors and healers. For this purpose, the

---

[75] National Institute of Traditional Medicine, Ministry of Indigenous Medicine http://www.indigenousmedimini.gov.lk/NITM.html (last retrieved 20 February 2019)

[76] National Institute of Traditional Medicine, Ministry of Indigenous Medicine http://www.indigenousmedimini.gov.lk/NITM.html (last retrieved 20 February 2019)

[77] National Institute of Traditional Medicine, Ministry of Indigenous Medicine http://www.indigenousmedimini.gov.lk/NITM.html (last retrieved 20 February 2019)

NITM coordinates and provides a platform for the inter-generational healers to host seminars and training programs to share their knowledge with other traditional doctors and healers.[78] Inter-generational healers are paid a very nominal honorarium for convening these programmes. The programmes are organised with the objective of sharing inter-generational healers' knowledge with other traditional healers and to document the informal knowledge system. The NITM believes that providing a platform for the inter-generational healers to share their knowledge and to document traditional knowledge systems in a systematic way safeguards the knowledge for future generations. The NITM's attempts to share inter-generational healers' knowledge openly with other traditional healing professionals questions the security and rights of the inter-generational healer's secret knowledge that was passed down from generation to generation and is their form of livelihood.[79]

Another program that threatens the security of the inter-generational healers is the placements for degree students in Ayurveda with traditional healers for residential internship of three months. The internships enable the students to get exposed to and develop practical knowledge, skills and attitudes in practising traditional healing. Yet the inter-generational healers are expected to accommodate the interns voluntarily. What has to be emphasised is that this knowledge has been their heritage and livelihood. Due to changes in the social systems, most of these inter-generational healers are from poor economic backgrounds. Requesting the inter-generational healers to share their knowledge for a minimal fee or as an honorary activity makes them very vulnerable. Chapter 6 on 'Inter-generational Healing and Loss of Culture' discuss characteristics of inter-generational healing, challenges faced by the healer and the implications of government intervention on inter-generational healing in detail.

The NITM also plays a gate-keeper role. More specifically the NITM updates the knowledge of the registered traditional medical doctors with Ayurveda, Siddha and Unani degrees practicing island wide.[80] The

---

[78] Based on National Institute of Traditional Medicine web page http://www.indigenousmedimini.gov.lk/NITM.html (last retrieved 20 February 2019)

[79] Interviews with the following inter-generational healers portray the secret knowledge of inter-generational healing is their form of livelihood Sunil Shantha (#25), R. P. Udayapala (#28), Rathnawathie (#29), W. A. Kusuma Wijesekera (#32), H. D. Karunawathie (#53), R. V. Piyadasa (#57), R. M. D. J. Gunasekera (#58), K. O. Rajarathna (#101), R. M. Premachandra (#113).

[80] Based on National Institute of Traditional Medicine web page

NITM also hosts regular training programs for the registered traditional medical doctors to update their knowledge.[81] An interesting fact about gate keeping role of the NITM is its focus is on Ayurveda and on the Ayurvedaisation of all traditional healers. For this purpose, they host training programs to induct inter-generational healers (who they call traditional healers) to Ayurveda. This attempt to assimilate the traditional healers' knowledge with the concept and theories of Ayurveda threatens diverse forms of traditional knowledge. Once the traditional healers are inducted to new knowledge of Ayurveda theories and principles, as the mainstream knowledge accepted nationally, they find it difficult to go back to the knowledge and healing systems they were practicing earlier.[82] Additionally, after a short-term training program, traditional healers may not possess sufficient knowledge to practice Ayurveda. The NITM's programme of education and training traditional healers in Ayurveda can be seen as adding to the isolation, confusion and loss of traditional cultural heritage non-Ayurveda inter-generational healers possess. A healer expresses his views in this regard:

> I come from an inter-generational healing background but as being an inter-generational healer alone is not recognised, I studied a Diploma in Ayurveda and got myself registered as a traditional healer. After being qualified as a traditional healer with an Ayurveda background, I find myself not using the inter-generational healing knowledge that often as I feel Ayurveda treatment is more accepted by the society. I fear our inter-generational knowledge in healing sarvanga (all bodily disorders) will die a natural death.[83]

Not all forms of indigenous medicine can be understood or interpreted through the lens of Ayurveda. In order to protect indigenous healing systems, it is important to understand and safeguard the theories and methods each healing system has been based on.

To register as a 'traditional healer' it is compulsory for an inter-generational healer to follow the three-day Ayurveda induction programme introduced by the NITM. Furthermore, the knowledge of traditional

http://www.indigenousmedimini.gov.lk/NITM.html (last retrieved 20 February 2019)

[81] Based on National Institute of Traditional Medicine web page http://www.indigenousmedimini.gov.lk/NITM.html (last retrieved 20 February 2019)

[82] See Chapter 6, 2.4.

[83] R. M. C. D. S. B Rajapakse (# 19)

healers[84] is screened by a panel of judges, who are mostly Ayurveda qualified doctors and have studied Ayurveda systematically. Traditional healers are required to undertake a written and an oral exam. Marks are given according to the knowledge they possess on their traditional healing system, ability to identify medicinal plants used to treat their specialty, and knowledge about the local medical techniques in general. This process raises some significant concerns. Foremost is whether the expertise and knowledge of the examinees should be measured by a person who may not be specialised in the same field of traditional healing. An inter-generational healer explains his experience with the process of registration as follows:

> I tried to sit for the traditional healer registration exam twice but failed. The knowledge they are testing is not the knowledge I have received from my inter-generational healing practice. My practice in *Kadum Bidum* (orthopedics) is quite popular not only among the villagers but outsiders too and it is very effective, but due to not having the registration as a traditional healer I cannot have a seal or produce official prescriptions/ sick letters.[85]

In this section I have argued, that although the NITM plays a vital role in regulating traditional medicine in Sri Lanka, its intervention often threatens the survival and livelihood of the inter-generational healers. This section has portrayed NITM's role of regulating traditional medicine through training programs for traditional physicians, medical officers, other staff and communities and by playing a gate-keeper role. Concerns about the training and gate keeping offered by the NITM are the focus on Ayurveda and Ayurvedisation of all traditional healers and the expectation of inter-generational healers to share their secret-knowledge, which is the means of their livelihood with other traditional healers.

3.3 Institute of Indigenous Medicine, University of Colombo

The Institute of Indigenous Medicine (IIM) is the first university affiliated institute for traditional medicine in Sri Lanka that provides a formal university education in Ayurveda and Unani. In the early 20th century, a government regulated system of traditional medicine was introduced to the British colony of Ceylon due to continued public demand.[86] The Government had a system of traditional medicine in place focusing mostly

---

[84] NITM reference of 'traditional healers' is to persons I have referred to as 'inter-generational healers'

[85] S. M. K. Nimal Karunaratne (# 93).

[86] See Chapter 5, part I.

on Ayurveda and to a lesser extent Siddha and Unani healing systems, but lacked a college to provide traditional medical education. Recognising the importance of formal traditional medical education, individuals interested in promoting traditional medicine[87] came up with a proposal to start a college that provided indigenous medical education. Interestingly, although the proposal refered to 'indigenous' medical education, it did not refer to the inter-generational or the cosmic healing systems that are indigenous to Sri Lanka, but instead to the more systematic healing systems such as Ayurveda and Unani systems that were adopted from other countries. As the Director of Institute of Indigenous Medicine, Sunimal Senaratne stated:

> our institute is a vocational training institute and our vision is to be the world's best Ayurveda Institute producing skilled Ayurvedic medical professional, teachers and researchers, and to promote the traditional knowledge in health and wellbeing.[88]

The process of establishing the IIM at the university level was influenced by three associations established in order to preserve the systems of traditional cures. These were: Sinhalese Medical Association in 1891, Sri Lanka Vaidya Maha Mandalaya in 1901 and the Sri Lanka Samaja Prathisanskarana Sangamaya in 1915.[89] In 1927, for the first time, the Committee on Indigenous Systems of Medicine proposed that a college be established,[90] and according to that proposal *Swadeshiya Vaidya Vidyalaya* (Indigenous Medical College) was established on 10th June 1929.[91]

Some important milestones that effected the Institute of Indigenous Medicine were the enactment of the *Indigenous Medical Ordinance no 17 of 1941* by the then Minister of Health, to uplift the education of indigenous medicine with the quality of teaching of the national standards; and the enactment of the *Ayurveda Act no. 31 of 1961*, repealing the *Ayurveda Act no. 71 of 1941*. According to the *Ayurveda Act no 31 of 1961*, the Institute was renamed as the College of Indigenous Medicine and was administered under the management of the college and hospital board. This change was adopted to uphold the quality of Ayurveda healthcare education. In 1963, Diploma in Indigenous Medicine and Surgery (DIMS) was changed to Diploma in Ayurveda Medicine and Surgery (DAMS) according to the new

---

[87] Including eminent professional such as Sir S. W. R. D. Bandaranayeke, F.R Senanayake, Ananda. Coomaraswamy, K. Balasingham and D. Wijesekara.
[88] Sunimal Senaratne (# 12).
[89] Sunimal Senaratna (# 12).
[90] Commission of Indigenous System of Medicine. Report of Indigenous System of Medicine. *Sessional Paper No. 1 of 1927.*
[91] History, IIM - http://iim.cmb.ac.lk/history (last retrieved 20 February 2019).

Ayurveda Act.[92] The College of Ayurveda that was first started in the island was subsequently upgraded and affiliated to the University of Colombo as the Institute of Indigenous Medicine in the year 1977 under the *University Act No. 1 of 1972*. In 1979 the *Indigenous Institute of Medicine Ordinance* was made under the *University Act No. 16 of 1978*, transferring the Siddha section to the University of Jaffna, Ayurveda and Unani remained in Colombo. Shifting the Siddha section to Jaffna limited the access for Siddha education mostly to the Tamil community in the Northern Province of Sri Lanka.

Presently the IIM is one of the premier higher educational institutes in Sri Lanka providing instruction in two streams for undergraduate and postgraduate students, namely, Ayurveda and Unani.[93] When selecting streams of education, it is apparent that the majority of the Sinhala students select Ayurveda and a majority of the Muslim students select Unani.[94]

The Management Committee of the IIM was established according to the section 10 (1) of the *Institute of Indigenous Medicine Act No 7 of 1979*. Education Committees established include Ayurveda Section Committee, Unani Section Committee, Research and Higher Degree Committee.

There are a range of degree programs offered by the Institute. All of these focus on Ayurveda and Unani. All other traditional healing practices are not taught and are, therefore, overlooked. First degrees and postgraduate qualifications in indigenous medicine are offered at the institute. The two degree programs currently available at are the Bachelor of Ayurveda Medicine and Surgery (BAMS) and Bachelor of Unani Medicine and Surgery (BUMS). A five-year program with one year internship training where there is theoretical and practical training (clinical) in the ward is included in this course. Students are also sent to traditional healers in their internship year according to their choice of healing systems (if they choose a traditional option). For example, one of the IIM students was sent to a monk practicing a popular cure, namely 'Pranajeeva Oushada' in Kiribathgoda. After the death of the monk, the student continued the healing tradition which is now internationally known.[95]

In addition to the Bachelor's degree programs, there are other courses offered by the Institute. A 2 year diploma course on Ayurveda Pharmacology offered by IIM gives an intensive training to government and private pharmacists where they are trained to identify native medicines

---

[92] History, IIM http://iim.cmb.ac.lk/history (last retrieved 20 February 2019).
[93] Based on IIM home page http://iim.cmb.ac.lk (last retrieved 20 February 2019).
[94] Dr. M. W. S. J. Kumari (# 11).
[95] Sunimal Senratne (# 12).

and learn about their value and usage.[96] One-year post graduate diploma courses in Ayurveda and Unani are offered by IIM increase the theoretical and practical knowledge of the medical professionals in the fields of Ayurveda and Unani.[97] As this post graduate diploma course in Ayurveda is a full time course, medical professionals working in the provincial councils and Ayurveda department are offered paid leave. This post graduate diploma has been made a compulsory qualification in order to obtain a promotion.[98] An Ayurveda doctorate MD (AYU) post-graduate program has also been offered at IIM since 2012, offering opportunities for Ayurveda qualified doctors to pursue higher academic qualifications.[99]

Although academic research is promoted by the institute and government funding is available for Ayurveda research through the Nawinna Ayurveda Research Institute, the research output of the academic staff seems limited. Details on research, new findings and publications of IIM staff in 2012 are provided in Figure 4.1:[100]

Subject	Expressed	Presented
No. of Experiments	25	14
New findings	01	-
No. of Journals	01	-
No. of books	-	-
No. of letters	02	-
Other	-	-
Total	29	14

Figure 4.1- Research, New Findings and Publications of IIM

Supporting the government vision of making Sri Lanka the international focal point in higher education by 2020, the IIM has implemented many plans. The plans include revising the education syllabi, developing infrastructure facilities, increasing the employability of the graduates by developing their job related skills, and networking with the

96 Sunimal Senratne (# 12).
97 IIM, PG Dip in Ayurveda/Unani IIM, PG Dip in Ayurveda/Unani http://iim.cmb.ac.lk/academic/postgraduate-studies (last retrieved 20 February 2019)
98 Sunimal Senratne (# 12).
99 IIM, Postgraduate Degree: Docotr of Medicine in Ayurveda http://iim.cmb.ac.lk/academic/postgraduate-studies/doctor-of-medicine-in-ayurveda-m-d-ayu (last retrieved 20 February 2019)
100 IIM Annual Report (2012), p 11.

government and the private sector in carrying forward the work of the IIM.[101] The new changes have also resulted in changing the medium of instruction from Sinhala (Ayurveda) and Tamil (Unani) to English. Currently the courses are conducted bilingually, but soon they will be converted to English.[102] Language is intimately tied with the cultural and traditional aspects of these medical practices.[103] It could be feared that changing the medium of instruction to English would lead to a biomedicalisation of traditional medical practices and alienating them from their roots. According to the interview with Dr. M. W. S. G. Kumari:

> it is necessary for our traditional healing practices to change with the modern trends and to internationalise. Using Sinhala or Tamil as the medium of expression limits the opportunities of the Ayurveda and Unani graduates to compete at the global level.[104]

According to Dr Kumari, knowledge is universal, and as an objective science regardless of the medium of expression, Ayurveda and Unani should be taught and applied.[105] Another great challenge faced at this transitional period is that most of the lecturers who teach Unani and Ayurveda are not very competent in English. There are also a very limited number of text books published in English.

Another concern with the IIM is that it only promotes Ayurveda and Unani systems of education, and it is, therefore, not contributing towards systematically imparting knowledge of indigenous medicine. Perhaps more importantly is that the IIM discourages other practices such as inter-generational healing and cosmic healing as they are not formal or structured knowledge systems and actively works against the development of the traditional cultural healing heritage of Sri Lanka.

3.4 Gampaha Wickramarachchi Ayurveda Institute

The Gampaha Wickramarachchi Ayurveda Institute is affiliated to the University of Kelaniya,[106] and is one of the two university institutes of Ayurveda education in Sri Lanka. The Institute has its origin in the well-known Gampaha Sidayurveda Vidyalaya founded by Ayurveda Cakrawarti Pandit G. P. Wickramarachchi in 1928, as a centre of learning Siddayurveda

---

[101] IIM Annual Report (2012).
[102] Sunimal Senaratna (# 12).
[103] Dr. E. A. S. C.S. Edirisuriya (#7); Dr. M. Chithra Nalini (#8).
[104] Dr. M. W. S. G. Kumari (# 11).
[105] Dr. M. W. S. G. Kumari (# 11).
[106] It is located in Kandy Road, Yakkala, Gampaha District, Western Province.

tradition of medicine.[107] It was established in Pandit G. P. Wickramarachchi's personal land in Yakkala. The Gampaha Sidayurveda Vidyalaya provided knowledge and competence in herbal drug preparation and *cikitsa* to traditional physicians.[108] The drug manufacturing unit, hospital and herbal garden were available to the institute at its inception. Most of the students who studied at the institution at the beginning were students from traditional healing families. They were keen to learn and keep the traditions alive. The uniforms worn by the students (white osari for ladies and white sarong and shirt for men) and the traditional teaching systems of memorising sloka, utmost respect towards the teachers, studying the ola leaves and learning in the mother tongue made it possible to keep the traditions alive.[109]

The institute was established with the vision of becoming 'a centre of excellence in education, research and outreach in Ayurvedic medicine and allied sciences.'[110] It strives to 'produce young men and women who possess knowledge and skills in Ayurvedic medicine and allied sciences and with enthusiasm, initiative, and wisdom to engage in health care provision to the society nationally and globally and to engage in basic and applied research and dissemination of research information with dual objectives of advancing core knowledge in Ayurvedic medical sciences and serving research and development needs of the society.'[111]

Declaring the Vidyalaya a state recognised institute in 1951, made the diploma holders of the Vidyalaya eligible to take up appointments in state sector Ayurveda hospitals.[112] The Vidyalaya was incorporated as

---

[107] Gampaha Wickramarachchi Ayurveda Institute http://www.kln.ac.lk/institutes/wickramarachchi/ (last retrieved 20 February 2019).

[108] Gampaha Wickramarachchi Ayurveda Institute http://www.kln.ac.lk/institutes/wickramarachchi/ (last retrieved 20 February 2019).

[109] Interviews with Dr. E. A. S. C.S. Edirisuriya, Dr. M. Chithra Nalini, Residential Medical Officers, Gampaha Wickremarachchi Ayurveda Institute (5 August 2013) and Dr. Saranadasa Devaraja, Siddhauveda Medical Institute, Siri Vajiraghanodaya Pirivena, (5 August 2013). The three doctors have been students in the Wickramarachi Ayurveda Institute before it was recognised as part of the State University system.

[110] Vision of the Institute – http://www.kln.ac.lk/institutes/wickramarachchi/index.php/department/vision-a-mission.html (last retrieved 20 February 2019).

[111] Mission of the Institute – www.kln.ac.lk/institutes/wickramarachchi/index.php/department/vision-a-mission.html (last retrieved 20 February 2019)

[112] Gampaha Wickramarachchi Ayurveda Institute http://www.kln.ac.lk/institutes/wickramarachchi/ (last retrieved 20 February 2019).

Gampaha Wickramarachchi Ayurveda Institute in 1982 under the Ministry of Indigenous Medicine by the *Parliamentary Act No 30, in 1982.*[113]

The human resources of the Institute comprise its 30 academic staff, 104 non-academic staff and 371 students.[114] The institution offers the Bachelor of Ayurveda Medicine and Surgery (BAMS) degree, a six year course including one year internship training in state hospitals.[115] The degree programme is conducted by five departments of study namely the Department of Ayurveda, Department of *Dravyaguna*, Department of *Shalya Shalaky*, Department of *Kaumarabhrity stree Roga* and the Department of *Cikitsa.*[116] Further to the degree programme, the institute offers Postgraduate Diplomas in Hospital Management that aims at upgrading the administrative capabilities of Ayurveda graduates.[117]

The Courses offered from the Institutein addition to the Bachelors degree programme is presented in Figure 4.2.[118]

In order to facilitate undergraduate and postgraduate educational programmes, Graduate Studies division, the Research and Publication Division, the Computer Centre and an Independent laboratory are in function. The staff of these divisions is appointed by the Board of management under the recommendation of the board of studies.[119]

The research contribution of the Institution still seems low. Statistics for 2011, are shown in figure 4.3:[120]

[113] The general objectives of the corporation include, '(a) to conduct and administer the Vidyalaya as a broad national institution oriented to impart instructions in the indigenous, Sidha and Ayurvedic systems of medicine; (b) to establish an Ayurvedic hospital to train medical students and provide free medical aid to patients; (c) to conduct examinations for the purpose of ascertaining the persons who have acquired proficiency in the field of Ayurveda; and (d) to construct, equip and maintain necessary buildings for the use of the Vidyalaya.' *Parliamentary Act No 30, 1982.*

[114] Gampaha Wickramarachchi Ayurveda Institute Annual Report (2011) p 4.

[115] Gampaha Wickramarachchi Ayurveda Institute Annual Report (2011) p 4.

[116] Gampaha Wickramarachchi Ayurveda Institute Annual Report (2011) p 4.

[117] Gampaha Wickramarachchi Ayurveda Institute Annual Report (2011), p 8.

[118] Gampaha Wickramarachchi Ayurveda Institute Annual Report (2011), p 8.

[119] History, Gampaha Wickramarachchi Ayurveda Institute http://www.kln.ac.lk/institutes/wickramarachchi/index.php/department/history.html (last retrieved 20 February 2019).

[120] Gampaha Wickramarachchi Ayurveda Institute Annual Report (2011), p 7.

Department	Course	Medium	Certificate	Diploma	Post-graduate	Masters
Shalya Shalakya	Kshara Sutra*	Sinhala	✓	-	-	-
Stree Roga and Kaumarabruthya	Ayurvedic Beauty Culture	Sinhala	✓	-	-	-
Dravyaguna Vignana	Ayurveda Pharmacy*	Sinhala	-	✓	-	-
Graduate Studies Division	Yoga and Relaxation Technique*	Sinhala	✓	-	-	-
	Management and Administration of Ayurveda Institutions*	English	-	-	✓	-
	Management and Administration of Ayurveda Institutions	English	-	-	-	✓
Total			03	01	01	01

*Ongoing courses.

Figure 4.2 - The Courses offered from the Gampaha Wickramarachchi Ayurveda Institute in addition to the Bachelors degree programme

Subject	Published	Commercialised	Presented
Number of Researches	Shalya Shalakya 04	01	01
	Dravyaguna Vignana	-	02
Innovations	-	-	-
Number of Magazines	-	-	-
Number of Books	-	-	-
Number of Articles	Dravyaguna Vignana Stree Roga 05	-	02
Other	-	-	-
Total		01	05

Figure 4.3 - The Research Contribution of Gampaha Wickramarachchi Ayurveda Institute

The government attempts to formalise and regulate the Institute has both positive and negative impacts. Some of the positive aspects of the Institute have been the recognition of the degree, and formal acknowledgement and promotion of the knowledge system. The negative impacts include the narrow focus on traditional healing practices, limiting access to the knowledge of healing, and losing the cultural heritage aspect of healing.

Since the Gampaha Wickramarachchi Ayurveda Institute was converted to a university institution, admission for the degree has been granted only for G. C. E. Advanced level Science students based on their Advanced level results (the Z score).[121] Almost all the students selected for the Institute were students who aspired to become Western medical doctors graduating from the Medical Faculty, but as a result of not being able to obtain the required marks they have selected the next best option of being an Ayurvedic doctor.[122] As a consequence, the opportunities for individuals coming from traditional healing backgrounds, or who are interested in serving as traditional healers, are limited.[123] Additionally, those students who are interested in studying at the institute are often excluded because of the Z-score entry requirement. The initial identity of a traditional doctor and the traditional Sri Lankan cultural identity developed through the dress, value systems and form of teaching and studying is no longer present.[124] The Ayurveda Institute has become one more institution offering academic qualification.

Another problem in the way in which the Ayurveda Institute is administered is language. In addition to the above mentioned changes, introducing Ayurveda teaching in English has resulted in the loss of the authentic nature of Ayurveda.[125] Of course these new initiatives have managed to universalise Ayurveda as another subject, but translations can never match the originals.[126] Teachers who had acquired Ayurveda knowledge in Sinhala have had to re-learn how to teach the subject in English. When learning a healing subject in a new language it is difficult to share the cultural connotations attached to that subject.

[121] Dr. E.A.S.C.S. Edirisuriya (# 7), Dr. M. Chithra Nalini (# 8).
[122] Dr. E.A.S.C.S. Edirisuriya (# 7), Dr. M. Chithra Nalini (# 8).
[123] Dr. Saranadasa Devaraja (# 9).
[124] Interview with A. D. H. Sudesh (# 50).
[125] Dr. E.A.S.C.S. Edirisuriya (# 7), Dr. M. Chithra Nalini (# 8).
[126] Dr. Sanjay Garg (# 45) in an informal conversation refers to translation as looking outside a window, where you can see everything but cannot feel and sense.

3.5 Diploma in Ayurveda

Another way that Ayurveda is prioritised by the Government is by supporting various institutions to prepare students to sit for the Diploma of Ayurveda examination. The Samastha Lanka Paramparika Ayurveda Vaidya Vidyalaya of Keraminiya located in Mawanella, and Pirivena Ayurveda medical institutes located all over the country can be identified as institutes preparing students for the government recognised Diploma in Ayurveda.

3.5.1 Samastha Lanka Paramparika Ayurveda Vaidya Vidyalaya of Keraminiya

The Palaka Sabawa or the Governing body of the institution was incorporated using the *Palaka Sabhawa of Samastha Lanka Paramparika Ayurveda Vaidya Vidyalaya of Keraminiya Mawanella (Incorporation) Act 1 of 1986.*[127] The corporation is constituted from the Act with the objectives of:

- conducting, maintaining and administering the Vidyalaya as a national institution providing instructions in the traditional Ayurveda system of medicine;
- establishing an Ayurveda hospital to train medical students and provide free treatment to patients;
- conducting with the approval of the Commissioner of Ayurveda, examinations for the purpose of ascertaining persons who have acquired proficiency in the traditional ayurveda system of medicine; and
- constructing, equipping and maintaining building that are necessary for the Vidyalaya.[128]

Due to less government interventions in the standardisation of the Keraminiya Institute, it has been able to maintain the cultural aspect of healing, which is also apparent from the practitioners of Keraminiya healing.[129] But less Government interventions has also meant less funding for the institute, posing a risk to the survival of its educational facilities.

---

[127] *Palaka Sabhawa of Samastha Lanka Paramparika Ayurveda Vaidya Vidyalaya of Keraminiya Mawanella (Incorporation) Act 1 of 1986.*

[128] *Palaka Sabhawa of Samastha Lanka Paramparika Ayurveda Vaidya Vidyalaya of Keraminiya Mawanella (Incorporation) Act 1 of 1986, s 3.*

[129] Interview and participant observation, Mr. R. M. P. Rathnayake (# 13).

3.5.2 Pirivena Ayurveda Medical Institutes

Centres for teaching traditional healing in pre-colonial Sri Lanka were Pirivena Ayurveda medical institutes and the homes of the traditional healers.[130] With the recent developments, Pirivena Ayurveda institutes have focused on training students to sit for the Diploma in Ayurveda (DA) examination organised by the Ministry of Indigenous Medicine.[131] The courses are usually advertised through the newspapers and students are admitted after a screening process, which includes calling for applications and interviews.[132] In earlier days, students were free to join the Pirivena Ayurveda institute, regardless of their qualifications. Most students who joined the Piriveda Medical institutes used to be children of traditional healers, with a background in Ayurvedic knowledge, belonging to the ancestral medical families.[133] With recent efforts for standardisation of the DA course, the minimum qualification to join the programme has become three passes in the Bio-Science stream in the G. C. E. Advanced level examination. Additionally, they must pass English and Mathematics subjects in the G.C.E Ordinary level examination.[134] The entry requirement limits many interested students in following the programme. The DA courses offered by Pirivena Ayurveda institutes are usually three years.[135] The teachings of the Pirivena Ayurveda institutes which used to focus mostly on traditional healing methods, now focuses mainly on Ayurvedic medicine. Most often these institutes follow old methods of teaching, such as reading the ola leaves and memorising. Students in most Pirivena Ayurveda institutes are also given practical training with private Ayurveda medical practitioners and indigenous medical professionals. Most students who join the DA programme are from low socio-economic families. Considering the economic constraints of the students, fees charged are very nominal. As Ven. Piyakeerthi says, 'we charge the students 300 rupees (LKR) for a month from a student.'[136] The number of students who undertake a DA in Ayurveda in Pirivena institutes has dropped remarkably as these students do not have any form of secure employment after completing their studies. The DA in Ayurveda students find it difficult to follow the traditional healing systems they have learnt from their families

[130] Ven. Kubulgama Piyakeerthi (# 55), and Dr. Saranadasa Devaraja (# 9).
[131] Ven. Kubulgama Piyakeerthi (# 55).
[132] Ven. Kubulgama Piyakeerthi (# 55), and Dr. Saranadasa Devaraja (# 9).
[133] Dr. Saranadasa Devaraja (# 9).
[134] Dr. Saranadasa Devaraja (# 9).
[135] Ven. Kubulgama Piyakeerthi (# 55), and Dr. Saranadasa Devaraja (# 9).
[136] Ven. Kubulgama Piyakeerthi (# 55).

due to the new knowledge they have been inducted into in Ayurveda. They become disoriented between the traditional healing and Ayurveda treatment systems.

Government patronage for Pirivena Ayurveda institutes is not sufficient. Due to the lack of funding, most Pirivena Ayurveda institutes find it difficult to pay fees for their teachers, maintain the buildings and provide materials for students.[137] As there is no strong state support system to fund the institutions adequately and to monitor the standards, the Ayurveda Pirivena institutions are struggling for survival.

3.5.3 Siddharyrveda Medical Institute, Siri Vajira, Ghanodaya Pirivena

Siddharyuveda Medical Institute in Siri Vajira Ghanadoya Pirivena is an attempt by few healers to protect the cultural heritage of traditional healing systems.[138] The Institute was established in 1997, by the alumni group of Siddhayurveda medical traditions introduced by Chakrawarti Pandit G. P. Wickramarachchi in 1928.[139] The institution strives to preserve the Siddhayurveda in a traditional context after Gampaha Siddhayurvedda Vidyalaya was incorporated as part of the University of Kelaniya, renamed as Gampaha Wickramarachchi Ayurveda Institute and traditional values and practices were replaced.[140]

There are 15 staff at the Institute.[141] All the staff members are graduates of the Gampaha Siddhayurveda Institute and all the staff members are dedicated to the ideology that traditional healing should be taught in a traditional context and the healers role is not only to learn a knowledge system but also acquire the cultural heritage of traditional healing, into which the staff members were inducted at the Gampaha Siddhayurveda Institute.[142] Figure 4.4 portrays a class in progress in the Gampaha Siddhayurvedda Vidyalaya where traditional attire is worn by the students. The women wear a white saree and the men wear a white shirt and a sarong.

---

[137] This is evident in Siddhayurveda Medical Institute and Sri Mahinda Pirivena case studies discussed below.
[138] Dr. Saranadasa Devaraja (# 9).
[139] Dr. Saranadasa Devaraja (# 9).
[140] Dr. Saranadasa Devaraja (# 9).
[141] Dr. Saranadasa Devaraja (# 9).
[142] Dr. Saranadasa Devaraja (# 9).

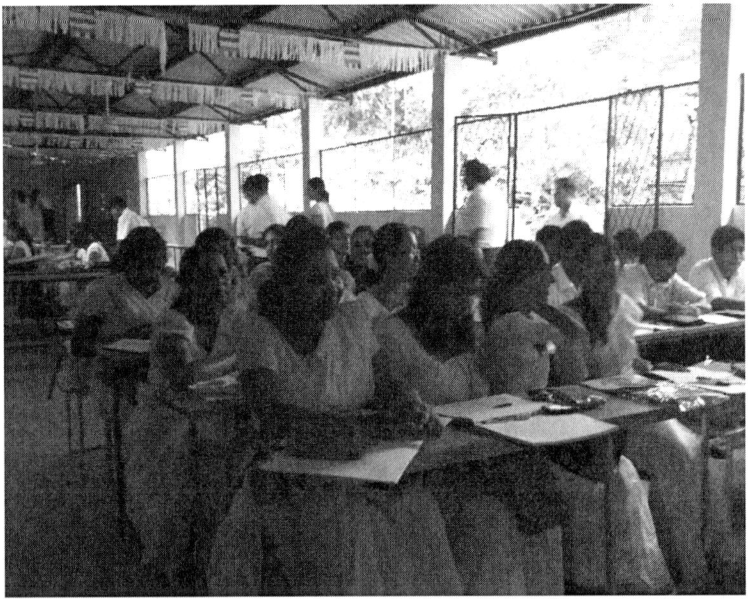

Figure 4.4 – Class in progress in Siddhaurveda Medical Institute

The total number of students currently registered is one hundred.[143] The institute recruits students by advertising in the newspapers and by interviewing them. A nominal course fee is charged for enrolling students. Most of the students in the Institute come from a traditional healing family background. The Institute trains students to sit for the Diploma in Ayurveda (DA) in three years. In addition to the Diploma in Ayurveda syllabus, students are also inducted to Astrology, *Bhoota vidya* and *Yantra mantra*.[144] The full training programme offered by the Institute is for five years. For practical training they are sent to inter-generational healers.[145] The institute faces difficulties in expanding or sustaining due to financing. The income the institute receives as tuition fees is very limited as the fees charged are very nominal. Government patronage for the institute is also very limited and the institute does not have external sponsors.

---

[143] Dr. Saranadasa Devaraja (# 9).
[144] Dr. Saranadasa Devaraja (# 9).
[145] Dr. Saranadasa Devaraja (# 9).

3.5.4 Sri Mahinda Pirivena, Ayurveda Medical Institute

Sri Mahinda Pirivena, Ayurveda Medical Institute, Kurunegala is an example of how the small institutes providing Ayurveda education struggle for survival.

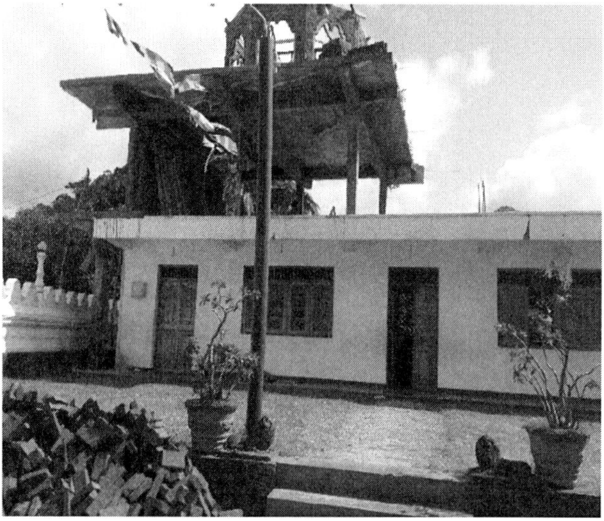

Figure 4.5 – The Sri Mahinda Pirivena building where classes are conducted

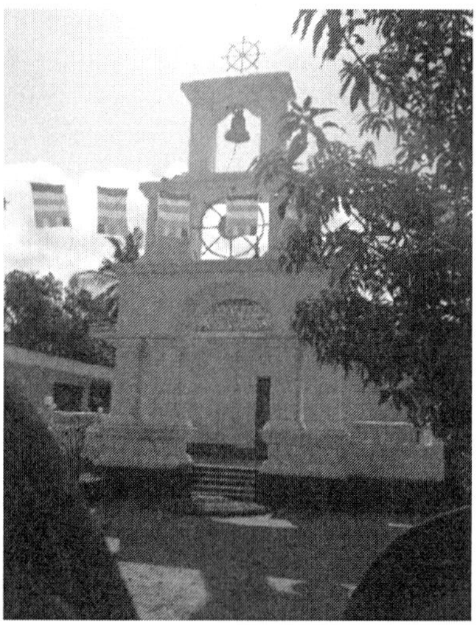

Figure 4.6 – Sri Mahinda Pirivena entrance

The Ayurveda Medical Institute of Sri Mahinda Pirivena (shown in Figure 4.5 and 4.6) was established by the late head monk of the temple who was also an indigenous healer.[146] The Institute trains students for the Diploma in Ayurveda (DA) in three years.[147] At the initial stage, this Pirivena medical institute was thriving. There were over two hundred students. The prosperity of the institute in the beginning had a lot to do with the commitment of the late head monk and the teaching faculty.[148] Now the student population has decreased to twenty. The reasons for the decreased interest according to Ven. Kubulgama Piyakeerthi include not having strong leadership, not having government patronage for the College and not having a secure career for the students who graduate with the Diploma in Ayurveda qualification.[149]

The '*Podi Hamuduruvo*' (young monks) in this Pirivena are interested in learning Ayurveda at the institution but they have to have passed the G.C.E Advanced level examination in the Bio-science stream.[150] Additionally they must pass English and Mathematics subjects in the G.C.E Ordinary level examination as well. Young monks who have an ancestral indigenous medical practice can also learn and pursue their practice from this college with a pass for Mathematics and English at the G.C.E Ordinary level examination.[151] This knowledge is tested because in order to learn Ayurveda students must be able to read and understand books. The Sanskrit language is taught as well because Ayurveda is an Indian healing system and its basics are written in Sanskrit. Most interested monks do not have the entrance educational qualification requirement and as a result are denied access to the training program.[152]

Students are recruited by paper advertisements and interviews.[153] The students are charged 300 rupees (LKR) for a month. [154] Classes are conducted three days of the week, from morning until mid-day. Women are required to wear a saree and the men have to wear white clothes (sarong and shirt or trouser and shirt).

---

[146] Ven. Kubulgama Piyakeerthi (# 55).
[147] Ven. Kubulgama Piyakeerthi (# 55).
[148] Ven. Kubulgama Piyakeerthi (# 55).
[149] Ven. Kubulgama Piyakeerthi (# 55).
[150] Ven. Kubulgama Piyakeerthi (# 55).
[151] Ven. Kubulgama Piyakeerthi (# 55).
[152] Ven. Kubulgama Piyakeerthi (# 55).
[153] Ven. Kubulgama Piyakeerthi (# 55).
[154] Ven. Kubulgama Piyakeerthi (# 55).

Part 4: Hospitals and Curative Services

This part of the chapter argues how hospitals and curative services sponsored by the Government have contributed to adopting Western styled venues for treatments using traditional healing and also how the focus of traditional healing curative services has been mainly on Ayurveda and to a lesser extent on Siddha and Unani. Given that the Sri Lankan Government recognises, supports and regulates education and training in Ayurveda, Siddha and Unani, it is perhaps unsurprising that hospitals and other curative services also focus mainly on Ayurveda and to a lesser extent Siddha and Unani. An added complication is that hospitals are structurally and administratively similar to Western-styled hospitals. In order to present the argument this part outlines some of the issues associated with Sri Lankan hospitals and curative services that treat patients using traditional knowledge and practices. As mentioned earlier (Part 2) curative services are administered under different structures. That is, curative services are centrally administered through the Department of Ayurveda established under the Ministry of Indigenous Medicine and at the provincial level curative services are administered by the Provincial Department of Ayurveda/Indigenous Medicine established under the Provincial Ministerial System in each respective province. The curative services are provided through teaching hospitals, provincial Ayurveda hospitals, district Ayurveda hospitals, rural Ayurveda hospitals, dispensaries and mobile units.

The treatment provided by the Ayurveda hospitals include,

- general medicine (*Sarvanga*);
- Orthopedics (*Kadum Bidum*);
- Ophthalmology (*Ass Vedakama*);
- Rheumatology (*Vatha Roga*);
- treatment for Snake Bites (*Sarpa Vedakama*);
- treatment for Rabies (*Pissu Balu Vedakama*);
- treatment for Mental Disorders (*Umathu Roga*);
- Dermatology (*Charma Roga*), Peadiatrics (*Bala Roga*);
- Gynecology (*Stri Roga*);
- Diarrhoea (Atheesara);
- Piercing and Heating (*Vidum Pilissum*);
- Abscess and Wounds (*Gedi Vana*);
- Treatment for Burning (*Pilissum*);
- Veterinary Science (*Harak Vedakama*);
- Occultism (*Abchichara*) and

- Panchakarma.[155]

Ayurveda and Siddha hospitals and dispensaries play an important role in Sri Lanka by providing free health care services to its people. About 11 percent of the Sri Lankan population seek treatment at government operated Ayurvedic hospitals.[156] Over 3 million people seek treatment at these hospitals annually.[157] Sixty-two Ayurveda hospitals offer residential curative services to nearly 2 500 patients per year,[158] while free of charge services are offered by the 230dispensaries administered by local government authorities.[159] The required drugs are provided by the Sri Lanka Ayurvedic Drug Corporation while the Provincial Departments of Ayurveda coordinates the distribution of drugs.[160]

Ayurveda hospitals have followed the same architectural structure as the other government hospitals that provide allopathic treatment. These structures, however, do not suit the concept and practice of Ayurveda treatment; where the treatment focuses on holistic wellbeing rather than treating a symptom. An ideal Ayurveda hospital should provide a relaxing ambience. Currently the treatment provided in Ayurveda/ Siddha hospitals are not integrative treatments.

One of the ways in which the government regulates hospitals is through the appointment and registration of staff. Professional permanent appointments in Ayurveda hospitals are limited to persons with the minimum degree qualification in Ayurveda, Siddha or Unani. On the one hand, this is an attempt to standardise the quality of treatment given.[161] On the other hand, this measure has limited the opportunity for other inter-generational and cosmic healers who come from diverse backgrounds and hold diverse knowledge systems to practise in hospitals. In some hospitals

---

[155] Palitha Weerakoon (# 3).

[156] Palitha Weerakoon (# 3).

[157] About us, The Ministry of Indigenous Medicine http://www.indigenousmedimini.gov.lk/About_us.html?&session-id=bf4e6b1982ea3f0348ebc843f9083fae (last retrieved 20 February 2019).

[158] About us, Ministry of Indigenous Medicine website http://www.indigenousmedimini.gov.lk/About_us.html (last retrieved 20 February 2019).

[159] About us, Ministry of Indigenous Medicine website http://www.indigenousmedimini.gov.lk/About_us.html (last retrieved 20 February 2019).

[160] About us, The Ministry of Indigenous Medicine http://www.indigenousmedimini.gov.lk/About_us.html?&session-id=bf4e6b1982ea3f0348ebc843f9083fae (last retrieved 20 February 2019).

[161] Palitha Weerakoon (# 3).

inter-generational healers are recruited as 'Special Doctors'. Their appointments are on a contract basis and there is no job security for these doctors. Their remuneration is not on par with the academically qualified Ayurveda, Siddha and Unani doctors. The government faces difficulties in recognising the diverse knowledge systems, particularly the traditional knowledge and the intangible cultural heritage of the country and giving a conducive platform for the inter-generational healers to practice in the hospitals due to difficulties in systematically regulating the knowledge systems.[162]

There are three teaching hospitals, namely Borella Ayurveda Teaching Hospital in Colombo, Kaitady Siddha Teaching Hospital in Jaffna and Gampaha Wickremarachchi Teaching Hospital in Yakkala. The teaching hospitals are administrated directly by the Department of Ayurveda that is by the Central Government of Sri Lanka. The nature of these teaching hospitals is briefly described below.

4.1 Borella Ayurveda Teaching Hospital

Borella Ayurveda Teaching Hospital was established in 1929 and it was moved to the current location in Cotta Road, Borella in 1931.[163] It is the main Ayurveda teaching hospital,[164] the oldest and the largest government Ayurvedic hospital in the country.[165] This hospital has 271 beds.[166] In addition to the regular cadre of Ayurveda physicians, the hospital employs specialists[167] for the treatment of snake bites, boils, fractures and dislocation, burns, mental diseases and children's diseases.[168] The Panchakarma

---

[162] For a detail discussion see Chapter 6, part 2.

[163] Department of Ayurveda introduction to Borella Ayurveda Teaching Hospital www.ayurveda.gov.lk/borella.html (last retrieved 20 February 2019).

[164] Practical training for the students of National Institute of Indigenous Medicine is provided at the Ayurveda Teaching Hospital.

[165] Palitha Weerakoon (# 3).

[166] 247 beds in non-paying wards and 24 beds in paying wards (12 for males and 12 for females). Ayurveda Hospitals, Ministry of Indigenous Medicine http://www.indigenousmedimini.gov.lk/Hospital.html (last retrieved 20 February 2019).

[167] Inter-generational healers are referred to as 'specialists' on the Department of Ayurveda website.

[168] Ayurveda Hospitals, Ministry of Indigenous Medicine http://www.indigenousmedimini.gov.lk/Hospital.html (last retrieved 20 February 2019).

treatment[169] offered at this hospital is the main attraction. Approximately 2000 out-patients are given Panchakarma treatment daily.[170]

4.2 Kaitady Siddha Teaching Hospital

Kaitady Siddha Teaching Hospital in Jaffna was founded in 1978, with five wards, a laboratory, and a pharmacy and out-patients unit.[171]In 1983, the services had to be limited to two wards (male and female) as most of the staff were displaced due to the civil conflict.[172] In 1990, the first batch that graduated with a Siddha Ayurveda degree from the Department of Siddha Ayurveda Medicine were employed at the Kaitady Siddha Teaching Hospital. With the new recruitments, the hospital re-established six wards including a maternity ward and surgery unit.[173] In 2000, the hospital was destroyed due to the civil conflict between the Liberation of Tigers of Tamil Eelam (LTTE) and the Government of Sri Lanka.[174] It functioned as a dispensary in its new location in Manipay.[175] Again in 2002, the hospital shifted to the remaining buildings and in 2004 the Department of Ayurveda started repair works.[176] Currently the hospital is functioning with 4 wards and an out-patient unit.[177] 36 staff members including six doctors (Siddha and Unani) are employed in the hospital.[178] The Medical Officer in charge of the Kaitady Siddha Teaching Hospital, Dr. Shivashanmugarajah, explained the structure, organisation and common treatments of the hospital.[179] The Kaitady Siddha Teaching Hospital has one Unani doctor, and all the others are Siddha doctors. The treatment provided by the hospital includes all the types of sicknesses, including minor surgeries. The most common sicknesses the hospital treats are arthritis (such as rheumatoid and osteo-arthritis), skin diseases (such as eczema), and the common cough and

---

169 The only government institution providing full-course of Panchakarma treatment.
170 See http://www.ayurveda.gov.lk/borella.html (last retrieved 20 February 2019).
171 Based on the Department of Ayurveda introduction to Kaitady Siddha Teaching Hospital www.ayurveda.gov.lk/kaithadi.html (last retrieved 20 February 2019).
172 Dr. Pema Shivashanmugarajah (#98).
173 Based on the Department of Ayurveda introduction to Kaitady Siddha Teaching Hospital www.ayurveda.gov.lk/kaithadi.html (last retrieved 20 February 2019).
174 Dr. Prema Shivashanmugarajah (# 98).
175 Based on the Department of Ayurveda introduction to Kaitady Siddha Teaching Hospital www.ayurveda.gov.lk/kaithadi.html (last retrieved 20 February 2019).
176 Based on the Department of Ayurveda introduction to Kaitady Siddha Teaching Hospital www.ayurveda.gov.lk/kaithadi.html (last retrieved 20 February 2019).
177 Dr. Pema Shivashanmugarajah (#98).
178 Dr. Pema Shivashanmugarajah (#98).
179 Dr. Prema Shivashanmugarajah (# 98).

cold.[180] The duration of treatment is a maximum of 45 days, unless the doctor prescribes further treatment. The daily count of in-house patients varies from 50 to 70 patients; about 200 patients come daily for clinics. All the medicines are given free of charge. Most of these medicines are brought from the Ayurveda Drug Corporation, Maharagama; some are produced in the hospital. It is difficult to obtain some ingredients such as opium that are needed to manufacture the medicine due to government regulations. All the vacancies for medical doctors have been filled, but the number of other staff members is not sufficient. Once in a while the hospital advertises for inter-generational healers to practice as 'Special Doctors' on contract basis. When advertised traditional healers have to apply and come. They are paid according to the days they serve. At this moment the hospital has only one 'Special Doctor' who does not have many patients.[181]

4.3 Gampaha Wickramarachchi Ayurveda Teaching Hospital

Pundit G.P Wickramarachchi established Gampaha Wickramarachchi Sidhayurveda Medical College in 1929 with the aims of improving Ayurveda medicine and providing free treatment.[182] The medical college was upgraded to a teaching hospital in 1984.[183] On 27th of February 2008 it was affiliated by the Department of Ayurveda.[184] This hospital can presently accommodate 120 in-house patients in the four wards.[185] The hospital also has an efficient out-patient unit and a pharmacy.[186] This Ayurvedic teaching hospital provides teaching and training facilities to undergraduate medical students attached to the Gampaha Wickramarachchi Ayurveda Institute.[187]

---

[180] Dr. Prema Shivashanmugarajah (# 98).
[181] Dr. Prema Shivashanmugarajah (# 98).
[182] Based on –Gampaha Wickramarachchi Ayurveda Teaching Hospital website www.kln.ac.lk/institutes/wickramarachchi/index.php/gampaha-wickramarachchi-ayurveda-teaching-hospital.html (last retrieved 20 February 2019).
[183] Based on –Gampaha Wickramarachchi Ayurveda Teaching Hospital website www.kln.ac.lk/institutes/wickramarachchi/index.php/gampaha-wickramarachchi-ayurveda-teaching-hospital.html (last retrieved 20 February 2019).
[184] Based on –Gampaha Wickramarachchi Ayurveda Teaching Hospital website www.kln.ac.lk/institutes/wickramarachchi/index.php/gampaha-wickramarachchi-ayurveda-teaching-hospital.html (last retrieved 20 February 2019).
[185] Dr. E. A. S. C. S. Edirisuriya (#7).
[186] Dr. E. A. S. C. S. Edirisuriya (#7).
[187] Dr. E. A. S. C. S. Edirisuriya (#7).

4.4 Government Homeopathy Hospital

In addition to government curative services facilities provided in Ayurveda, Siddha and Unani as discussed above, there is one government homeopathy hospital[188] in Sri Lanka. The Sri Lankan Government has approved this medical system under the *Homeopathy Act No 8 in 1970.*[189] Homeopathy treatment is an easy and affordable system that can prevent and eradicate sickness. The Government Homeopathy hospital was established with the idea of promoting this traditional alternative healing system among the Sri Lankan community.

Homeopathic treatment is used to cure all viral diseases (influenza, viral eye diseases, viral disorders, contagious diseases), paediatric disorders (influenza, common colds, coughs, asthma, fever, diarrhoea, rheumatic disease), disorders associated with females (problems associated with menstruation, diseases of the womb, disorders during pregnancy), skin diseases (*'pothu kabara,' 'sudu kabara,'* boils, leprosy), geriatric diseases (diabetes, joint aches and pains, high blood pressure), diseases associated with the stomach, and long term headaches and nervous diseases.

Services provided by the hospital include, the out-patient unit that treats about 150-200 patients a day; conducting programs on maintaining a healthy lifestyle and education on mental wellbeing; an active, 24-hour indoor patients department; organising mobile clinics and conducting educational programs for patients; providing homeopathic medicines; organising homeopathic medical clinics and mobile clinics; promoting foreign homeopathic programs; and providing facilities for practical work for graduates. Currently, only three doctors are working at this hospital in Welisara, although there is a great demand for this natural treatment system.[190]

Part 5: Medicines and Drugs

This part of the chapter argues that Ayurveda medicines and drugs receive prominence by Government of Sri Lanka in standardising, sponsoring production and freely distributing to government hospitals and dispensaries

---

[188] located in 94, Shelton Jayasinghe Mawatha, Welisara.

[189] Kurugala, P (4 January 2013) Homeopathy hospital completes first decade. Daily News. http://archives.dailynews.lk/2013/01/04/news41.asp (last retrieved 20 February 2019).

[190] Kurugala, P (4 January 2013) Homeopathy hospital completes first decade. Daily News. http://archives.dailynews.lk/2013/01/04/news41.asp (last retrieved 20 February 2019).

under the purview of Ministry of Indigenous Medicine. The argument is presented by analysing the role of the main bodies that regulate medicine and drugs in Sri Lanka, namely, the Formulary Committee and Sri Lanka Ayurvedic Drug Corporation.[191]

5.1 Ayurveda Formulary Committee

One of the ways in which Ayurveda medicine is recognised, supported and regulated is by the Ayurveda Formulary Committee. *Ayurveda Pharmacies Regulation* section 21(1) states that 'every formula for the preparation of any drug to be sold to the public shall be first approved by the Formulary Committee set up for the purpose' and section 21(2) states that 'any alteration or addition made to or any omission from any formulae already approved shall require the approval of the Formulary Committee.' The Ministry of Indigenous Medicine has appointed a Formulary Committee consisting of nine members to implement the above regulation.[192]

5.2 Sri Lanka Ayurvedic Drugs Corporation

The Sri Lanka Ayurvedic Drugs Corporation is the other body that recognises, supports and regulates Ayurveda medicine in Sri Lanka.[193] The Sri Lanka Ayurvedic Drugs Corporation was incorporated in 1969 under the provision of *State Industrial Corporation Act no. 49 of 1957*.[194] The vision of the Sri Lanka Ayurvedic Drugs Corporation is to fulfil the national and international medicinal needs with high standards by preserving the identity of the indigenous medical science.[195] The Sri Lanka Ayurvedic Drugs Corporation's role includesmanufacturing, importing, distributing, researching and supplying of services of Ayurvedic drugs with high standards.[196]

Currently the Sri Lanka Ayurvedic Drugs Corporation is the pioneer and main institute to manufacture and market Ayurvedic drugs to

---

[191] Herein after Formulary Committee.
[192] L. H. Thilakaratne (# 4).
[193] Sri Lanka Ayurvedic Drugs Corporation Website – http://www.ayurvediccorp.gov.lk/web/ (last retrieved 20 February 2019).
[194] Government extra ordinary gazette notification no. 14853/1 dated 11 May 1969. Also see Sri Lanka Ayurvedic Drugs Corporation Website – http://www.ayurvediccorp.gov.lk/web/ (last retrieved 20 February 2019).
[195]Overview, Sri Lanka Ayurvedic Drugs Corporation- http://www.ayurvediccorp.gov.lk/web/index.php?option=com_content&view=article&id=1&Itemid=109&lang=en (last retrieved 20 February 2019)
[196] Mission of the Ayurveda Drugs Cooperation.

the government hospitals, Ayurvedic physicians and the private sector.[197] The medicines produced at the Ayurvedic Drugs Corporation are based on *Ayurveda Sammithi Sangrahaya*.[198] As the drugs and medicine that are accessible for the healers through the government are Ayurvedic and as some inter-generational healers find it difficult to get the ingredients or medicine to prepare the drugs and medicines according to their ancient prescriptions, sometimes they have to prescribe Ayurvedic medicine and drugs to the patients.[199]

Being the prime government body in disseminating traditional drugs and medicine, it is through the Ayurvedic Drugs Corporation that inter-generational healers have to obtain some of the required medicine and medicinal herbs.[200] The process of obtaining some of the medicinal herbs (which are called *thahanam oushada* (prohibited herbs)) is not an easy task for the inter-generational healers. It takes at least three weeks for an inter-generational healer to obtain the clearance to purchase prohibited herbs. In this example, an inter-generational healer expresses his feelings of restrictive laws: 'there should be a law to prevent abuses, but it should not restrict the freedom of using ingredients for traditional healing.'[201]

The Ayurvedic Drugs Corporation has registered suppliers to provide medical ingredients. Most suppliers find it difficult to provide for the requirement as they usually pick the herbs from the jungle.[202] The Department of Wildlife Conservation, however, has restricted picking medicine from the jungles.[203] The suppliers have to find herbs while complying to these restrictions. As the Ayurvedic Drugs Corporation does not have access to sufficient medical ingredients to produce all the drug

---

197 L. H. Thilakaratne (# 4).

198 Dr. P. Ekkanayake (# 49).

199 S. D. M. Mahipala (# 51), H. D. Karunawathie (#53), R. M. D. J. Gunasekera (#58).

200 Dr. P. Ekkanayake (# 49).

201 Based on an interview with an inter-generational healer. As requested, due to confidentiality purposes I am not quoting the name.

202 *Fauna and Flora Protection (Amendment) Act No. 22 of 2009* is a legislation to protect animal species and wild flora. This act regulates access and usage of fauna and flora.

203 One of the main functions of Dempartment of Wildlife Conservation is to implement the *Fauna and Flora Protection (Amendment) Act No. 22 of 2009* and other regulations to minimize illegal exploitation of wildlife resources. See: Overview of Department of Wildlife Conservation. http://www.dwc.gov.lk/index.php/en/aboutdwc/overview (last retrieved 20 February 2019).

requirements, some medicines have to be exported from India.[204] The Unani medicine is imported by the Ayurvedic Drugs Corporation from Middle-Eastern countries.[205]

Part 6: Research and Herb Gardens

This part of the chapter argues that the Sri Lankan Government focuses on Ayurveda in both research and the maintenance of herb gardens, and the government sponsored research has adopted a Western research framework to support the Western concepts of universalisation and standardisation of knowledge.[206] In doing so, this part first discusses the historical development of government sponsored Ayurveda research in Sri Lanka. Then the role of the Ayurveda Research Committee is presented. Subsequently the role Bandaranaike Memorial Ayurveda Research Institute is discussed. Afterwards the contribution of herbal gardens and herbal farmer village projects are analysed. This discussion on the role of government institutions and programmes on research in traditional health care shows the Sri Lankan Government's role in recognising, supporting and regulating research and gardens.

In order to systematically promote traditional healing as a healing system, in a country where biomedical framework for administration and regulation is adopted, conducting and validating healing methods and medicine according to Western parameters became an important concern. Until policy makers' interest in rationalising and explaining the reasons for the Ayurvedic research arose in Sri Lanka, systematic research was not conducted on Ayurveda in Sri Lanka.[207] The reason for not conducting Ayurveda research prior to policy makers' influence was due to the theory of the divine origin of the Ayurvedic science, where Ayurveda has developed a character of sacredness and demanded that its teachings be accepted on faith. [208] Recommendation 17 of the *Ministry of Health Proposal for the Revival and Development of Indigenous Medicine in Ceylon* from 1955 is an example of applying a biomedical framework for Ayurveda:

---

[204] Dr. P. Ekkanayake (# 49).
[205] Dr. P. Ekkanayake (# 49).
[206] Dr. M. W. S. J. Kumari (# 11).
[207] Ministry of Health (1955) p.7 http://www.ayurveda.gov.lk/Research.html (last retrieved 20 February 2019).
[208] Dr. Parakrama (#15).

> Immediate action must be taken to provide adequate facilities for research in Indigenous Medicine. As this research has to be up to the standards acceptable to Western Science, it is necessary that it should be done by persons fully acquainted with modern methods of scientific investigation and under the supervision and guidance of Scientists and Doctors qualified in Western Medicine...[209]

6.1 The Ayurveda Research Committee

The Ayurveda Research Committed has been established according to section 33 of *Ayurveda (revised) Act no 31 of 1961* as a working group to promote Ayurveda research. As required by the Act, the responsibilities of the committee include advising the Minister on conducting research on Ayurveda, including on Ayurveda literature, Ayurveda concepts, Ayurveda treatment and Ayurveda medicine; and based on the Minister's request, establishing and maintaining libraries, museums, herbariums (*Oushada Nidi*), laboratories; publishing information on Ayurveda, including handbooks, Ayurvedic books, Ayurvedic magazines, papers and Ayurveda *Oushada Sangrahaya*; and standardising Ayurvedic medicine.[210] The responsibilities of this committee are limited to protecting and promoting Ayurveda, not other forms of traditional, inter-generational and cosmic healing practices.

6.2 Bandaranaike Memorial Ayurveda Research Institute

Bandaranaike Memorial Ayurveda Research Institute[211] was established on 14 October 1962,[212] recognising the need for Ayurveda research with a

---

[209] Ministry of Health (1955) rec. 17.

[210] Department of Ayurveda (2013) p 42.

[211] Bandaranaike Ayurveda Research Institute is located in Old Kottawa Road, Navinna, Maharagama, Western Province of Sri Lanka. TP 094-011-2850333.

[212] The history of establishing the Ayurveda Research Institute can be traced back to 1928, where the Board of Indigenous Medicine was created with the instructions among other things to foster research. Due to the inadequacy of funding, the Board couldn't fulfil this objective. The recommendation by the Executive Committee of Health in 1936 to establish an Institute for Research in Indigenous Medicine was approved by the State Council but wasn't implemented. The Gupta Commission's report in 1947 also identified the lack of facilities for research in Indigenous medicine in the island and recommended that 'the steps to be taken to organise research under the direction of a qualified Western medical practitioner and in collaboration with the Medical Research Institute.' (Ministry of Health: 1955: p8) Despite the high level commission recommendations, no concrete action was taken till 1956, where Nagarjunaa managed to capture Hon. Prime Minister S. W. R. D.

Western framework.[213] As the title of the institution suggests, the scope of the institution is limited to 'Ayurveda' research and does not provide for research on all forms of traditional, inter-generational and cosmic healing practices. The research activities presently carried out by the Institute could be clustered as clinical research, drug research and botanical research. Special weekly clinics conducted by the Institute include, rheumatoid arthritis, eye diseases, bronchial asthma, gynaecology, panchakarma, vitiligo, paediatrics, diabetes mellitus, anorectal disease.[214]

When establishing the Bandaranaike Memorial Ayurveda Research Institute, the policy makers did not take into account that the diversity of existing traditional healing systems in Sri Lanka could not be limited to Ayurveda. Also that it is difficult to cover inter-generational and cosmic healing methods using a Western research framework because the ethics and value systems are different from the Western scenario.[215] Inter-generational and cosmic healing methods are developed through experimentation by individuals.[216] These healers are not interested in publicising the methods of treatment or the recipes of medicine, as the healing system is their livelihood and their heritage.[217] Introducing the

---

Bandaranaike's attention by commenting on the need to establish Ayurvedic Research Institute in Sri Lanka on the Editorial of the Ayurvedic Journal in India. Based on the suggestion Hon. S. W. R. D. Bandaranaike directed Pandith Shiva Sharma an eminent Ayurvedic Physician from India to produce a report on the development of Ayurveda in Sri Lanka. The Bandaranaike Memorial Ayurveda Research Institute was setup based on the recommendations of Pandith Shiva Sharma. (See: http://www.indigenousmedimini.gov.lk/Research_institute.html (last retrieved 20 February 2019).

[213] Ministry of Health (1955) 7. Here, Western framework refers to a biomedical framework.

[214] Based on the interview with Dr. Parakrama, Bandaranaike Ayurveda Research Institute (7 May 2012).

[215] Dr. E. A. S. C. S. Edirisuriya (# 7), Dr. M. Chithra Nalini (#8).

[216] Ms. Rathnawathhie (#29), Ms. W. A. Kusuma Wijesekera (#32), Ms. B. V. Punchimanike (#42), Mr. P. Weerasinghe (# 52), Mrs. H. D. Karunawathie (# 53), Mrs. W. M. Anulawathie (# 56), Mr. R. M. D. J. Gunasekera (#58), Mr. Wanasinhe Mudiyanselage Sudu Banda (# 59), Mr. Ajith Liyanage (# 96), Mr. Je Jeyalan (#100), Mr. S. Paranasivamullai and Mr. R. L. Kularatne (#110) have informed how experimentation play a significant role in developing their respective fields of healing.

[217] Some of the healers that stated they are not interested in sharing their inter-generational knowledge system publicly include, VishwakeerthiVanaspathi UruWalige Wanniya Attho (#18), Mr. R. M. C. D. S. B. Rajapakse (#19), Mr. Sunil Shantha (# 25), Mr. S. K. Liyanarachchige (# 27), Ms. Rathnawathie (# 29), Ms. B. V. Punchimanike (#42), Mr. S. D. M. Mahipala (#51), Mr. P. Weerasinghe (# 52),

Western form of research to Ayurveda is a means of imposing an alien system and westernising the traditional medical system.[218] The traditional social structure and values gets lost when the world is looked at in a western framework.[219]

6.3 Herbal Gardens

The Ministry of Indigenous Medicine has taken measures to establish herbal gardens in Sri Lanka to protect and promote hereditary medicinal plants.[220] The roles of the herbal gardens are, to establish national level medicinal plants, to preserve ancient medicinal plants and to propagate medicinal plant cultivation.[221] The five herbal gardens established by the Department of Ayurveda in Sri Lanka are at Haldummulla (65 acres) and Girandurukotte (165 acres) in Uva province; Pattipola (25 acres) and Pallekele (5 acres) in Central parts and Navinna (12 acres) in the Western province.[222] The functions and services of the herbal gardens project include, providing extension services, conducting nurseries, conducting awareness programmes for school children and Ayurveda physicians, conducting plant exhibitions, implementing research on plants and cultivation and non-formal education on plants for the community.[223]

6.4 Herbal farmer village project of the Ministry of Indigenous Medicine

The Ministry of Indigenous Medicine has been bearing huge costs for importation of dried herbs such as katuwelbatu, amukkara, asamodagam,

---

Mrs. H. D. Karunawathie (# 53), Mrs. W. M. Anulawathie (# 56), Mr. R. V. Piyadasa (#57), Mr. Wanasinhe Mudiyanselage Sudu Banda (# 59), Mr. Ajith Liyanage (# 96), Mr. R. M. D. J. Gunasekera(#58), Mr. Je Jeyalan (#100), Mr. S. Paranasivamullai and Mr. R. L. Kularatne (#110), Mrs. C. Kularatne (#111).

[218] Dr. E. A. S. C. S. Edirisuriya (# 7), Dr. M. Chithra Nalini (#8).

[219] Mr. A. D. H. Sudesh (# 50).

[220] In Sri Lanka, approximately 1500 species of medicinal plants are used. Out of them, 208 species of medicinal plants are frequently used. (Ministry of Indigenous Medicine).

[221] Prof. Piyal A. Marasinghe (#41).

[222] Herbal Gardens, Ministry of Indigenous Medicine http://www.indigenousmedimini.gov.lk/Herbal_Garden.html (last retrieved 20 February 2019).

[223] Herbal Gardens, Ministry of Indigenous Medicine http://www.indigenousmedimini.gov.lk/Herbal_Garden.html (last retrieved 20 February 2019).

welmee, pathpadagam and dewadara.[224] The annual estimated cost for imported dried herbs is Rs 125 million according to a survey conducted in 2000.[225] The herbal farmer village project, also called the medicinal plant cultivation programme, started on 28 March 2005,[226] with the aim of minimising the cost of imported dried herbs.[227] The progress and the impact of this project are not well established.

Part 7: Programmes to Develop Community Healthcare and Inter-Generational Healing

The Ministry of Indigenous Medicine has introduced programmes to develop community healthcare and inter-generational practices of healing. This part argues all community healthcare programmes and inter-generational healing programmes promoted by the Ministry of Indigenous Medicine are not well established. To make this argument, part 7 describes how the community healthcare programmes initiated by the Ministry of Indigenous Medicine are in their infancy: all of them have been pilot projects and some of them have been failures. The Sri Lankan Government's focus mainly targeting traditional curative healthcare and overlooking traditional community healthcare has been a reason for this. This part presents and discusses the community healthcare pilot project in Anuradhapura; and two programmes were implemented to develop the practice of inter-generational healing, namely, *Hela Weda Gedera*, and Preserving Vedda Culture and Medicinal Plants Cultivation. It is suggested that the government initiatives to develop inter-generational healing

---

[224] Dr. Ekanayake (# 49) endorsed the extensive import of dried herbs.

[225] Development programme of the Ministry – Medicinal Plant Cultivation http://www.indigenousmedimini.gov.lk/Development_Program.html (last retrieved 20 February 2019).

[226] Development programme of the Ministry – Medicinal Plant Cultivation http://www.indigenousmedimini.gov.lk/Development_Program.html (last retrieved 20 February 2019).

[227] Other objectives of the project include: 'to identify herbs which are locally cultivatable and turn out a new farmer community for the cultivation of herbs to popularise this cultivation as a source of income generation; to establish and maintain of herbal cultivation among youth; to develop herbal gardens; to expand herb cultivation in association with Divi Neguma; to extend herbal cultivation programme to the villages affected by terrorist menace in concurrence with national programme.' See: Development programme of the Ministry – Medicinal Plant Cultivation http://www.indigenousmedimini.gov.lk/Development_Program.html (last retrieved 20 February 2019).

programmes are at an early stage because the government has not duly recognised and given patronage and commitment towards such practices.

7.1 Community Health Care Pilot Project in Anuradhapura

Government interventions in preventive health and community health care services have played a role since 1926.[228] Yet, the Ministry of Indigenous Medicine's focus of community health care has only started since 1 October 2004, with the community health care pilot project in Anuradhapura. The community health care pilot project covers 22 Divisional Secretariats in the Anuradhapura district.[229] Under this service, 22 community health promotion Ayurvedic medical officers and 210 community health promotion officers were appointed. The main focus of the project was to introduce food items with nutritional and medicinal value to reduce the health expenditure of the community.[230] To implement the project, the project coordinators sought to obtain support of the community. Other sub-programs implemented under this project aimed at controlling contagious and non-contagious diseases, eradicating drug menace, preventing renal failure and diabetes, improving sanitation among school children, popularising local grains and conduct first aid training programs and mobile clinics.[231] A community health pilot group has been appointed to carry out these programs. The programmes introduced include:

- Medicinal Plant Cultivation, where 146 selected farmers from Anuradhapura district were given assistance (agro wells and water pumps) to cultivate medicinal plants; and[232]
- Establishing Poshana Mandira *(*nutritious food centres). Since 2011 as part of the community healthcare programme the Ministry

---

[228] Department of Medical and Sanitary Services (1948).
[229] Development Programme of the Ministry, Medicinal Plant Cultivation. http://www.indigenousmedimini.gov.lk/Development_Program.html?&session-id=bf4e6b1982ea3f0348ebc843f9083fae (last retrieved 20 February 2019)
[230] Development Programme of the Ministry, Medicinal Plant Cultivation. http://www.indigenousmedimini.gov.lk/Development_Program.html?&session-id=bf4e6b1982ea3f0348ebc843f9083fae (last retrieved 20 February 2019)
[231] Development programmes of the Ministry. http://www.indigenousmedimini.gov.lk/Development_Program.html (last retrieved 20 February 2019)
[232] Development programmes of the Ministry. http://www.indigenousmedimini.gov.lk/Development_Program.html (last retrieved 20 February 2019)

of Indigenous Medicine has been making arrangements to establish two permanent nutritious food centres in identified locations.[233] The nutritious food centres are aiming to popularise local foods and herbal drinks among the Sri Lankans and improve their nutrition standard. In addition, 10 mobile nutritious food centres have been arranged as a self-employment of selling herbal drinks. At present 20 mobile nutritious food centres are being prepared and the youths of low-income groups are provided with vehicles such as carts and bicycles to start self-employment.[234]

7.2 *Hela Weda Gedera*

Hela Weda Gedera is a term referring to traditional healing homes. Traditionally, the healers used to treat patients as a service, without expecting economic advantages in return.[235] In a capitalist economy healing practitioners are facing financial viability issues.[236] In order to support inter-generational healers to continue the practice of healing, the Ministry of Indigenous Medicine has initiated the *Hela Weda Gedera* programme. Under this programme, a selected inter-generational healer from each of Sri Lanka's provinces (a total of 9 selected traditional healers) is supported to establish a building in their own land to provide residential treatment for up to ten patients.[237] Inter-generational healers interviewed for the purpose of this research felt that there was political influence in selecting recipients for

---

[233] Development programmes of the Ministry.
http://www.indigenousmedimini.gov.lk/Development_Program.html (last retrieved 20 February 2019)

[234] Development programmes of the Ministry.
http://www.indigenousmedimini.gov.lk/Development_Program.html (last retrieved 20 February 2019)

[235] VishwakeerthiVanaspathi UruWalige Wanniya Attho (#18), Mr. Sunil Shantha (#25), Ms. Rathnawathie (#29), Ms. B. V. Punchimenike (# 42), Mr. S. D. M. Mahipala (#52), Mrs. W. M. Anulawathie (#56), Mr. Wansinghe Mudiyanselage Sudu Banda (#59), Mr. T. Herath Banda (#108) have discussed traditionally practicing inter-generational healing as a service rather than a means of income.

[236] Inter-generational healers views on financial viability is discussed in Chapter 6, 2.1 Limited Employment Opportunities

[237] Rs. 12 million has been allocated for the total project (to build nine residential care treatment facilities in the land of 9 identified healers). Development programmes of the Ministry.
http://www.indigenousmedimini.gov.lk/Development_Program.html (last retrieved 20 February 2019)

the *Hela Veda Gedara* and that the criteria used in selecting suitable candidates was not transparent.[238]

7.3 Preserving Vedda Culture and Medicinal Plants Cultivation

The programme to preserve Vedda culture and medicinal plant cultivation is another programme implemented by the Ministry of Indigenous Medicine with the aim of developing the practice of inter-generational healing. The Vedda healing system is a prominent inter-generational healing system in the country and is discussed in Chapter 5.[239] Recognising the vanishing art of Vedda healing and the need to safeguard it, the Ministry of Indigenous Medicine in collaboration with the Ministry of Cultural Heritage has introduced a program to improve the traditional systems of healing in Sri Lanka by preserving the Vedda culture, cultivating medicinal plants and providing an opportunity to practice their own medical practices. Figure 4.7 and 4.8 show the centre established by the program.

The program on preserving Vedda culture and medicinal plants cultivation was given wide publicity through the websites of Ministry of Indigenous Medicine and Ministry of Cultural Heritage, as a very large project conducted in collaboration with the indigenous community in Dambana (Veddas).[240] During discussion with several members of the Vedda Community in Dambana it became apparent that the programme was not as significant or collaborative as the Ministry claimed.[241] The interviewees said:

> Ministry officials visited the Vedda community in Dambana for about a month and stopped after the officials got the publicity what they wanted from being engaged with us. The Government has cheated us saying that they were going to preserve traditional Vedda medicines and the forests and use them in the Ayurveda Institute. The officials of the Ministries

---

[238] This is the opinion of traditional healers in Matara in Southern Province; Badulla in Uva Province; Gampaha in Western Province; Kurunegala in Wayamba Province; Anuradhapura in North Cenral Province and Kandy in Central Province. I am not quoting names due to confidentiality purposes.

[239] Chapter 6, 3.2 Assimilation of Vedda Community.

[240] For a write up on the net see, Lankadesha E-Magazine (August 27, 2011) Ayurvedic Medical Centre for the Sri Lanka's Indigenous People in Dambana. http://www.lankadesha.com/ayurvedic-medical-centre-for-the-sri-lankas-indigenous-people-in-dambana/ (last retrieved 20 February 2019).

[241] Based on interviews with the Vaddha Community Members in Kota Bakina, Dambana including VishwakeerthiVanaspathi UruWalige Wanniya Attho (# 18), Dambane Gunawardena (# 17), Gunapala Wanniya Attho (# 16).

> requested us to collect herbs. Taking their word, we collected herbs worth more than two million rupees. They haven't even seen the medicines we collected. The life time of the herbs has now expired. [Figure 4.9 portrays some of the expired herbs] All the herbs have been destroyed and attacked by termites so we have had to burn them. We collected the medicine by 9 August 2012, as requested by the officials. This action portrays that the Government is cheating us, we have spoken to everyone we can, ministers and other leaders, and no one takes any interest. The Government has not taken any other steps to uphold the health and wellbeing of the Vedda community. Under this programme, the Government has promised training in Ayurveda medical treatment to be given to the descendants of the Veddas but that too has not been implemented up to date.[242]

Traditionally, a Vedda leader disseminates his knowledge of indigenous healing systems to about ten selected disciples of the Vedda community.[243] This training takes about 3-4 months. Vedda knowledge in healing is an indigenous form of knowledge learnt through interactions with the natural world. It is different from Ayurveda. Inter-generational knowledge sharing has been the way Vedda community has preserved their healing systems. According to Vishwakeerthi Vanaspathi Uru Walige Wannia Attho:

> This knowledge is shared only within the Vedda community in Damabana and not even with the ones who were dispersed since we cannot trust them to keep our healing systems within our community.[244]

As planned by the government, if they had trained the Vedda healers in Ayurveda,[245] it would have been another attempt of Ayurvedisation of an inter-generational practice of healing. Such a programme would have threatened the existence of indigenous knowledge of Vedda healing. Vishwakeerthi Vanaspathi Uru Walige Wannia Attho says, 'In order to preserve and improve the traditional healing systems of the Vedda community, one must change the attitudes of the Vedda community

---

242 Based on interviews with the Vaddha Community Members in Kota Bakina, Dambana including VishwakeerthiVanaspathi UruWalige Wanniya Attho (# 18), Dambane Gunawardena (# 17), Gunapala Wanniya Attho (# 16).

243 Vishwakeerthi Vanaspathi Uru Walige Wannia Attho (# 18).

244 Vishwakeerthi Vanaspathi Uru Walige Wannia Attho (# 18).

245 Vishwakeerthi Vanaspathi Uru Walige Wannia Attho (# 18) and Dambane Gunawardena (# 17) stated one of the programmes suggested by the officials of Ministry of Cultural Heritage and Ministry of Indigenous Medicine was to train selected Vedda member on Ayurveda by conducting short courses.

members and the state.[246] Dambane Gunawardena adds, that the value system and the lifestyles of the Vedda community need to be restored.[247]

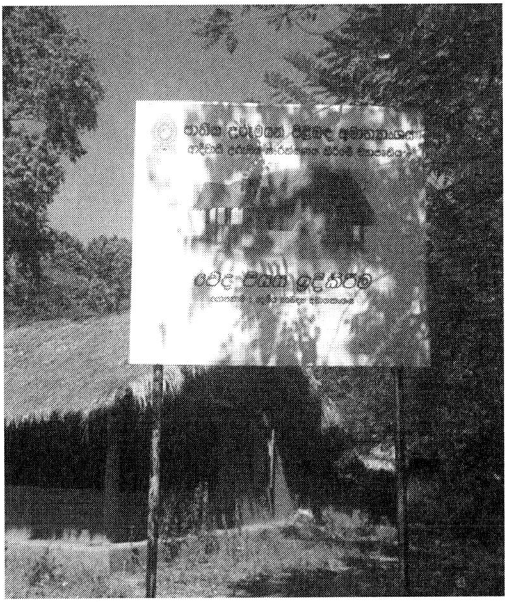

Figure 4.7 – Board by Ministry of Cultural Heritage (Project to protect Indigenous Heritage, Establishment of 'Veda Piyasa' (Indigenous Healing Centre) Project proposed by Ministry of Indigenous Medicine)

[246] Vishwakeerthi Vanaspathi Uru Walige Wannia Attho (# 18).
[247] Dambane Gunawardena (# 17).

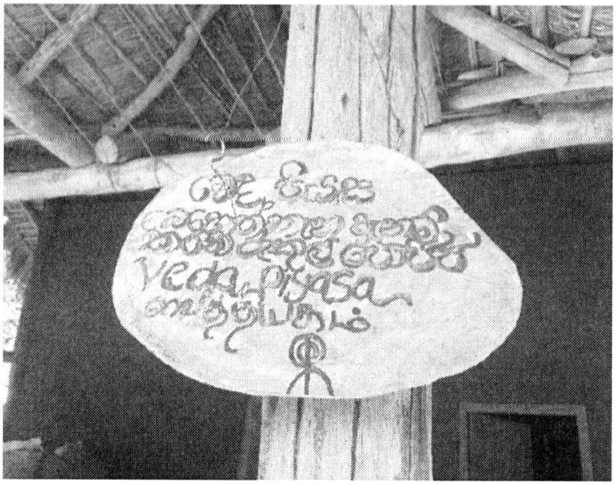

Figure 4.8- 'Veda Piyasa' (Indigenous Healing Centre)

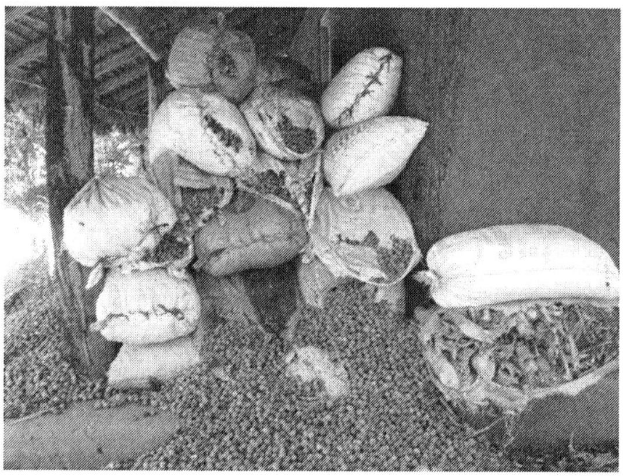

Figure 4.9 – Herbs collected by the Vedda community as requested by the Government officials. The lifetime of all these herbs has now expired.

Conclusion

The history of healthcare in Sri Lanka shows how public demand for non-Western healing systems has led colonial and post-colonial Sri Lankan governments to recognise, support and regulate traditional healing practices. In so doing the government has developed a range of mechanisms including:

- A wide spread government administrative structure. As discussed in part 2 of the chapter, the Ministry of Indigenous Medicine plays a key role at the national level in administrating traditional medicine in Sri Lanka. The main arm of the Ministry that supports in administration is the Department of Ayurveda. The Ayurveda Medical Council also plays a vital role in regulating traditional medicine and influencing the administration of traditional medicine. Administration of traditional medicine at the provincial level is supported by the Provincial Administrative structures in the respective provinces;
- Government sponsored education in traditional medicine has contributed towards introducing diplomas, degrees, post-graduate diplomas and PhDs in Ayurveda, Siddha, Unani in Sri Lanka. The process of formalising traditional medical education is supported by the Ayurveda Education and Hospital Board. The National Institute of Traditional Medicine, Institute of Indigenous Medicine, University of Colombo, Gampaha Wickramarachchi Ayurveda Institute and the Diploma in Ayurveda programme as discussed in part 3 are examples of government sponsored education in traditional medicine. Free curative services and medicine are available all over the county. The diverse range of facilities available for curative services as discussed in part 4 of the chapter include teaching hospitals, provincial Ayurveda hospitals, district Ayurveda hospitals, rural Ayurveda hospitals, dispensaries and mobile units. The medicine and drugs are regulated mainly by the Formulary Committee and provided by Sri Lanka Ayurvedic Drug Corporation as discussed in part 5 of the chapter;
- Government sponsored research, as discussed in part 6 of the chapter suggests that research is regulated by the Ayurveda Research Committee, and implemented mainly by the Bandaranaike Memorial Ayurveda Research Institute. The herbal gardens maintained by the government also contribute towards Ayurveda herbal medicine and drug research;
- Community health care programs and programmes introduced to develop the practice of inter-generational healing are in at an early stage or have been failures due to lack of commitment by the government.

While the government's efforts have gone some way to support and safeguard traditional practices in Sri Lanka this has been informed and influenced by Western and biomedical frameworks. This means that the Sri Lankan Government has taken rather a narrow approach to healing practices. The result of this narrow approach is that the government's involvement in the protection and promotion of traditional healing has formalised and standardised adopted traditional healing practices. The government's focus on traditional healing has been mainly on Ayurveda, and to a lesser extent Siddha, Unani, Acupuncture and Homeopathy. In all the government sponsored traditional healing systems emphasis is placed on the curative services and the Ayurvedisation of indigenous and traditional healing practices. There is a significant trend in the loss of cultural value in the process of standardisation and formalisation.

Due to the Government's conceptualisation of traditional healing practices (as formal practices of healing such as Ayurveda, Siddha, Unani, Homeopathy and Acupuncture that were adopted from other countries and to a lesser extent inter-generational healing practices) certain types of healing practices have been, and continue to be neglected, overlooked or threatened in the process of Ayurvedisation. The government also uses the words 'indigenous' and 'traditional' inter-changeably to refer to the traditional healing system adopted. Yet government support, recognition and regulation for inter-generational and cosmic healing is very limited. Due to the diversity and informal nature of the inter-generational and cosmic healing systems in the country, this 'traditional knowledge' in healing has been overlooked by the Sri Lankan Government. In chapter 5 and 6 the book discusses inter-generational healing practices and cosmic healing practices respectively to show how these healing practices have been overlooked or have not given due attention by the Government of Sri Lanka. In so doing it draws upon extensive interviews with inter-generational healers, cosmic healers and observations of healing practices.

CHAPTER 5

INTER-GENERATIONAL HEALING AND LOSS OF CULTURE

Introduction

This chapter examines inter-generational healing in Sri Lanka, and argues it is facing the threat of losing the cultural heritage aspects of healing due, in large part, to government interventions in recognising, supporting and regulating healing practices. More specifically this chapter presents cases of inter-generational healing practices of Sri Lanka which are partially recognised by the Sri Lankan Government such as *Sarvanga* (Physicians), *Kedum Bidum* (orthopaedic), *Akshi Roga* (eye disease), *Anshabaga* (stroke and paralysis), *Pilika* (cancer), *Visa* (toxicology), and *Adivasi Vedakama* (tribal medicine), to illustrate the cultural heritage aspect of healing and role of government in recognising, supporting and regulating healing practices This adds to the analysis of the history and nature of the recognition, support and regulation of traditional healing practices in Sri Lanka presented in Chapter 4. While the discussion in Chapter 4 was focused on healing practices that have received the full attention, recognition, support and regulation of the Government of Sri Lanka, Chapter 6 focuses on inter-generational healing practices that have only received partial recognition, support and regulation.

The chapter is organised into three parts. Part 1 argues that inter-generational healing is diverse, unstructured, informal and part of the intangible cultural heritage of Sri Lanka.This argument is illustrated through the case studies of *Visha Vaidya* (poison healer) Rathnawathie, and *Ansha Baga Vaidya* (stroke and paralysis healer) Wanasinghe Mudiyansalage Sudu Banda and *Kadum Bidum* healer, Sunil Shantha. Part 2 argues that largely due to the diverse, unstructured and informal character of inter-generational healing, inter-generational healers are faced with many challenges including lack of employment opportunities, secretive knowledge, and inappropriate treatment by the government and formal education. Part 3 further argues that government intervention in inter-generational healing threatens the rich and diverse cultural heritage of healing as a result of the assimilation which occurs through systematising and mainstreaming this diverse healing system, and also as a result of the tension and competition created between 'Western Doctors,' 'Ayurveda Doctors' and 'intergenerational healers.' The conclusion of the chapter analyses how inter-generational healing practice could be strengthen in the country in a way where the healing system and the cultural aspects are protected.

Part 1: What is intergenerational healing?

This part of the chapter argues that inter-generational healing is diverse, unstructured, informal and part of the cultural heritage in Sri Lanka. In presenting the argument it is necessary to set out the different 'kinds' of inter-generational healing and attempt to define inter-generational healing. It is then necessary to discuss the nature of inter-generational healing. Case studies are used to understand what 'inter-generational healing is.'

As defined in Chapter 3, inter-generational healing practices can be broadly defined as 'beliefs, knowledge and practices of local and indigenous community in Sri Lanka that have been used in healing through medical practices and have been passed down from generation to generation.' This is not always from parents to children. Sometimes the knowledge is passed down from an uncle, aunt, grandparents or a healer without a family lineage. Although inter-generational healing is known as beliefs, knowledge and practices of local and indigenous community, due to government interventions in regulating the knowledge, it is very much influenced by Ayurveda. There are diverse forms of inter-generational healing practices. Even within a practice, there is diversity. Some of the inter-generational healing systems practiced in Sri Lanka, as identified in Chapter 3 include:[1]

- *Sarvanga* (are physicians. It includes arthritis, diabetes, blood pressure, dysentery, fever, typhoid, haemorrhoids, goitre diseases,

[1] The list of healing practices is based on healing practices I came across during field research, the healing practices listed in Institute of Indigenous Medicine 'Deshiya Chikithsa' http://iim.cmb.ac.lk/ayurveda/deshiya-chikithsa, (last retrieved 4 September 2015) and Gampaha Wickramarachchi Ayurveda Institute 'Deshiya Chikithsa' http://www.kln.ac.lk/institutes/wickramarachchi/ (last retrieved 20 February 2019).

stokes and paralysis. Some Sarvanga physicians specialise in treating one or few forms of these diseases);[2]

- *Kadum Bidum* (orthopaedic);[3]
- *Akshi Roga* (eye disease);[4]
- *Devum Pilissum* (traditional treatment for burns); [5]
- *Visa* (Toxicology);[6]
- *Peenasa* (sinusitis);[7]
- *Vata Roga* (is one of the three doshas in Ayurveda, condensed from the elements air and space. It is the principle of kinetic energy in the body, is concerned with the nervous system and with circulation, movement and pathology, and is eliminated from the body through defecation);[8]
- *Gedi Vana Pilika Chikitsa* (wound management);[9]

---

[2] H. D. Karunawathie (#53) practices general *Sarvanga*. R. M. D. J. Gunasekera (# 58) is specialised in diabetics, cholesterol and pressure. Wanasinghe Mudianselage Sudu Banda (#59) is specialised in stroke and paralysis.

[3] *Kadum Bidum* inter-generational healers interviewed include Sunil Shantha (#25); W. M. Anulawathie (#56), R.V. Piyadasa (#55), Ariya (#84), S. M. K. Nimal Karunarathne (#93), R.A. Sudath Priyantha (#94), Sandan (#106).

[4] Healing system practiced by S. K. Liyanarachchige (# 27) and P. Weerasinghe (# 52).

[5] Based on the Deshiya Chikitsa subjects covered for the Course Curriculum for Bachelor of Ayurveda Medicine and Surgery (2011) at the Institute of Indigenous Medicine of the University of Colombo, p76 See http://iim.cmb.ac.lk/wp-content/uploads/2010/08/BAMS-CURRICULUM-2011.pdf (last retrieved 20 February 2019)

[6] *Visa* healers interviewed include Rathnawathie (#29); W. A. Kusuma Wijesekera (#32); S.D.M. Mahipala (#51); Ven. Kapugama Somalankara (#54).

[7] Based on the Deshiya Chikitsa subjects covered for the Course Curriculum for Bachelor of Ayurveda Medicine and Surgery (2011) at the Institute of Indigenous Medicine of the University of Colombo, p76 See http://iim.cmb.ac.lk/wp-content/uploads/2010/08/BAMS-CURRICULUM-2011.pdf (last retrieved 20 February 2019)

[8] Explained by Dr. E. A.S.C.S. Edirisuriya (#7) and Dr. M. Chithra Nalini (#8) *Vata Roga* is also a Deshiya Chikitsa subject covered for the Course Curriculum for Bachelor of Ayurveda Medicine and Surgery (2011) at the Institute of Indigenous Medicine of the University of Colombo, p76 See http://iim.cmb.ac.lk/wp-content/uploads/2010/08/BAMS-CURRICULUM-2011.pdf (last retrieved 20 February 2019)

[9] Based on The Centre for Traditional Knowledge of University of Kelaniya list of Sir Lanka's indigenous or traditional medicine: See http://www.kln.ac.lk/institutes/wickramarachchi/ayurex2014/ (last retrieved 20 February 2019).

- *Vidum Pilissum* (burning and penetrating skin with special tools);[10]
- *Nila Chikitsa* (accupressure treatment);[11]
- *Adivasi Vedakama* (tribal Medicine);[12]
- *Pashu Chikitsa* (traditional veterinmary medicine);[13]
- *Vrukshayurveda* (traditional treatments for trees and plants).[14]

This list of inter-generational healing highlights the diversity within and between inter-generational healing practices. For example, there are many forms of Sarvanga healers in the country. While some Sarvanga healers treat all bodily disorders[15] others specialise in one or few forms of ailment such as diabetes, kidney problems, pressure, cholesterol and arthritis,.[16] The treatments given by traditional eye healers as well as the forms of disease or defects treated by the eye healers differ from one traditional practice to another.[17] *Kadum bidum*, the indigenous method of orthopaedics also has different schools.[18] Although the treatment method

---

[10] Based on The Centre for Traditional Knowledge of University of Kelaniya list of Sir Lanka's indigenous or traditional medicine: See http://www.kln.ac.lk/institutes/wickramarachchi/ayurex2014/ (last retrieved 20 February 2019).

[11] Healing system practiced by R. M. Premachandra (#113).

[12] Healing system practiced by the Vaddha Community of Sri Lanka comes under this category. VishwakeerthiVanaspathi UruWalige Wanniya Attho (#18).

[13] Ajith Liyanage (#96) practice healing for elephants. The Centre for Traditional Knowledge of University of Kelaniya also list *Pashu Chikitsa* in the list of Sir Lanka's indigenous or traditional medicine: See http://www.kln.ac.lk/institutes/wickramarachchi/ayurex2014/ (last retrieved 20 February 2019).

[14] Based on The Centre for Traditional Knowledge of University of Kelaniya list of Sir Lanka's indigenous or traditional medicine: See http://www.kln.ac.lk/institutes/wickramarachchi/ayurex2014/ (last retrieved 20 February 2019).

[15] For example, Mrs. H. D. Karunawathie (#53) practices Sarvanga for all bodily disorders.

[16] R. M. D. J. Gunasekera (# 58) is specialised in diabetics, cholesterol and pressure. Mr. Wanasinghe Mudiyanselage Sudu Banda is specialised in stroke and paralysis.

[17] Dr. P. Weerasinghe (# 52), a very famous eye healer in Anuradhapura who treats eye patients by applying medicine to the toes and Dr. S. K. Liyanarachchige (# 27) traditional eye healier practicing at Aparakka Ayurveda Hospital in Matara Dr. Liyanarachi applies oils, ointments directly to the eyes.

[18] Horiwila Kadum Bidum (Mr. S.M. K. Nimal Karunarathne (#93), Mr. R. A. Sudath Priyantha (#94) and Mr. S. M. H. Seneviratne (#95), Eladuwe Kadum Bidum (Mr. R. V. Piyadasa (#57)), Pallewela Kadum Bidum

followed by different schools of *Kadum bidum* is quite similar in the sense that they demobilise the limb with the fracture or dislocation, apply oil and tie it with a medicinal bandage, *thel paththuva,* then this bandage is removed in 2-3 days and observed to see whether there are any changes in the alignment; then the *thel paththuva* is repeated. The oil and the herbal pack used by different schools differ.[19]

The diversity and the characteristics of inter-generational healing is shown by interviews with healers. The following are two case studies of *Visha Vaidya* (poison healer) Rathnawathie, and *Ansha Baga Vaidya* (stroke and paralysis healer) Wanasinghe Mudiyansalage Sudu Banda that illustrate the diverse forms of acquiring knowledge, the informal, unstructured nature of inter-generational healing and cultural beliefs associated with the healing practices. The third case study of *Kadum Bidum* healer, Sunil Shantha reflects on some of the intangible cultural heritage aspect of inter-generational healing practice.

1.1 *Visha Vaidya* (Poison healer) Rathnawathie

Rathnnawathie[20] hails from a family of healers where the healing lineage can be traced back to ancient times. Their inter-generational healing specialty is treatment for poison. Rathnawathie has acquired the healing knowledge by observing and helping her father since childhood.[21] The training Rathnawathie has received as a poison healer has involved learning how to make poison (from organic, mineral compounds, and words – mantra) and to get the poison out of the body using organic, mineral compounds and words- mantra.[22] The type of treatment is decided by observing the symptoms and understanding the type of poison.[23] The *manthra* are based on Buddhism and Hinduism. Some symptoms of being

(http://pallewelaayurvedic.com/ (last retrieved 20 February 2019) are some of the famous inter-generational schools of Kadum Bidum. There are many inter-generational practitioners of Kadum Bidum without a specific name for the school of practice. For example Mr. Sunil Shantha (#25), Mr. Sandan (#106), Mrs. W. M. Anulawathie (#56), Ariya Vedamahathaya (#84).

[19] Based on the explanation of the practice of *Kadum Bidum* by healers: Mr. S.M. K. Nimal Karunarathne (#93), Mr. R. A. Sudath Priyantha (#94) and Mr. S. M. H. Seneviratne (#95), Mr. R. V. Piyadasa (#57), Mr. Sandan (#106), Mrs. W. M. Anulawathie (#56), Ariya Vedamahathaya (#84), Mr. Sunil Shantha (#25).

[20] Rathnawathie (# 29), practices as a 'Special Doctor' in the district hospital, Trincomalee, in the Eastern Province of Sri Lanka.

[21] Rathnawathie (# 29).

[22] Rathnawathie (# 29).

[23] Rathnawathie (# 29).

poisoned are constant stomach aches, dehydration, headaches and backaches.[24] She can heal all forms of poison: the poison as a result of animal bites, food poisoning, or evil acts performed by humans (*kodi vina, hooniyam).*[25] Rathnawathie believes:

> one can acquire knowledge on sicknesses, methods of diagnosis, and ways of preparing medicine by learning from a text book or a teacher, but becoming a full-fledged healer is much more than learning. One who aspires to be a healer should be blessed with healing hands from birth. He/she should possess loving kindness to other human beings and a sixth sense to understand the illness, the cause and how to cure it. A healer should experience the nature and develop a strong understanding of different forms of plants, places they grow, the medicinal value of the plant based on the environment it grows in (the proximity to other plants, mineral contents of the soils, etc.). Some healers although belonging to healing families and having access to learn the traditional knowledge, are not interested in experiencing and experimenting with the nature, nor do they possess the power and qualities needed for healing.[26]

Rathnawathie has identified her son (16 years-old), as possessing healing attributes.[27] She has started training him to take this traditional healing knowledge forwards to the next generation. Changing social circumstances and economics have caused Rathnawathie to change the cultural practice of healing, where the service is offered freely to charge a fee from the patients. She says that although her father and other ancestors did not demand money for their treatment now it is not possible to afford to practice without charging a fee, as the healers need money to survive and to make the medicine.[28] Rathnawathie charges a nominal price for treatment but for the poor she gives treatment for free.[29]

The nature of the healing practiced by Rathnawathie is elaborated in the story she shares as her first experience as a healer:

> One night, when I was 15 years, two people came to our home saying that a young man in our village had passed away and they were preparing for the funeral. We were living in a very rural village, and we were the only healing family. My father and my brother who were the only practicing healers at that time were out of the village for few weeks. As a result,

---

[24]Rathnawathie (# 29).
[25]Rathnawathie (# 29).
[26]Rathnawathie (# 29).
[27]Rathnawathie (# 29).
[28]Rathnawathie (# 29).
[29]Rathnawathie (# 29).

> without consulting us, they had taken the patient to the nearest hospital, where they had certified the patient as dead. Yet, my conscious said, I will be able to give life to this man. It was about 10 at night. The messengers accompanied me to the patient's house that was few kilometres away, by foot. As soon as I saw the patient, I realised the patient had been poisoned by a human spell (*visa badala*). The spell had affected the head and the throat. He has been unconscious for 24 hours and the black pupil in the eyes wasn't there and his body was cold and stiff like a log. The family has already given up hope with the patient and was preparing for the funeral.
>
> I requested five people to gather forty-eight ingredients to make the medicine. I wanted them to bring the ingredients before the sun rose. While they got the ingredients, I shaved the patient's head. Then I made the body sit up. As the body was like a log, it was hard to do so. However, we kept him against a wall. Then I asked them to burn 25 coconut shells with palm leaves, in close proximity to the body. After the ingredients were brought, I mixed appropriate quantities and prepared a paste. Afterwards, I marked four lines on top of the head. Blood started pouring out like water. The paste was kept on the head. Saliva came out of the mouth and he started sweating. He regained consciousness and I continued to treat him for 7 days. What I did was I got the poison out of the head (*visa bassuwa*).
>
> The Western doctors do not understand the impact of the *Visa bandanaya*,[30] and what areas it affects and how to get it out of the system. This event was my coronation as a healer. Since then, I was also well-respected and became popular as a healer.[31]

Rathnawathie's case illustrates a number of key aspects: how she has acquired the knowledge of healing inter-generationally from her father, her belief that a healer should possess healing attributes to practice healing, Rathnawathie's ambition to pass down the inter-generational practice of healing to her son, how changing social circumstances and economics have caused Rathnawathie to change the cultural practice of healing, and the nature of the healing practice practiced by Rathnawathie. The next case study also reveals the diverse, informal nature of the practice of inter-generational healing.

---

[30] *Visa Bandanaya* refers to human spell.

[31] Rathnawathie (# 29).

1.2 *Ansha Baga Vaidya* (Stroke and Paralysis healer) Wanasinghe Mudiyansalage Sudu Banda

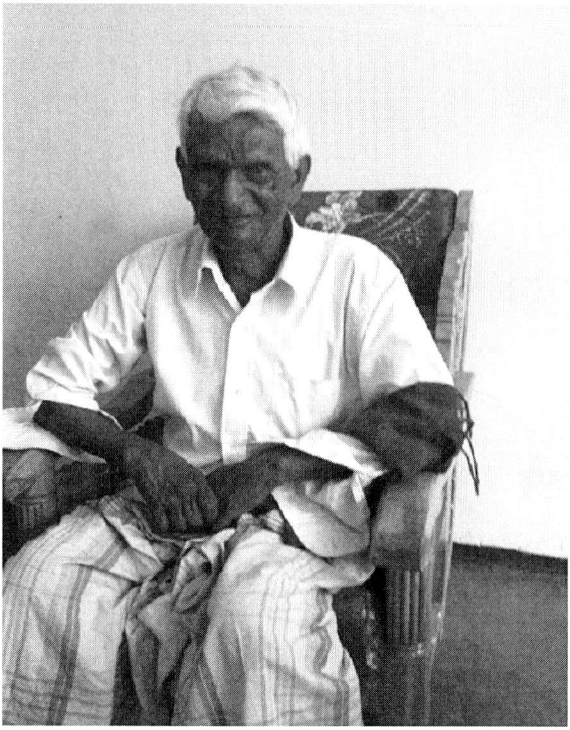

Figure 6.1 - Indigenous Healer Wanasinghe Mudiyanselage Sudu Banda at his home. Image taken by Author.

Wanasinghe Mudiyansalage Sudu Banda in Figure 6.1,[32](hereafter referred to as Sudu Banda) has learnt traditional stroke and paralysis healing by studying under a practitioner monk for ten years. Although in Sudu Banda's case the indigenous healing practice is not passed down from family lineage, it has been passed down from one generation to another, also possesses the informal, unstructured characteristics, and is part of the cultural heritage. I am discussing Sudu Banda's case, therefore, as an inter-generational healing

[32] Based on the interview Wansinghe Mudiyanselage Sudu Banda (# 59), Healer specialised in – stroke and paralysis, Siri Siddhartha Oushadalaya Maligathanna, Pattiyegedera in Sabaragamuwa Province.

method because of the similarities it shares with diverse cases of inter-generational healing.[33]

Sudu Banda is a renowned healer for stroke and paralysis who has cured thousands of patients during 59 years of service.

Sudu Banda says:

> Like a child learns in school, systematically we learn this specialty, as we grow, we learn more about sicknesses, we refer to the book *Madavi* to learn to identify various sicknesses, and another book *Siri Siddhartha* to learn about various medicines. We master the knowledge and practice of healing by continuing in the practice and our experiments every day.[34]

Sudu Banda learned the art of healing strokes and paralysis from a Buddhist monk, fifty years ago. Explaining the healing knowledge Sudu Banda says:

> The subject of healing and the skills one needs to master to practice as a healer is vast. This knowledge and skills cannot be mastered by reading books. One should develop a strong sense of understanding of healing, how human bodies work, nature including plants and minerals and their effects on human body.[35]

In order to grasp the knowledge of healing, Sudu Banda believes one should be in a Pirivena (a place of learning for Buddhist Monks) or understudy the healing master for at least 8 to 10 years. 'Traditional medicine comes down from generations, but is also taught in the 'Pirivena' by learned Buddhist monks'[36] says Sudu Banda. There are many 'Pirivena' which teach medicine.

Sudu Banda lives in a remote area in the hill country, which is barely accessible with public transport, yet his patients for *Ansabaga* treatment (stroke and paralysis) come from all over the island. Sudu Banda says he has cured thousands of patients of stroke and paralysis during the 59 years of his service.[37] Although Sudu Banda's specialty is *Ansabaga*, he would treat any patient who comes for Sarvanga treatment (any form of

---

[33] Similarities Sudu Banda's case shares with inter-generational practices such as Rathnawathie (#29), W. A. Kusuma Wijesekera (#32), S. D. M. Mahipala (#51), P. Weerasinghe (#52), H. D. Karunawathie (#53), W. M. Anulawathie (#56), R. V. Piyadasa (#57), R. M. D. J. Gunasekera (#58), Ariya (84), Sandan (#106), T. Herath Banda (# 108), include knowledge being passed down from one generation to another, informal and unstructured characteristics.

[34] Wansinghe Mudiyanselage Sudu Banda (# 59).

[35] Wansinghe Mudiyanselage Sudu Banda (# 59).

[36] Wansinghe Mudiyanselage Sudu Banda (# 59).

[37] Wansinghe Mudiyanselage Sudu Banda (# 59).

bodily disorder).[38] Sudu Banda's patients for other bodily disorders come from the local community.[39]

Sudu Banda prepares some of the medicines at home, while some medicines he prescribes he requests the patients to prepare by instructing them on the ways of finding the herbs, the exact quantities required and the method of preparation. Sudu Banda says:

> The oils are prepared by grinding medicinal herbs and straining the water out, and then after adding other medicines, you leave the moisture to vaporise and collect the remaining oil. '*Arishta*' is prepared by grinding all the medicines together, mixing with water and boiling it to ¼ its original level of water.[40]

Sudu Banda believes medicine alone cannot cure Ansabaga. Proper diet and healthy life style also should be adopted. Sudu Banda says he finds the herbs for the medicine from the jungles or purchases them from herbal shops.[41] He charges a nominal fee for the oils and *Arishta* he prepares in order to cover the cost.[42]

In order to secure the traditional knowledge of healing Sudu Banda agrees that he must share his knowledge with interested disciple(s). He says he has groomed one healer who is practicing the profession now. Sudu Banda is not interested in teaching the healing practice in formal educational institutes. He says, 'students need to be mentored in healing, not taught by giving lectures.'[43]

Despite being 85 years-old, Sudu Banda still practices daily at his healing centre, treats patients who come to his home after hours and also looks after his fields, which are his main source of livelihood.[44] Although Sudu Banda has adopted a simple lifestyle, he practices healing as an honorary profession rather than a means for survival.[45]

Sudu Banda's case reveals how he has learnt the indigenous tradition of healing by understudying a monk for ten years. Although his healing practice was not passed down from family lineage, due to the similar characteristics it shares, such as being passed down from one person to another, informal, unstructured and being part of the cultural heritage, Sudu

[38] Wansinghe Mudiyanselage Sudu Banda (# 59).
[39] Wansinghe Mudiyanselage Sudu Banda (# 59).
[40] Wansinghe Mudiyanselage Sudu Banda (# 59).
[41] Wansinghe Mudiyanselage Sudu Banda (# 59).
[42] Wansinghe Mudiyanselage Sudu Banda (# 59).
[43] Wansinghe Mudiyanselage Sudu Banda (# 59).
[44] Wansinghe Mudiyanselage Sudu Banda (# 59).
[45] Wansinghe Mudiyanselage Sudu Banda (# 59).

Banda's practice of healing can be categorised as inter-generational healing. Another feature revealed in Sudu Banda's case is the continued practice of healing as an honorary profession rather than charging a fixed amount, despite the fact that the income from this inter-generational healing practice is not sufficient for a livelihood. The next case study focuses on the intangible cultural heritage aspect of inter-generational healing.

1.3 *Kadum Bidum* healer, Sunil Shantha

Due to the traditional knowledge, practices, expression and skills[46] aspects of inter-generational healing, it realises a part of Sri Lanka's intangible cultural heritage.[47] *Kadum Bidum* healer, Sunil Shantha reflects on some of the intangible cultural heritage aspects of inter-generational healing practice:

> *Kadum Bidum* treatment has a medicinal and spiritual component to it. The medicine is prepared using herbs and a mantra. When preparing an oil, powder or a paste for treatment, you first look at an auspicious time (*nakath kalaya*), then using *mantra* you give life to the medicinal preparation (*jeewan karanawa/ dahan karanawa*).[48]

Sunil explains the need for purity and precautions in preparing medicinal oils:

> When making medicine, we have to protect the oils from spirits. There are negative effects of spirits (*bhootha balapaam*) on oils. So, we have to be very careful in the process of oil refinery to taking it off the stove. The spirits can get into the oil (*piliya ahu wenawa*) and topple the oil pot or lose the effectiveness of the oil. In order to protect the oil from getting caught by the *piliya*, the healer should be very clean and avoid impurities

---

[46] *UNESCO Convention for Safeguarding the Intangible Cultural Heritage (2003), A 2 (1)* the definition of 'intangible cultural heritage' includes 'the practices, representations, expressions, knowledge, skills – as well as the instruments, objects, artefacts and cultural spaces associated therewith – that communities, groups and, in some cases, individuals recognize as part of their cultural heritage. This intangible cultural heritage, transmitted from generation to generation, is constantly recreated by communities and groups in response to their environment, their interaction with nature and their history, and provides them with a sense of identity and continuity, thus promoting respect for cultural diversity and human creativity.'

[47] Also known as living heritage. See UNESCO 'Intangible Cultural Heritage' http://en.unesco.org/themes/intangible-cultural-heritage (last retrieved 20 February 2019).

[48] Sunil Shantha (# 25).

> (*killi*). That is, he/she should bathe before preparing the medicine, should not consume any meats, fish or alcohol, cannot visit funerals or puberty parties, and if it is a woman they should not prepare medicine when she has her menstruation.[49]

Sunil elaborates his experience of growing up in a healing family. He says:

> I was exposed to the healing practice since early childhood. As a child I was inducted to the different types of herbs, how to find them in the jungle, how and at what time to pick them and ways to pick. The real herbs can be identified only by the indigenous healer who has experience. Commercially manufactured Ayurveda healing products do not have the same effect as the medicine carefully prepared at home, considering the quality and value of the herbs as well as the spiritual influences. I also learnt how to diagnose the patients, how to treat them and how to talk to them by observing my grandfather and father. Learning to be a healer is a life-time of learning. It is hard to practice indigenous healing only through the knowledge gathered through books.[50]

Sunil highlights some of the traditional cultural aspects attached to the inter-generational healing practice, such as having a medical as well as spiritual component, the role of beliefs in the practice of healing and how the knowledge is acquired informally from the family background.

Part 2: Challenges for Inter-generational Healers

This part of the chapter argues that inter-generational healers are faced with many challenges. As we will see these challenges include lack of employment opportunities, secretive knowledge, inappropriate treatment by the government, and formal education for recognition. Each of these challenges will be discussed in turn.

2.1 Limited employment opportunities

A lack of employment opportunities has challenged the survival of inter-generational healing and practices. There are many causes that have threatened the employment opportunities of the inter-generational healers. These include, with the past influence of caste-based social system[51] healers

---

[49] Sunil Shantha (# 25).

[50] Sunil Shantha (# 25).

[51] Caste is a system of social stratification. It is characterized by endogamy, hereditary transmission of a lifestyle including an occupation, ritual status in a hierarchy and customary social interaction and exclusion based on cultural notions of purity and

considered healing as a duty, an honorary act or act that is performed in addition to their regular means of income. With the adoption of capitalist economy[52] and changes in social systems to a class-based social system,[53] the idea of reciprocating healing via formalising, structuring[54] and monetary payments has caused a debate over healing. That is whether healing should exist as disinterested, selfless and pure act or whether it should emerge as an interested, selfish, impure act. For traditional healers the act of healing needs to be disinterested, informal and pure for it to be effective, and they consciously contrast with the healing of those who charge money, who they say are ultimately acting out of self-interest.[55] Due to these controditional ideologies healers are faced with limited employment opportunities and the subsequent struggle for survival. This section focuses on two case studies: S. D. M. Mahipala and W. M. Anulawathie.

S. D. M. Mahipala[56] in Figure 5.2 is an inter-generational healer for poisoning from animals (specialised in *Jalabithika*[57] *and Sarpavisha).*[58] His case provides an example of the limited employment opportunities for healers such as him. More specifically it shows how S. D. M. Mahipala has struggled to secure a means of livelihood from inter-generational healing

---

pollution. (Scott and Marshall: 2005: p 66)- Sri Lanka's caste system had a service and occupational role. Traditional knowledge on occupation was passed down from generation to generation based on the caste system.

[52] Capitalist economy is a system of private ownership of capital and production of goods and services for profit. For more on capitalist economy and impact on society see, Braudel (1982-4), de Soto (2000), Sayer (1991), Wood (1999), Chandler (1990), Coates (2000), Gray (1998), Shiva (2000), Fulcher (2004).

[53] A class based society is divided according to social, economic and educational status. (Princeton University. Social Class- http://wordnetweb.princeton.edu/perl/webwn?s=social+class&sub=Search+WordNet&o2=&o0=1&o8=1&o1=1&o7=&o5=&o9=&o6=&o3=&o4=&h=0 (last retrieved 20 February 2019) Hereditary transmission of a lifestyle does not play an important role in a class based society.

[54] Here formal, structured health care systems are healing systems that have codified the knowledge, that have a formal curriculum for training, and knowledge available to public regardless of family heritage. Examples of such healing systems in Sri Lanka are Ayurveda, Siddha, Unani, Homeopathy and Acupuncture. Inter-generational healing remains informal and unstructured due to the diverse form of knowledge, knowledge not been systematically documented or codified and limits in access to knowledge.

[55] The distinction of acts along these polarized lines is an outcome of Capitalism. Parry (1986).

[56] S. D. M. Mahipala (# 51).

[57] *Jalabithika* treatment refers to treatment for dog bites.

[58] *Sarpavisha* treatment is treatment for serpent poisoning.

that had resulted in looking for alternative means of earning and has threatened the continuation of his inter-generational healing practice.

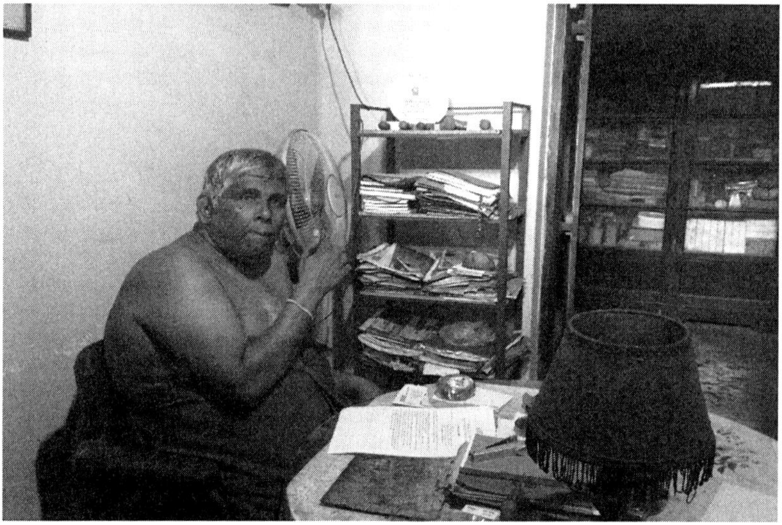

Figure 5.2 - S. D. M. Mahipala, Indigenous healer for Jalabithika and Sarpavisha at his healing centre in Yakkala. Image taken by Author

Mahipala is continuing the ancestral practice he has learnt from his aunt and uncle and treats patients with poisoning from all forms of animal bites.[59] His most popular treatments are for rabies (*Jalabithika*) and reptile bites (Sarpavisa). According to Mahipala:

> humans can be infected with the rabies virus from any mammal carrying the virus. Most common rabies transmitters for humans according to my experience is bites of dogs, followed by monkeys, rats and cats. I can identify the animal that has bitten by looking at the wound, the pulse and the physical characteristics of the patient. The '*Vattoru*', (medicines) differ according to the type of bite, the different age groups, physical characteristics and the symptoms of the patient.[60]

Mahipala says, one needs to have a good understanding of the sickness, causes for sickness and remedies in order to practice healing.[61]

---

[59] S. D. M. Mahipala (# 51).
[60] S. D. M. Mahipala (# 51).
[61] S. D. M. Mahipala (# 51).

Due to the dilemma of financial stability and his ideology of practicing indigenous healing as a form of social service, Mahipala has had to depend on other forms of income to make a living.[62] Mahipala is engaged in a ceremony furniture renting business. As part of the business, he has to attend funerals. As a result of the *killi* (impurity) he cannot chant certain *gatha* and *mantra that* he needs to chant to prepare medicine or to treat patients until three days after attending a funeral.[63] Avoiding *killi* is a requirement for the indigenous medical practice. If he breaks these rules, and disregards these basic practices Mahipala says the patients can be affected negatively.[64] Mahipala's healing practice has severely been affected due to his livelihood.[65]

Explaining the changes in society and how it had impacted on Mahipala's practice of healing, he says:

> In the ancient times up to the twentieth century due to the scarcity of Western medical systems to treat all forms of animal bites and the painful process, many people sought the indigenous medical option. Those days herbs for medicines were also freely available. Now it is different, the Western medical practice is flourishing and there is easy access, effective and painless methods of treatment for animal bites.[66]

Elaborating on difficulties of sustaining indigenous healing practice Mahipala says:

> Now there is a practical difficulty to give indigenous medical treatment as well. There is no government patronage to the indigenous medical practice. If a patient seeks help of the indigenous healer as the last resort (which is the usual case) and dies under the supervision of the healer, the healer is held responsible. The healer can even be remanded for this.[67]

The inter-generational medical practice is being destroyed because due to current socio-economic conditions the practitioners seek financial stability in the inter-generational healing profession whereas traditionally this was practiced as an honorary profession. Mahipala believes that this should not be the case, and that indigenous healing should be practiced as a

---

[62] S. D. M. Mahipala (# 51).
[63] S. D. M. Mahipala (# 51).
[64] S. D. M. Mahipala (# 51).
[65] S. D. M. Mahipala (# 51).
[66] S. D. M. Mahipala (# 51).
[67] S. D. M. Mahipala (# 51). As per the *Ayurveda Act, s 67*, it is only the registered Ayurveda practitioners (here the legal definition cover registered inter-generational healers) will have legal protection.

form of social service.[68] If the financial states of the indigenous medical professionals are secured there is a chance for genuine practitioners to flourish.[69]

Mahipala regrets he has not been able to transmit his knowledge of healing to anybody. He has only been able to share a little bit of his knowledge with one of his nephews.[70] But unfortunately none of the family show any interest in learning the traditional knowledge or practices of the profession due to its financial instability as well as the current low status of social recognition for indigenous healing.[71]

Another case that portrays difficulties of economic survival in practicing inter-generational healing is the case of W. M. Anulawathie[72] in Figure 5.3, who practices treatment for *Iru Rudhawa* (headaches due to the effects of the sun) and *Kadum Bidum* (orthopedics).

Anulawathie's sole intention in being an indigenous healer practicing treatment for *Kadum Bidum* and *Iru Rudawa* is to be of use to people and to obtain merit for the good deeds.[73] She has learnt the practice from her mother.[74] Daily she treats about 7-8 patients. She can cure a sprained ankle within 6 treatments and headaches due to the effects of the sun within three days.[75]

Anulawathie finds the required ingredients for the medicine from the jungle and makes the medicines by mixing the ingredients and chanting *mantra*.[76] When preparing medicine, the *mantra* has to be chanted before the cock crows in the morning. She does not charge money for the treatment.[77] Even when she receives a gift of money, she uses it for religious purposes, or to make the medicine, but not for her personal use.[78] She believes healing should be practiced only as a service not as a living.[79] Due to this mentality, she lives in poverty and is totally dependent on her son for support for daily living.[80] Knowing the limited economic benefits of traditional healing, Anulawathie's son shows no interest in learning healing

---

68 S. D. M. Mahipala (# 51).
69 S. D. M. Mahipala (# 51).
70 S. D. M. Mahipala (# 51).
71 S. D. M. Mahipala (# 51).
72 W. M. Anulawathie, (# 56).
73 W. M. Anulawathie, (# 56).
74 W. M. Anulawathie, (# 56).
75 W. M. Anulawathie, (# 56).
76 W. M. Anulawathie, (# 56).
77 W. M. Anulawathie, (# 56).
78 W. M. Anulawathie, (# 56).
79 W. M. Anulawathie, (# 56).
80 W. M. Anulawathie, (# 56).

for a profession.[81] She has not written down or passed her knowledge on healing to anyone. As Anulawathie says, 'When I die, there's nobody to continue this profession.'[82]

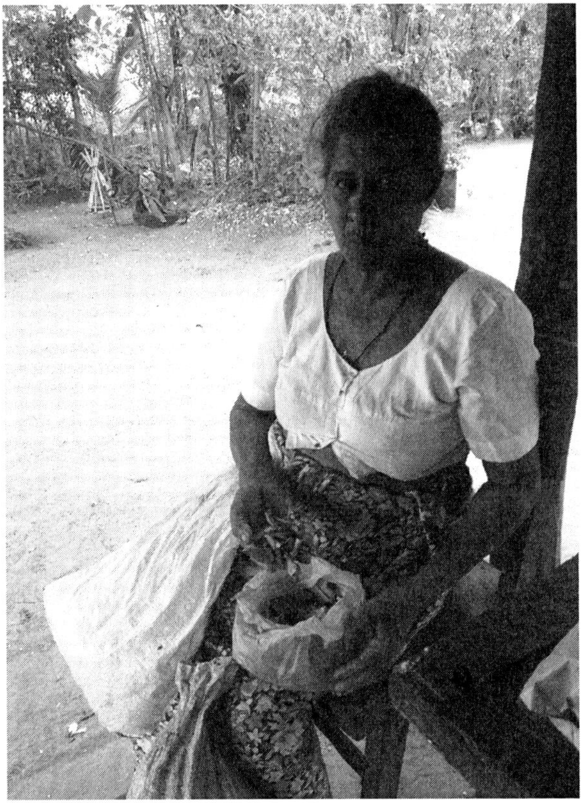

Figure 5.3 – W. M. Anulawathie holding herbal ingredients collected from the jungle. Image taken by Authour

Mahipala and Anulawathie's cases portray some of the causes for lack of economically productive employment opportunities. These include a clash in ideologies between disinterested vs. interested, informal vs. formal and pure vs. impure. This is due in large part to the influence of capitalist values of responding to healing. The two case studies have

[81] W. M. Anulawathie, (# 56).
[82] W. M. Anulawathie, (# 56).

portrayed how changes in ideologies have further threatened employment opportunities for traditional healers by showing how inter-generational healing was previously regarded as an honorary profession to a society but now where the healer cannot exist without giving a monetary value for their services, difficulties of finding herbs for medicinc, recognition and prominence given to biomedicine and no appropriate government patronage. The following section provides an exploration of the secretive nature of inter-generational healing practices

2.2 Secretive Knowledge

Inter-generational knowledge is considered a secretive knowledge system that is passed down to the identified inherent from generation to generation. Sometimes the knowledge is also passed down from a healing monk, or inter-generational healer to a carefully identified student without family lineage[83] but even in this case, the healer is expected to protect the knowledge system. Protecting the secret knowledge system has made it possible to keep these knowledge systems alive for many generations. These secret inter-generational knowledge systems worked well when the caste system was alive in Sri Lanka as families followed the family trade for livelihood. In an open economic social system where the caste does not have a significant impact on career and where the knowledge systems are formalised and accessible to all interested persons; Where the price of a good or service is determined by the market, the efforts on protecting secretive knowledge is no longer a viable option. Yet, the interviews with the inter-generational healers clearly portray their commitment towards safeguarding their secretive knowledge.

In R. M. D. J. Gunasekera's family, out of the six children, only Gunasekera has received the blessings to practice healing.[84] He has learned the healing practice from his father, who started practicing in 1975.[85] Gunasekera agrees that the main cause for the decline of inter-generational indigenous healing system is because the ancestors did not let the secrets of the medical systems out of the family.[86] Yet he says, 'even I will train only one person, my child to take this specialty forward'[87] as he believes this

[83] For example, it was a healing monk that inducted Wansinghe Mudiyanselage Sudu Banda to inter-generational knowledge. (Wansinghe Mudiyanselage Sudu Banda # 59).

[84] R. M. D. J. Gunasekera (# 58).

[85] R. M. D. J. Gunasekera (# 58).

[86] R. M. D. J. Gunasekera (# 58).

[87] R. M. D. J. Gunasekera (# 58).

profession should be carried out very carefully with a dedication towards wellbeing and respect towards family traditions.[88] Gunasekera does not like to lecture on the treatment methods he practices in a formal or informal institute or gathering because he cannot reveal the secrets of the medicines, that he has promised his forefathers not to reveal, and he cannot discuss the subject matter with an audience without revealing the secrets.[89]

The need to protect secrecy of traditional knowledge is endorsed by H. D. Karunawathie:

> In order to protect traditional knowledge in healing, its secrecy should be maintained and should be carefully handed down to a person in the next generation who is willing to respect the traditions and customs followed for many generations.[90]

As Gunasekera and Karunawathie articulate, they are determined to protect the traditional knowledge in healing as a secretive knowledge. Keeping it as a secretive knowledge, however, limits the possibilities of formalisation, independent testing of its veracity and making it available in the mainstream for anyone interested in pursuing it. The secretive and informal nature of the knowledge and passing it down from generation to generation is the cultural heritage aspect of traditional knowledge. Revealing the secrets also threatens the cultural heritage aspect of the practice of inter-generational healing.

2.3 Inappropriate Treatment by the Government

Another threat to intergenerational healing comes from limited, or non-existent government recognition, support and regulation. As Chapter 4 has portrayed government focus is mostly on Ayurveda and there is a trend of Ayurvedisation of inter-generational healing systems due to government sponsored training schemes and the registration scheme introduced to register inter-generational healers (traditional healers as called by the government). In this part, I will start with R. M. D. J. Gunasekera's views on reasons for inappropriate government treatment, then discuss the role of Ayurveda Sanrakshana Sabhawa, registration of inter-generational healers and discriminatory treatment towards Special Doctors in government hospitals to portray the inappropriate treatment by the government that have

---

[88] R. M. D. J. Gunasekera (# 58).
[89] R. M. D. J. Gunasekera (# 58).
[90] H. D. Karunawathie (# 53).

threated the inter-generational healing and the cultural heritage aspect of healing.

Inter-generational healer R. M. D. J. Gunasekera gives three reasons for inter-generational medical systems to be disregarded:

i. the privileges and recognition given to the biomedical profession;
ii. the healing systems promoted by the Ministry of Indigenous Medicine, such as Ayurveda, Siddha and Unani being systematic and organised;
iii. the opposition within the community where although the inter-generational healers strive to improve their systems of healing, there are people who oppose inter-generational healers.[91]

Gunasekera's views on improving the practice of inter-generational healing is as follows:

> in order to bring our inter-generational forms of healing to a higher level of acceptance we must educate the people more, we must introduce the concepts to the people and instil in them the fact that even though our systems take time, we are able to holistically heal.[92]

Government initiated initiatives to recognise, support and regulate inter-generational healing practices also have not been able to successfully promote and protect the inter-generational healing systems and traditional cultural aspects of healing. Following is a discussion of the case of *Ayurveda Sanrakshana Sabhawa*.

2.3.1 *Ayurveda Sanrakshana Sabhawa*

Ayurveda Sanrakshana Sabhawa (translation – Ayurveda Protection Committee) is a government initiative with the intention of protecting and promoting traditional healing practices and traditional healers. Although *Ayurveda Sanrakshana Sabhawa* is established in good faith, the Committee's name, inefficiency of the activities, lack of commitment of its members and the practical requirement of economic stability criteria to become a member of the district level committee can be seen as challenges in protecting inter-generational healing.

The name itself Is misleading as it refers to 'Ayurveda' not 'traditional healing' or 'inter-generational healing' and most of the members

---

[91] R. M. D. J. Gunasekera (# 58).
[92] R. M. D. J. Gunasekera (# 58).

of this committee are not Ayurveda physicians but inter-generational healers.

Activities conducted by the Committee vary significantly from division to division and district to district based on the commitment of the committee member. The range of activities vary from holding Ayurveda clinics, engaging in social work, to maintaining a funeral fund to support if a healer passes away. Only the members of the committee, in other words, the healers who are registered in this committee, would be considered for funding allocations from the budget, if there are any. From an inter-generational healer's perspective, the main benefit of being a member of the committee is the support it provides during times of hardship.[93]

Most inter-generational healers subscribe to the view that *Ayurveda Sanrakshana Sabhawa* has not been effective in solving the issues of inter-generational healers. This is partially due to lack of commitment of the committee members. There are approximately 200 inter-generational healers in each of the '*District Ayurveda Sanrakshana Sabhawa*' (District Ayurveda Protection Committee) but it is hard to gather at least 10 members to come for a meeting because they would rather stay at home and see patients and derive an income than attend a meeting which they know will not benefit them.[94] Other reasons are difficulties in coming into any agreements and lack of political will in implementing programs based on the decisions of the committee members.[95]

It is noteworthy that economic stability is one of the major requirements for an inter-generational healer to be a representative at the district level Ayurveda Protection Committee. Due to the long distances to travel for meetings, owning a personal vehicle has become an un-written pre-requisite for the inter-generational healer that represents at the district committee.[96] Also a mobile or land phone number is a necessity for the representative due to the need to be contactable.[97] Most inter-generational healers are not in an economically advantageous position to be able to afford personal vehicles or telephones, and therefore as a result of the economics involved in being part of the government decision making process, many inter-generational healers get left out.

Government initiated committees at the divisional, district and national levels to promote and protect traditional healing systems in Sri

---

[93] P. Weerasinghe (# 52).

[94] This opinion was expressed by many Inter-generational healers belonging to different districts.

[95] Kumari (# 71).

[96] Sunil Shantha (# 25).

[97] Sunil Shantha (# 25).

Lanka could be an effective mechanism if the government was to rethink the name of the committee, its agenda, inclusiveness of healers regardless of economic stability and if there was political will and funding to support the activities of the committees. Yet another challenge for intergenerational healing and healers relates to registration.

2.3.2 Registration of inter-generational healers (as Traditional Healers)

Government requires healers to register with the Ministry of Indigenous Medicine. The criteria set up for registration of inter-generational healers challenges the knowledge base of the inter-generational healers and results in their Ayurvedaisation. As discussed in Chapter 4, under the National Institute of Traditional Medicine, all inter-generational healers are expected to register as traditional healers after passing a test administered by the Ayurveda Medical Council and following a three-day Ayurveda induction programme. Only registered traditional healers can officially practice healing, can have a seal and provide medical certificates.[98] To illustrate issues faced by inter-generational healers in registration, this part will present the views of Sunil Shantha, R. M. D. J. Gunasekera, Karunawathie and Weerasinghe.

Sunil Shantha[99] (Figure 5.4) expresses his view on the exam convened for the registration of traditional healers. He says,

> The exam does not directly test our indigenous healing knowledge; as a result, we had to study Ayurveda. It is only after passing this test on Ayurveda that an indigenous healer can legally register and practice his family traditions. It is ironic that the test does not really test our knowledge in indigenous healing. Of course, the government is not in a position to certify that knowledge as we learnt it from our forefathers and it is not the formal knowledge available in the public domain. Although we get the permission to legally practice our vocation after registering as traditional healers, we do not have any form of job security or retirement allowance by the government.

---

[98] Chapter 5 2.4 has discussed role of Sri Lanka Ayurveda Medical Council in registering Paramparika (traditional) physicians and privileges of registered practitioners.

[99] Sunil Shantha (# 25).

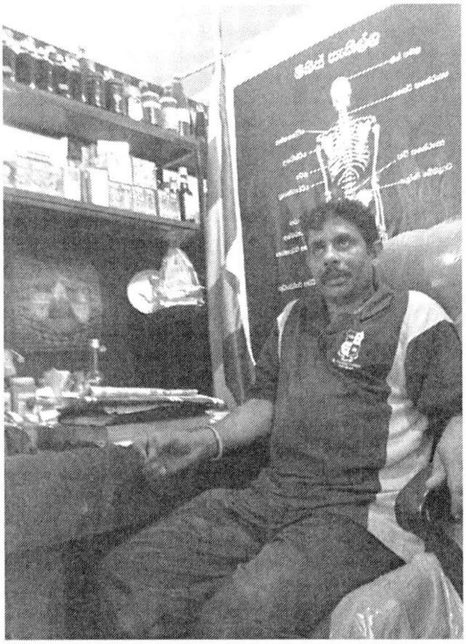

Figure 5.4 - Sunil Shantha, Kadum Bidum healer at his desk. Image taken by Author

R. M. D. J. Gunasekera's view on practicing his inter-generational healing practice as a distinct practice rather than assimilating with Ayurveda and ascribing to government requirements of a healer is not to register. As Gunasekera expresses:

> I am not a registered healer and I do not believe it is necessary to register. My father didn't have the need to be registered and nor do I, we don't seek financial stability nor government recognition through this profession. Our healing systems don't need a law to protect it, if there is no jealousy we can thrive.[100]

Karunawathie[101] is a registered traditional healer.[102] According to her, traditional healers do not get any benefits from the government as a result

[100] R. M. D. J. Gunasekera (# 58).
[101] H. D. Karunawathie (# 53).
[102] A registered traditional healer is a person who is registered with the Ayurveda Medical Council. Documents to be provided for registration are given on http://www.ayurvedicmedicoun.gov.lk/web/index.php?option=com_content&view=article&id=89&Itemid=54&lang=en (last retrieved 20 February 2019).

of being registered. [103] Weerasinghe also subscribes to Karunawathie's view. As he puts it:

> I am registered as a traditional eye healer with the Ayurveda Medical Council. There are no benefits for being registered as an eye healer. It is only the politicians that benefit from the healers. Politicians have given promises for allowances for healers during elections to get the votes of the healers, but these promises are not fulfilled.[104]

The registration program introduced for healers by the Ministry of Indigenous Medicine threatens the healers and their knowledge system by inducting them to Ayurveda and alienating the healers from their inter-generational forms of healing. Also, registration does not bring many additional benefits to the healer. However, what these case studies have not been able to capture is that by registering as a healer, they are some benefits, such as the are government recognition allowing the use of a seal permitting them as being able to issue sick certificates.[105] Unregistered healers do not have formal, government sourced authority to represent as a healer in Sri Lanka.[106] Registered inter-generational[107] healers are entitled to practice Ayurveda,[108] to sue for and recover in due course of law by action in a court of competent jurisdiction any reasonable sum claimed by Ayurveda practitioner as (a) fees for any services rendered or advice given or work done in his professional capacity; (b) charges for any medicine, medicinal preparations or appliances or medicated articles of food or drink, supplied by him; or (c) expenses incurred by him in connection with or for the purposes of the medical treatment of any patient.[109]

---

[103] H. D. Karunawathie (# 53).

[104] P. Weerasinghe (#52).

[105] *Ayurveda Act no 31 of 1961,* art 64 only a registered person can legally practice Ayurveda. Legally practicing Ayurveda includes the privileges of using an official seal and issuing sick certificates.

[106] According to *Ayurveda Act no 31 of 1961,* art 64(1) only a registered ayurvedic practitioner, shall be entitled to use the title "Vaidyacharya" either before or after his name; and art 64(2) states a person who does not abide by the provisions of subsection (1) is committing and offence.

[107] Ayurveda practitioner has been referred to as a generic term in *Ayurveda Act* to refer to all registered doctors and healers registered under the Ayurveda Act. This includes Ayurveda Doctors, Siddha Doctors, Unani Doctors, Homeopathy practitioners, Acupuncture practitioners and registered Intergenerational healers.

[108] *Ayurveda Act,* art 67(1) Here the use of the word 'Ayurveda' is confusing. It not only covers Ayurveda but also other adopted traditional and inter-generational practices of healing recognised by the Government of Sri Lanka.

[109] *Ayurveda Act,* s 67 (2).

2.3.3 Discriminatory Treatment towards 'Special Doctors' in Government Hospitals

In Sri Lanka, healers are given different titles and are treated differently by the Government. Inter-generational healers, for example, are often referred to, and appointed as, 'Special Doctors' in government Ayurveda/ Siddha hospitals.[110] The healers with inter-generational knowledge, who practice in the government hospitals, on temporary contract appointments are called 'Special Doctors.' The appointment of intergenerational healers as 'Special Doctors' is different to the Ayurveda, Siddha, Unani 'doctors' with a university degree, or the 'specialists/consultants' who possess post-graduate qualifications from their field. Although there are provisions to accommodate, traditional healers as Special Doctors, there are only very few healers who practice under this category. The salaries are comparably lower and, in most cases, they are given contracts for part-time consultations not a permanent position. The reasons given by the senior administration in hospitals include, there are not sufficient funding to accommodate such healers and there are only very limited number of patients interested in the services of a Special Doctor.[111] The case study of S. K. Liyanarachchige is presented to portray why and how he has decided to be a Special Doctor and the discriminatory treatment he received.

S. K. Liyanarachige has practiced healing since the 1970's; the main reason that made him interested in applying for a government position is the economic insecurities.[112] Liyanarachige has acquired the inter-generational knowledge of Sarvanga from his father and received mentoring from a Buddhist monk practicing healing for five years.[113] The monk was Liyanarachchige's uncle. Liyanarachchige has practiced as a Sarvanga healer for many years but he has struggled financially.[114] Learning about being a Special Doctor (having a specialisation in one area rather than a general Sarvanga practitioner) he applied for government registration as a Special Doctor (eyes).[115] Afterwards, seeing a paper advertisement for Special Doctors, he applied to Aparaka Ayurveda Hospital in Matara. Liyanarachchige has been employed in the hospital since 2011.[116] He works on a contract and it is not a permanent position like the university qualified

[110] For a discussion see Chapter 4, Part 4: Hospitals and Curative Services.
[111] Dr. Pema Shivashanmugarajah (# 98).
[112] S. K. Liyanarachige (# 27).
[113] S. K. Liyanarachige (# 27).
[114] S. K. Liyanarachige (# 27).
[115] S. K. Liyanarachige (# 27).
[116] S. K. Liyanarachige (# 27).

Ayurveda, Siddha and Unani Doctors.[117] His salary scale is also much lower. [118]

S. K. Liyanarachchige's case demonstrates how due to economic difficulties inter-generational healers seek positions in government hospitals, but do not find job security or similar benefits as the university qualified Doctors.

2.4 Formal Education for Recognition

Obtaining formal education for recognition challenges the informal, unstructured knowledge base of inter-generational healers by inducting them to the formal knowledge of traditional healing, that is mainly Ayurveda and to a lesser extent, Siddha, Unani, homeopathy and acupuncture. In order for the knowledge to be recognised inter-generational healers who have acquired knowledge from family traditions seek formal educational qualifications of a diploma or a degree. Siva Paranasivamullai's[119] case illustrates why he had to obtain formal education to be recognised as a healer.

Siva Paranasivamullai, (Figure 5.5) is a practitioner of Sarvanga healing specialised in rheumatism.[120] Siva comes from a healing background, where he has been mentored in healing from childhood by his parents.[121] For many generations his family members have been practicing Sarvanga healing based on the secret knowledge passed down from generation to generation. His ancestors have not had any formal education in healing.[122] However, due to lack of recognition given to healers with only an inter-generational healing background, Siva's parents have guided him to acquire a formal education in healing in order to be recognised as a healer in today's society.[123] As a young man, after completing high-school, Siva has pursued studies at the Siddha-Ayurveda College in Jaffna because of his passion for healing. He graduated from the college in 1970, and joined the government Ayurveda hospital from 1978 and worked there until the year 2000;then from 2000 to 2008 he has worked as a visiting lecturer at the Siddha-Ayurveda College.[124] Now he practices at home from 6.00am to 9.00am in

---

[117] S. K. Liyanarachige (# 27).
[118] S. K. Liyanarachige (# 27).
[119] S. Paranasivamullai (# 102).
[120] S. Paranasivamullai (# 102).
[121] S. Paranasivamullai (# 102).
[122] S. Paranasivamullai (# 102).
[123] S. Paranasivamullai (# 102).
[124] S. Paranasivamullai (# 102).

the morning and in his dispensary in Jaffna from 4.00pm to 5:30pm in the evening.[125] Siva believes his formal education on Siddha-Ayurveda and working as a lecturer at the Siddha-Ayurveda College has given legitimacy and more recognition for his practices of healing.[126]

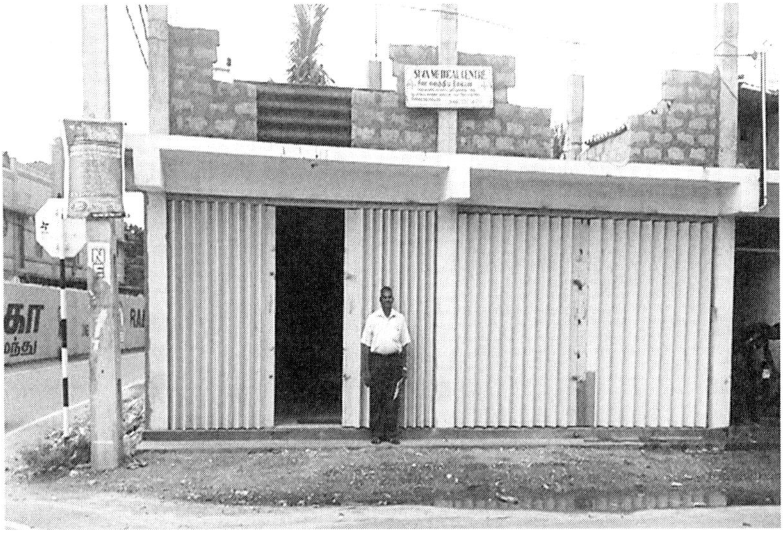

Figure 5.5 - Siva Paranasivamullai in front of his dispensary in Jaffna. Image taken by Author

An interesting revelation in Siva's case is that his formal education in Siddha-Ayurveda medicine had brought recognition for Siva and he has been able to hold government positions as a healer. However, after the training, what Siva has been practicing is the Siddha-Ayurveda medicine from this formal education. Although Siva has continued research and writing on healing, it is based on his formally acquired knowledge in Siddha-Ayurveda. This case study also implies that when an inter–generational healer acquires a formal education in healing, the healer can no longer be called an inter-generational healer.

---

[125] S. Paranasivamullai (# 102).
[126] S. Paranasivamullai (# 102).

Part 3: Impacts of Government intervention on Inter-generational Healing: Assimilation and Loss of Cultural Diversity

The characteristics of and challenges for intergenerational healers discussed in part 2 has portrayed how inter-generational healing is highly fragmented, dispersed, not always documented and most often remains only in the memory of local groups in remote areas. These characteristics and the challenges faced by inter-generational healers have resulted in many consequences such as assimilation and loss of cultural diversity. In part 3, I argue that government intervention in inter-generational healing creates tension and competition between 'Western Doctors', Ayurveda and intergenerational healers[127] As a result, traditional cultural aspects of healing are being threatened in Sri Lanka. To show this, this part shows how healers are forced into Ayurveda. Then a personal experience to illustrate the competition and tension between Western doctors and the inter-generational healers is narrated. A case study of the Vedda community then presents how a naturalisation process and loss of cultural heritage has threated the cultural aspect of healing due to government interventions. Finally, the chapter discusses some possibilities of protecting the cultural heritage of diverse inter-generational healing practices.

3.1 Healers forced in Ayurveda

Inter-generational healers are forced into Ayurveda in direct and indirect ways. Direct ways the Sri Lankan Government force healers into Ayurveda as discussed above include testing the knowledge of Ayurveda in the examination to be recognised as a traditional healer,[128] compulsory induction in Ayurveda for registered traditional healers,[129] and naming the committees set-up for inter-generational healers (in government terms – traditional healers) as *Ayurveda Sanrakshana Sabhawa* (Ayurveda Protection Committee).[130] Indirect ways of forcing into Ayurveda include the introduction of Diploma in Ayurveda programme focusing on inter-generational healers[131] and the formal recognition of the diploma programme, and difficulties for healers to access ingredients for healing.

---

[127] As discussed in Siva Paranasivamillai's (#102) case in 2.4 of this Chapter.
[128] As discussed in Chapter 2.3.2.
[129] Also discussed in Chapter 2.3.2.
[130] As discussed in Chapter 2.3.1.
[131] See Chapter 2.4.

The direct and indirect forms of colonisation by Ayurveda discussed above do not contribute to the protection of inter-generational healing practices. They have had a negative impact on inter-generational knowledge systems, as when healers are inducted to a new knowledge system, they find it difficult to access their former knowledge system. As the inter-generational healers believe, inter-generational healing knowledge can only be acquired by mentoring of a healer. The next, section of the chapter explores the competition and tension between Western doctors and the inter-generational healers.

3.2 Competition and Tension between Western Doctors and the Inter-generational Healers

Another challenge for the inter-generational healers is the competition and tension between the inter-generational healers and Western Doctors. In presenting the argument, my experience with inter-generational eye healer P. Weerasinghe[132] and Consultant Ophthalmologist Dr. M. Nandakumar,[133] is narrated to portray this competition and tension.

The art of healing eyes is a family heritage Weerasinghe has inherited from his father. He treats almost all forms of eye diseases. In cases where he is not competent to treat, he informs the patient during the first consultation visit. He treats close to one hundred patients per day on weekends and twenty five to thirty patients on weekdays. Weerasinghe says he has to limit his practice on week days as he works in the Department of Archeology in Anuradhapura to make a living. Patients come from all over the island. Some come the previous night and camp out at his premises, while others come as early as 3 – 4 in the morning to get a number for

---

[132] P. Weerasinghe (# 52). Obtaining an interview with healer P. Weerasinghe was not easy. The first day I visited the healing centre was a Sunday and the place was over crowded. When I asked the assistant for an appointment he said the next available appointment was in one month's time, he refused to give the contact number of the healer. As I was determined to complete the interview during this field visit I opted to stay in the queues and try my luck. A patient told me on weekday mornings you might have a chance as there is less number of patients. So I went back on Monday morning and stayed for three hours but he could not even complete the patients in the queue before he left for work. I decided to go to his office at the Department of Archaeology to seek a possible time for an appointment. Then he suggested I come in the evening on 17 July 2012. Even in the evening there was a queue. I stayed for two hours before I got the opportunity to interview him.

[133] Dr. M. Nandakumar practices at Lanka Hospitals, 578, Elvitigala Mawatha, Narahenpita, Colombo 5. http://www.lankahospitals.com/index.php (20 February 2019).

treatment. He usually gives medicine sufficient for one month for the patients who come from distant places.

Weerasinghe starts treating infant patients when they are three months old. His most common treatment method is to wrap medicine on the toe. If he is treating the left eye, the medicine is wrapped in the right toe on alternate days for 3-4 hours. After one hour of removing the medicine wrapped on the toe, the patient is required to have a bath. On the days medicine is not wrapped on the toe, the patient is given an oil to apply in his/her head. Weerasinghe says he tries to avoid treating directly in the eye as the patients don't favour it much, but there are unavoidable instances that require stitches in the eye or the direct application of medicine to the eye.

Western practice does not have treatment for nerve weaknesses such as colour blindness, night time blindness (*raththri andathawaya*) and side complications which arises for the offspring of blood relations, says Weerasinghe. He continues, 'The Western doctors only protect the vision that is left and have the idea that it cannot be bettered. They prescribe glasses for children who are long distance blind saying they cannot be corrected, but we cure them.'

Seeing the popularity of the healer and the great respect he receives from patients all over the island, I decided to try out an eye treatment for my son who was 4 and a half years at the time who had been diagnosed with astigmatism and was wearing spectacles. Healer Weerasinghe gave me the medicine to wrap on the toes and the oil. I continued the medicine for four months and brought him to Anuradhapura each month for treatment. After four months of continuous treatment, I wanted to check Anuk's eyes with Dr. M. Nandakumar, the Consultant Ophthalmologist at Lanka Hospital, to see whether there was an improvement. During this time, I stopped him wearing the eye patches and the spectacles as had been recommended by Healer Weerasinghe. After the usual testing Dr. Nandakumar asked me, has Anuk been wearing his spectacles and eye patches as recommended by me? I said no Doctor. Dr. Nandakumar was furious. He asked me what are you thinking? Then I told him my experience with the eye healer. He threw away the file and asked me to leave immediately. He said how foolish one could be. According to Dr. Nandakumar's testing Anuk's vision has not improved at all. With tear-filled eyes I said sorry to Dr. Nandakumar. He asked me to make a firm decision and that if I wanted Anuk's vision to improve not to do any experiments with his eyes. Since that day I have stuck with spectacles and eye patches for Anuk.

The above story is an example that illustrates the tension between inter-generational healers and Western doctors where Western doctors do not believe in or accommodate inter-generational practices of healing. Due to tension between different forms or healers and doctors sometimes patients have to choose between the available forms of healing practices. The following case study examines how assimilating policies towards the Vedda community has impacted on their system.

3.3 Assimilation of Vedda Community

The Vedda community is an indigenous community in Sri Lanka. Historically the Vedda population lived as part of the environment and did not alienate themselves from nature. As Dambane Gunawardena expresses it, 'we lived with nature, faced and adapted to the environment and its changes, as it came. If it rains, we get wet; when it is sunny, we enjoy the sunshine. We depend on our environment for our wellbeing.'[134]

The Vedda community had their own healing system based on their beliefs on supernatural spirits and the understanding of the need to be one with nature. Types of healing adopted by the Vedda community varied from various rituals, such as spirit worship[135], Shanthi Karma[136], *Kem Krama,*[137] *Manthra,*[138] to herbal medicine.[139]

---

[134] Dambane Gunawardena (# 17).

[135] Veddhas believe in spirits (*Na Yakku* - the spirits of relatives who have passed away. The word *Yakku* is derived from the *Yaksha gothra* or *Yakksha* clan. It is not devil, it is the ancestry of the Veddhas.) They believe the evil spirits cause mental and physical illness while the good spirits protect them from danger. They performed various forms of healing and wellbeing rituals for the spirits, to overcome illness, to celebrate milestone events in life and to obtain blessings for day to day activities.

[136] There are three famous types of Shanthi Karma performed by the Veddha Community to invoke the blessings of the super natural powers. They are, *Hethme* ritual, *Kiri Koraha* ritual, and *Deva Danaya.*

[137] *Kem Krama* are practices conducted based on faith, for protection. The commonly practiced *Kem Krama* include, for *Goyam Massa* and *Veli Panu Rogaya.* The term '*Kem*' is derived from the Sanskrit '*Kshema*,' it means protection. Warusawitharane (2012) *Krama*' is a Sinhalese term that refers to systems.

[138] The Veddha community uses various forms of mantra to control and get protection from wild animals. It is believed that Mantra contains mystical potentialities. Mantra refers to 'sacred verbal formula repeated in prayer, meditation, or incantation, such as an invocation of a god, a magic spell.' (Mantra definition is based on www. thefreedictionary.com/mantra (last retrieved on 20 February 2019) Some of such mantras[138] are chanted to chase bears, to chase elephants, to chase *Yak* (wild buffalo), to ease the pain caused by centipede bites. (Mantras chanted for each of the examples cited have been documented in detail in De Silva and Punchihewa (2011) p 339-344.

[139] Traditional Vaddha medicine has treatment for hypertension, cholesterol, diabetes, bacterial treatment, bear bite, snake bite, worm treatment, urinary tract

Although the Veddas still conduct the practices and rituals that come from their ancestors, the faith is slowly diminishing, due to mainstreaming policies adopted by the government. Transformation undergone by the community is clear in Dambane. As a result of the Mahaweli Project, the government relocated 13 Vedda villages in Heranegala, Ampara District in 1983.[140] Vedda children were introduced to the national education system. Schooling was made compulsory for all children and they had to follow the national, main-stream syllabus. The medium of instruction in Dambana and Sinhalese majority areas was Sinhala, while in areas with majority of Tamil population was Tamil.[141] The dominant language assimilation process distanced them from the Vedda creole.[142] The religion taught in schools in areas with a Buddhist majority population was Buddhism, while Hinduism was taught in areas with a Hindu majority population.[143] The new religion has distanced the Vedda children from their traditional religious practice of spirit worship.[144] The assimilation approaches that led to socio-cultural change and the negative impact on the Vedda community are summarised in Gunawardena's novel, *Dadabimen Dadabimata* where he describes how the hunters (Vedda community) culture has become the hunted (destroyed) by the government policies. A Vedda community member expressing the sentiments regarding their situation says,

> Hunting is prohibited from the law; if our community had the capacity to fight, we would have fought for our rights, and ended in war. Our means of making a living has been banned. Vedda population is known for their hunting, it is all we know how to do; therefore, we are left without a choice. Our identity has been destroyed; the Vedda Head is now only a representative figure, who has no power.[145]

---

infection, wasp sting, stomach ache, fever/ headache, stomach ache induced by worms (Gulumaya gahanava), diarrhea, and orthopedic issues (fractures and dislocations) (Details of Traditional Medicine used by the Veddha community has been documented in De Silva and Punchihewa (2011), pp 339 - 342).

[140] Based on the History of Veddha Community briefing at the Indigenous People's Heritage Centre, Kota Bakina, Dambana, by Gunapala, Wanniya Attho Community Member. 12 August 2013.

[141] De Silva and Punchihewa (2011).

[142] Dharmadasa (2011).

[143] De Silva and Punchihewa (2011), p 6; and Dambane Gunawardena (#17).

[144] Vishwakeerthi Vanaspathi UruWalige Wanniya Attho (#18).

[145] Gunapala Wannia Attho (#16).

The lifestyle of Vedda community was based on living with nature. From childbirth to death, Vedda community members followed a naturalisation process. There was no bias between male and female; they both worked very hard for a living. There was no registration by law or grand celebrations for marriage. Now marriage has to be registered by the law, as the child cannot obtain a birth certificate or enter school otherwise. Child birth is now assisted by western medical systems. From the time a woman is pregnant she has to register with the Family Health Worker. The pregnant woman should take the tablets recommended for her. Unless the child is born in a hospital, a birth certificate will not be issued. As a result of the domination of Western practices, natural pregnancies and child birth without the influence of any additional tablets, non-indigenous nutrition, and injections are not common. This process of transitioning to artificial environments and food from the time of pregnancy is causing problems for Vedda children. The natural indigenous food items consumed have been replaced by non-indigenous food stuffs imported into the region. Limiting the area they can live in and prohibiting hunting has limited physical exercise. They are brought up to be children with no connection to the natural environment, and they are unable to cope with even the slightest environmental change as they grow.[146]

There is a distinct difference between the current situation where the Vedda community is inducted to non-indigenous food and nutrition and their connection to the natural environment is limited versus the traditional systems previously followed by the Vedda community where the lifestyle of the community was closely connected to the natural environment they inhabited. The concept of 'sickness' as conceptualised by the Vedda healers means,

> that the person is unable to cope with the environment, either he is going before the environment or the environment is above him, he is unfit to survive, thus he should be allowed to perish naturally if our healing systems fail.[147]

As all children are inducted to non-indigenous food and nutrition thus becoming distant from their natural environments from the beginning, the traditional healing system based on the process of naturalisation will not work efficiently on them.[148] A Vedda community member expressed the current situation as:

---

[146] Dambane Gunawardena (# 17).
[147] Dambane Gunawardena. (# 17).
[148] Dambane Gunawardena. (# 17).

> Our people must first identify what is happening to them, this is what they lack… they look for convenience and don't see the destruction beyond that.[149]

Another issue in practicing traditional healing systems is, unless registered as a traditional healer with the state, one is not allowed to practice traditional healing. In order to qualify for registration, one should face an exam and an interview. This is apparent with the Vedda healers. Most Vedda inter-generational healers who have learnt the craft from their families are not sufficiently literate or possess the conceptual framework to sit for the state exam. Uruwarige Wannila Aththan[150] is the only registered traditional healer of the Vedda community in Dambana and only he can practice the craft officially. According to Wannila Aththan, he will share his knowledge only with the Vedda community in Dambana. He considers this knowledge as the heritage of the community and feels it is necessary to protect the confidentiality of the knowledge. He feels he cannot trust even the people who belong to the Vedda community but who were relocated, when it comes to sharing traditional knowledge in healing.[151] Wannila Aththo is willing to practice healing and give medicine to anyone interested. Almost all visitors who visit Wannila Aththo in Dambana are inducted to available medicine which they can purchase for a reasonable price.

The case of the assimilation of the Vedda community has portrayed how government interventions and the introduction of mainstream culture to the Vedda community has challenged the survival of the Vedda community's cultural heritage including traditional healing and wellbeing systems and their lifestyles. The assimilation policies have alienated the Vedda community from their language, religion and occupation that played an important role in indigenous Vedda healing systems. The Vedda community's healing system was based on the theory of naturalisation or being one with nature and thus their lifestyle was directly linked to the natural environments they inhabited. Limiting the habitat of the Vedda community and introducing them to non-indigenous food and nutrition has

---

[149] Gunapala Wannia Attho (#16).

[150] Uruwarige Wannila Attho is the eldest son of Uruwarige Tissahamy Aththan. He became the chief leader of the aborigines under the traditional customs of the generation, after the demise of his father on 29th May 1998. His Lordship is the chief aboriginal leader of the pleasant, picturesque hamlet of Dambana, Gurukumbura, Katabakina, Watayana etc. and the regional aboriginal village of Bibile, Mahiyangana, Ampara, Dehoattakandiya, Mahaweli Villages, Dimbulagala etc. He has been most honourably conferred with the honorary title '*Visva Keerthi Vanaspatta*' by the most venerable Maha Sanga Nayaka Theros of the three Buddhist sects.

[151] Vishwakeerthi Vanaspathi UruWarige Wannila Attho (# 18).

caused a negative impact on Vedda healing practices. The next section of the chapter focuses on some possibilities for protecting the diverse cultural heritage of inter-generational healing practice.

3.4 Possibilities of protecting the diverse cultural heritage of inter-generational healing practice

In order to protect the inter-generational healing system, the government must take initiative to systematise the inter-generational healing systems, without losing the cultural values and acceptance. The government also must focus on increasing the quality of life of the inter-generational healing practitioners, and patronise their traditional healing systems and the cultural heritage associated with the healing system.

In order to systematise and develop a curriculum of inter-generational medical practice, and to bring it to the level of the recognised traditional medicine in the country (i.e., Ayurveda, Siddha, Unani) one must first recognise and understand it well. This is a gradual process. When developing a system of imparting the knowledge, one must concentrate on developing the informal systems of education that transmit not only the knowledge of healing but also the traditional cultural aspects related to healing. Traditional systems of imparting knowledge and modern technological developments should be taken into account in developing an educational programme. Simply developing the degree programs is not the correct approach.[152]

In inter-generational knowledge of healing in Sri Lanka is passed from generation to generation by the traditional practitioners of healing based on the methods adopted by themselves, without any advanced technological support.[153] The teaching, learning and research systems for inter-generational knowledge is quite different from the western methodologies of similar disciplines.[154] The differences in teaching, learning and research contributed towards the uniqueness and diversity of healing practices.

Sri Lanka's inter-generational medical system is not recognised internationally because it is not organised nor well-preserved like the Ayurvedic medial system. Types of *Kasaya vattoru*, (method of preparation of medicine) and other healing systems have come from word of mouth and some written in ola leaf inscriptions. In order to preserve this knowledge, it

---

[152] Prof. Piyal A. Marasinghe (# 41).

[153] Director's Message, IIM http://iim.cmb.ac.lk/directors-message (last retrieved 20 February 2019).

[154] Director's Message, IIM http://iim.cmb.ac.lk/directors-message (last retrieved 20 February 2019).

has to be transferred to a form of tangible knowledge (by writing books etc). Most of the inscriptions in the ola leaves are very difficult to understand as the language is advanced and different. It is a very difficult task, therefore, to formalise the inter-generational medical system. An interesting question to ask is that if inter-generational knowledge is handed to a government, or private research or archival institute, can it be protected?

The drawback of the current generation to carry out their inter-generational healing practice and the reluctance of the indigenous healers to share their knowledge outside family has caused the downfall of inter-generational healing systems in Sri Lanka. Inter-generational medical knowledge belongs to healing communities or families associated with the healing practices. For example, *Neelammahara, Rathtalgoda, Banagala,* or *Horiwila* comes down from generation to generation, through ancestry, but it has not been preserved properly and is being destroyed. Children nowadays like to follow the latest trends. They do not like to go to the jungles and collect plants, roots and leaves and make their medicines at home. They prefer options with a more stable income and better quality of life. The indigenous medical professionals do not have anyone to give their knowledge to and thus the ancestry ends there. This is how the healing system is being destroyed. We must find a way to preserve and improve this medical practice.

It is necessary to systematically support the inter-generational healers to overcome the struggle for survival. Some suggestions to promote and strengthen the indigenous healers are as follows:

One suggestion would be to strengthen the *Ayurveda Sanrakshana Sabhawa*. The government should consider changing the name of Ayurveda Protection Committee to District Indigenous Healing Protection Committee as the name is misrepresentative. This committee should be strengthened by giving financial allocations and support in developing and implementing a long-term sustainable plan in protecting inter-generational healing systems in the community.

Another suggestion to consider is a reasonable price for herbal ingredients. Inter-generational healers should be given easy access and concessionary prices to purchase herbs including prohibitive medicines. An inter-generational healer expresses his views on prices of herbs as follows:

> Sometimes the prices of herbs at the Ayurveda Department are more expensive than in outside shops (A Rs.150 herb will be sold at 175 rupees at the Department) Most of us (indigenous healers) don't charge for the medicine as customary practice. We accept whatever the amount is given

> on the betel leaf. But how could we continue such practice when we have to pay high prices to obtain the ingredients for medicine?[155]

Yet another suggestion is to introduce a social security network for inter-generational healers, including a retirement scheme. Currently there is no suitable retirement scheme. There was a proposal for the indigenous healers to deposit some money for a retirement scheme,[156] however this was not a feasible system as most inter-generational healers are very poor and they struggle for their daily existence.

Conclusion

This chapter has argued that the inter-general healing systems of Sri Lanka, which is part of the cultural heritage of the country is facing the threat of losing the cultural heritage aspect of healing due to government interventions. The argument has been made in three parts.

Part 1 of the chapter has argued that inter-generational healing is diverse, unstructured, informal and part of the intangible cultural heritage in Sri Lanka using cases of Rathnawathie, Sudu Banda and Sunil Shantha. Rathnawathie's and Sudu Banda's cases have portrayed diversities in acquisition of knowledge of inter-generational healing. Rathnawathie's case has also depicted how changing social circumstances and economics have caused her to change the cultural practice of healing, and the nature of the healing she practices. Sudu Banda's case revealed the informal, unstructured, traditional cultural aspects of healing where the healer does not charge a fixed amount for healing but practices healing as an honorary profession. This has resulted in the income received from inter-generational healing practice not being sufficient for a livelihood. *Kadum Bidum* healer, Sunil Shantha's case has reflected on aspects of traditional knowledge, traditional practices, traditional expressions and traditional skills that makes inter-generational healing part of the intangible cultural heritage of Sri Lanka.

The second part of the chapter has argued that inter-generational healers are faced with many challenges. The first challenge identified in this part is the lack of employment opportunities for inter-generational healers. Causes for the lack of employment opportunities have been identified as a clash in ideologies between disinterested vs. interested, informal vs. formal and pure vs. impure, due to influence of capitalist values of reciprocating healing. The two case studies have portrayed how changes in social

---

[155] S. K. Liyanarachige (# 27).

[156] A.M.P. Abeysinghe (#2), P. Weerasinghe (#52), H. D. Karunawathier (#53).

circumstances, ideologies and values have threatened employment opportunities for healers. Inter-generational healing system remain informal and unstructured, without much government sponsorship while formal, structured health care systems receive extensive government sponsorship. The second challenge identified in this part is the secretive nature of inter-generational knowledge. It is argued that while it was possible for inter-generational healing system to exist and thrive as a secretive knowledge system in a caste-based society, the secretive nature of inter-generational knowledge challenges the existence of inter-generational healing systems in an open economic society. Inappropriate treatment towards inter-generational healing practices by the Government of Sri Lanka has been identified as yet another major threat. This section has focused on the role of *Ayurveda Sanrakshana Sabhawa*, the registration system in place for inter-generational healers and discriminatory treatment towards Special Doctors in government hospitals to portray inappropriate treatment by the government. The final challenge identified in this part was how inter-generational healers' efforts in obtaining formal education for recognition has challenged the existence of the informal, unstructured knowledge base of inter-generational healing.

Part 3 of the chapter focused on the impacts of government intervention in recognising, supporting and regulating inter-generational healing systems of Sri Lanka. In this part I have argued that government intervention in inter-generational healing has created tension and competition between Western doctors, Ayurveda and intergenerational healers and in some instances has forced healers into Ayurveda, causing traditional cultural aspects of healing to be threatened in Sri Lanka. To do so I have portrayed how healers are been forced into Ayurveda, and then a personal experience with an inter-generational healer and a Western doctor has been narrated to highlight this competition and tension., and finally the case study of the Vedda community have been presented to portray how a naturalisation process and loss of cultural heritage has threated the cultural aspect of healing due to government interventions. The final section of this part of the chapter has focused on some possibilities of protecting the diverse cultural heritage of inter-generational healing practices.

CHAPTER 6

CONCLUSION

Introduction

This book has argued that there are diverse healing and wellbeing practices in Sri Lanka and that the Government only recognises, supports and regulates some of these. Further, it proposes that the Sri Lankan Government's interventions have had direct effects on traditional cultural aspects of healing and wellbeing. This concluding chapter will, in part 1 summarise the findings in this book and in part 2 discuss some observations based on those findings. Part 3 focuses on the main concerns related to protecting and promoting diverse living practices on health and wellness in Sri Lanka.

Part 1: Summary of Findings

This book has argued that the recognition, support and regulation of the Government of Sri Lanka in healing and wellbeing practices plays an important role in determining, promoting, protecting or destroying the cultural aspect of healing. This argument has been made in four stages in this book. In the first stage it has examined the diversity of healing and wellbeing practices in Sri Lanka. In the second stage this book has argued that structured, formal healing systems, such as Western allopathic healing, Ayurveda, Siddha, Unani, Acupuncture and Homeopathy are more likely to be recognised, supported and regulated by the Government of Sri Lanka while informal healing systems such as inter-generational healing and cosmic healing practices are less likely to be recognised, supported and regulated. In the third stage of the argument, the book has questioned the definitions of traditional knowledge and its practical application in the Sri Lankan context, and, more broadly, the use of traditional knowledge as legal, social and cultural categories. In the fourth stage the book has highlighted the issues related to protecting the traditional cultural aspects of healing in the process of systematic regulation by discussing inter-generational healing practices.

Chapter 1 of the book has shared four short stories about traditional healers and practitioners in Sri Lanka. In so doing it has brought to light the diverse forms of living practices in health and wellbeing in Sri Lanka, as well as some of the themes and issues that are associated with the culture of healing and wellbeing practices, such as, the role of religion, language, social systems, customs, education, payment, organisation and duty. Chapter 1 then has briefly considered why Sri Lanka matters: why it is necessary to examine, in detail, some of the traditional practices related to health and wellbeing in Sri Lanka. The chapter also outlines the methodology used in conducting the research.

Chapter 2 recognised the regulating practices related to health and wellbeing in Sri Lanka. To do so, the chapter has first traced the development of the protection regime in traditional knowledge from the recognition of rights to self-determination of indigenous peoples to calls for the safeguarding and protection of traditional knowledge, expression and practice, as well as for sharing the benefits resulting from the exploitation of traditional knowledge, expression and practice. Then Sri Lanka's attempts to recognise and regulate traditional practices related to health and wellbeing were discussed by examining Sri Lanka's role in international institutions, Sri Lanka's domestic laws related to health and wellbeing and how the regulation of health and wellbeing has been affected by colonialism, globalisation and current revival efforts.

Taken together, Chapters 3 to 5 of this book highlighted the Sri Lankan Government's role in recognising, supporting and regulating the diverse forms of healing practices existing in the country and the impact on culture. These chapters revealed that healing practices matter not only because of their value in the health and wellbeing of the community, but also because they strongly contribute towards intangible forms of cultural heritage, including rich and diverse knowledge systems, belief systems, values, rituals, customs and identity of the healers and community. It also has highlighted the needs of existing regulatory mechanisms to broaden their scope in protecting the diversity of healing practices in Sri Lanka.

Chapter 3 has described and discussed the complexities of a range of living healing practices in Sri Lanka. In Chapter 3 it was argued that only some healing practices are recognised by the Government of Sri Lanka. It examined the government recognised traditional healing practices in Sri Lanka namely, Ayurveda, Siddha, Unani, Homeopathy, Acupuncture, and Deshiya Chikithsa. The second part of this chapter established the wider scope of healing practices in Sri Lanka, recognising that current healing practices in the country are far more extensive and richer than those recognised by the Government of Sri Lanka. To obtain a broader understanding of the healing practices in Sri Lanka, the diverse forms of healing were clustered into 5 categories drawing on discussions and analysis from interviews, namely: inter-generational healing, cosmic healing, adopted traditional healing, western healing and integrated healing. This classification helped identify what healing practices the Government has recognised, supported and regulated in Sri Lanka and the impact of their involvement or non-involvement in culture and practices of healing in Sri Lanka. The third part of that chapter explored and analysed, the complexities and dynamics of different forms of healing practices. The analysis of diverse healing systems has illustrated that the distinctions of these systems are mainly based on: (1) how a healing system has been influenced by science vs. religion and rituals; and (2) whether the healing system being practiced is in a formal, public domain vs. informal, private domain.

Chapter 4 examined the history and nature of the recognition, support and regulation of traditional healing practices in Sri Lanka. It traced the history of healthcare in Sri Lanka to illustrate how public demand for non-Western healing systems has led colonial and post-colonial Sri Lankan governments to recognise, support and regulate traditional healing practices. The chapter then examined the range of mechanisms developed by the Government to recognise, support and regulating traditional practices related to healing which included: the widespread government administrative structure; government sponsored education in traditional medicine; government sponsored research; and community health care programs; and programs introduced to develop the practice of inter-generational healing.

Chapter 4 has argued that while the Government's efforts have gone some way to support and safeguard traditional practices in Sri Lanka, this has almost always been informed and influenced by Western and biomedical frameworks. This has meant that the Sri Lankan Government takes a rather narrow approach to healing practices. The result of this narrow approach to traditional healing practices is that the Government's involvement in the protection and promotion of traditional healing has formalised and standardised traditional healing practices.

The second argument made in Chapter 4 was, that the Government's focus on traditional healing has been mainly on Ayurveda, and to a lesser extent Siddha, Unani, Acupuncture and Homeopathy. In all the government sponsored traditional healing systems emphasis has usually been placed on the curative services and the Ayurvedisation of indigenous and traditional healing practices. The third argument made in the chapter was that there is a significant trend in the loss of cultural value in the process of standardisation and formalisation. Due to the Government's conceptualisation of traditional healing practices (as formal practices of healing such as

Ayurveda, Siddha, Unani, Homeopathy and Acupuncture adopted from other countries and to a lesser extent inter-generational healing practices) certain types of healing practices have been, and continue to be neglected, overlooked or threatened in the process of Ayurvedisation.

Chapter 4 also points out that the Government uses the words 'indigenous' and 'traditional' inter-changeably to refer to the traditional healing systems they adopt. Yet the Government's support, recognition and regulation for inter-generational healing is very limited. Due to the diversity and informal nature of the inter-generational healing systems in the country, the real 'traditional knowledge' in healing has been overlooked.

Chapter 5 has argued that the inter-general healing systems of Sri Lanka are facing the threat of losing their cultural heritage aspects of healing due to government interventions. The argument has been made in three parts. Using cases of Rathnawathie, Sudu Banda and Sunil Shantha, part 1 of the chapter showed that inter-generational healing is diverse, unstructured, informal and part of the intangible cultural heritage in Sri Lanka.

In part 2 of Chapter 5, it is argued that inter-generational healers are facing many challenges. The first of these is the lack of employment opportunities for inter-generational healers. The reasons for lack of employment include the adoption of capitalist economy; changes in the social systems; changes in the value systems; informal and unstructured nature of inter-generational healing; and lack of government sponsorship. A second challenge identified in this part was the secretive nature of inter-generational knowledge. It is argued that while it is possible for practitioners of inter-generational healing systems to exist and thrive as a secretive knowledge system in a caste-based society, the secretive nature of inter-generational knowledge challenges the existence of their practices in an open economic society. Inappropriate government actions and initiatives aimed at inter-generational healing practices were identified as yet another major threat. Discussion of this third challenge has focused on the role of the *Ayurveda Sanrakshana Sabhawa* registration system in place for inter-generational healers and the discriminatory treatment towards special doctors in government hospitals to reveal the Government's inappropriate treatment of these types of healers. A final challenge discussed in this part is how the efforts of inter-generational healers in obtaining formal education for their recognition has impacted on the informal, unstructured knowledge base of inter-generational healing.

Part 3 of Chapter 5 has focused on the impacts of government intervention in recognising, supporting and regulating inter-generational healing system of Sri Lanka. This part argues that government intervention in inter-generational healing has created tensions and competition between

'Western Doctors,' Ayurveda and intergenerational healers and in some instances has forced healers into Ayurveda, causing traditional cultural aspects of inter-generational healing to be threatened in Sri Lanka. Interviews revealed how intergenerational healers had been forced to be treated through Ayurveda. Finally, the case study of the Vedda community was presented to expose how a naturalisation process and loss of cultural heritage has threated their cultural aspect of healing as result of government interventions. The last part of Chapter 6, drawing on interview data, has focused on some possibilities for protecting the diverse cultural heritage of inter-generational healing practice.

Part 2: Observations Based on Findings

In this part, two main observations based on the findings in this book are discussed. They are related to factors that are important in ensuring that traditional knowledge in healing and wellbeing practices continue to thrive, and the problems and dangers in the loss of cultural heritage.

2.1 Factors in Determining the Survival and Thriving of Traditional Knowledge Systems in Healing

An observation based on chapters 3, 4 and 5 of the book is the Sri Lankan Government's recognition, support and regulation of traditional practices in healing as a main factor that contributes towards the survival and vibrancy of healing practices. The formal[1] and informal[2] nature of the healing practices and the political will towards promoting a healing practice plays a key role in determining what healing practice would be given government recognition.

Another related observation based on the findings is that written forms of traditional knowledge in healing has a better opportunity to survive and thrive as a knowledge system. The history of government recognition, support and regulation discussed in Chapter 5 has revealed that it is the written form of traditional knowledge that is usually acknowledged as the cultural heritage of a country. Acknowledging the Government trends in recognising written and formal forms of healing practices, section 3.4 of

[1] Chapter 4 discussions suggested that formal, structured knowledge systems have received full government recognition.

[2] The analysis in Chapter 5 indicated that the informal inter-generational healing practices have received the partial attention of the Government.

Chapter 5 flagged the need to transfer inter-generational knowledge to a tangible form in order to protect this knowledge system.

How individual initiatives and political will has led to government recognition of healing practices are discussed in part 1 of Chapter 3. The political dynamics and complexities of diverse forms of healing practices are discussed in part 3 of Chapter 3. In these parts how politically supported knowledge systems in healing generally thrive while suppressed knowledge in healing struggles to exist openly is discussed. Reasons for politically supported knowledge to thrive include: the knowledge is advocated by organised groups; legal and policy initiatives to recognise, support and regulate such knowledge's are initiated; practitioners are given recognition in the community; and initiatives are taken to promote and formalise such knowledge systems by developing syllabi and establishing training courses.[3] On the other hand, politically suppressed knowledge does not have a strong voice to advocate,[4] financial support[5] or power to develop syllabi and establish training courses.[6] Thus, not having the power to systematically advocate a politically supressed knowledge system weakens the knowledge system.

2.2 Loss of Cultural Heritage

Diverse healing practices contribute towards the richness of intangible cultural heritage[7] of Sri Lanka. In Chapters 4 and 5 it has been argued that the cultural heritage aspect of healing is threatened in the process of their recognition, support and regulation by the Government of Sri Lanka. This section presents four aspects related to government intervention and loss of cultural heritage. The first is how government interventions in education have threatened the loss of cultural heritage by introducing Ayurveda training for inter-generational healers, formalising

---

[3] See, Chapter 3, section 1.4 Homeopathy and Chapter 3, section1.5 Acupuncture for examples of how organised advocacy and support for the knowledge systems resulted in the knowledge system to thrive.

[4] R. L. Kularathne (#110), Dr. T. Weerarathne (#40).

[5] R. M. D. J. Gunasekera (#58), H.D. Karunawathie (#53), P. Weerasinghe (#52) S. D. M. Mahipala (#51).

[6] Prof. Piyal A. Marasinghe (#41).

[7] Characteristics of intangible cultural heritage are, traditional, contemporary and living at the same time, inclusive, representative and community based. See UNESCO, *What is Intangible Cultural Heritage?* http://www.unesco.org/culture/ich/index.php?pg=00002 (last retrieved 20 February 2019).

and standardising knowledge of traditional healing in Ayurveda, Siddha and Unani at university level, and changing the language of instruction for traditional healing at university level. The second aspect is how the limited government intervention in education has resulted in maintaining traditional cultural aspects of healing but how lack of support and funding for the institutions has caused struggle for survival. The third aspect is how the lack of government recognition for the diverse forms of living healing practices threatens the survival and thriving of the non-recognised forms of healing practice. The fourth is how government approaches to assimilation of inter-generational healers to Ayurveda has threatened the protection of diverse cultural heritage of healing.

How the Government's intervention in the process of formalisation and standardisation of healing practices through education results in the loss of cultural heritage has been argued in section 3 of Chapter 4. The example of the National Institute of Traditional Medicine[8] illustrates how the attempt to standardise and formalise the knowledge of the inter-generational healers, by introducing a short programme of education and training in Ayurveda, can add to the isolation, confusion and loss of traditional cultural heritage of non-Ayurveda inter-generational healers. The example of the Gampaha Wickremarachchi Ayurveda Institute[9] has exposed how formalisation and standardisation by the Government has resulted in changing the traditional cultural aspects of healing. Here it is argued that the initial identity of a traditional healer/doctor and the traditional Sri Lankan cultural identity developed through the dress, value systems and form of teaching and studying is no longer present.[10] Section 3.4 of Chapter 5 also argues that the change in the medium of instruction from Sinhala to English has had a negative impact on culture as it is difficult to share the cultural connotations attached to the subject when it is taught in a foreign language. Change of language has caused teachers who had acquired the knowledge in Sinhala to teach the subject in English.[11] Teaching Ayurveda in English makes it a more formal, impersonal, objective subject for study at the university level and makes it difficult to transmit the values, beliefs and practices associated with the knowledge.

Limited interventions by the Government in education have made it possible for traditional healing educational institutions to maintain and transmit knowledge in traditional cultural aspects of healing. This has been revealed in the examples of Samastha Lanka Paramparika Ayurveda Vaidya

---

[8] See, Chapter 4 section 3.2.

[9] Chapter 4, section 3.4.

[10] Interview with A. D. H. Sudesh (# 50).

[11] Chapter 3, section 3.3.4.

Vidyalaya of Keraminiya[12] and Siddharyuveda Medical Institute in Siri Vajira Ghanadoya Pirivena.[13] Both examples are private initiatives for traditional healing education. The two examples also revealed that although less government interventions of formalisation and standardisation has made it possible for these institutions to maintain traditional cultural aspects related to training healers, due to lack of government support and funding these institutions are struggling for survival.

Lack of government recognition for the diversity of healing practices that are part of cultural heritage also threatens the existence of the non-recognised healing practice. This was illustrated by the discussion of the role of the Sri Lanka Ayurveda Medical Council[14] and the Institute of Indigenous Medicine (IIM).[15] It is argued, the Sri Lanka Ayurveda Medical Council adopting a limited approach to traditional healing has threatened the existence of the traditional knowledge of healing in Sri Lanka, which are the inter-generational and cosmic healing systems. This discussion has shown how the IIM is only promoting Ayurveda and Unani systems of education, and it is, therefore, not contributing towards systematically imparting knowledge of indigenous medicine. Section 3.3 of Chapter 4 also pointed out that the IIM discourages other practices such as inter-generational healing and cosmic healing as they are not formal or structured knowledge systems. Not recognising the diverse practices of healing actively works against the development of diverse intangible cultural healing heritage of healing in Sri Lanka.

How the Government's approach to assimilation of inter-generational healers to Ayurveda has threatened the protection of diverse cultural heritage of healing is discussed in section 3.7 of Chapter 5. This section points out that Ayurverdisation of healing is evident in government administration, government sponsored education, government supported hospitals and curative services, government sponsored medicines and drugs and government sponsored research.[16] The efforts of government intervention in systematising and mainstreaming diverse healing practices by Ayurvedisation of healing results in loss of diversity of healing practices that it turn causes the loss of intangible cultural heritage of healing.

---

[12] Chapter 4, section 3.5.1.
[13] Chapter 4, section 3. 5. 2.
[14] Chapter 4, section 2.2.4.
[15] Chapter 4, section 3.3.3.
[16] Chapter 4, section 3.3.7.

Part 3: The Main Concerns Relating to Protecting and Promoting Diverse Living Practices on Health and Wellbeing in Sri Lanka

The above section has pointed out the observations on current trends on diverse healing practices of Sri Lanka and government intervention. This section focuses on challenges for the Government in protecting diversity and the traditional cultural aspects of living practices on health and wellbeing.

3.1 Limited Legal Protection

Chapter 2 of the book has discussed multi-cultural legal pluralism prevalent in Sri Lanka, yet when it comes to protection of traditional healing in Sri Lanka, the main legal document is *Ayurveda Act No 31 of 1961.* Yet it is unclear from the *Ayurveda Act No 31 of 1961* whether or what other indigenous medicine systems are covered by it. Part 1 of Chapter 4 argues that indigenous methods of healing are assumed by the policy makers to be included in the legal definitions of Ayurveda. The *Ayurveda Act No 31 of 1961*, which is the main legal document for protecting indigenous medicine in Sri Lanka, refers only to Ayurveda. That is, all traditional and indigenous healing practitioners are referred to as 'Ayurveda practitioners.' All traditional/indigenous dispensers of medicine are referred to 'Ayurveda pharmacists,' and all nurses practicing in traditional healing are called 'Ayurveda nurses.' Not recognising the differences and diversities of healers and healing practitioners in legal documents challenges the possibility for the Government to support and regulate the diverse healing practices in a way that safeguards the differences between healing practices.[17] This also threatens the institutional recognition of diverse emergence of indigenous identities that is important in promoting traditional knowledge and cultural heritage.

3.2 Narrow Scope in Government Recognition

Chapter 4 has argued that Government recognition, support and regulation towards healing practices determine what healing practices and traditional cultural aspects will be protected, promoted or otherwise adversely affected. There are two main concerns about government recognition, support and

[17] See Chapter 5, section 3.1 for a discussion on how limited legal protection for diverse forms of healing has resulted in healers being forced in Ayurveda.

regulation of healing practices. One concern is that although there are a diverse range of healing practices as revealed in part 2 of Chapter 3 only a few healing practices in Sri Lanka are recognised by the Government as traditional healing practices. Part 1 of Chapter 3 has presented healing practices that are recognised by the Government of Sri Lanka as: Ayurveda, Siddha, Unani, Homeopathy, Acupuncture and Deshiya Chikithsa. The conclusion of Chapter 4 has also pointed out that Sri Lanka has adopted a narrow approach to traditional healing practices, where more formal practices are protected in a 'bio-medical' framework and where there is a tendency towards the 'Ayurvedisation' of traditional healing practices. This narrow approach adopted to protect traditional healing threatens the protection of diverse healing practices and traditional cultural aspects related to those healing practices. The second concern which was illustrated in part 3 of Chapter 3, is that to grant government recognition, support and regulation it is necessary to obtain a more nuanced understanding of the prevailing diverse forms of healing practices including socio-cultural and political dynamics of healing practices.

3.3 Inappropriate treatment by the Government challenges the survival and traditional cultural aspect of inter-generational healing practices

Section 2.3 of Chapter 5 has argued that the inappropriate treatment of the Sri Lankan Government of inter-generational healing practices is a threat to the survival of inter-generational healers, their practices and traditional cultural aspects of healing. To elaborate this point section 2.3 of Chapter 5 has cited the examples of the *Ayurveda Sanrakshana Sabhawa*,[18] a government mechanism in place to register inter-generational healers (as traditional healers),[19] and discriminatory treatment towards 'Special Doctors' in government hospitals.[20] Part 3 of Chapter 5 has presented the negative impacts of Government interventions on inter-generational healing. In this part it has been argued that healers have been forced into practising Ayurveda[21] and that the competition and tensions between Western doctors and inter-generational healers[22] have resulted in assimilation and a loss of cultural diversity.

[18] Chapter 5, section 2.3.1.
[19] Chapter 5, section 2.3.2.
[20] Chapter 5, section 2.3.3.
[21] Chapter 5, section 3.1.
[22] Chapter 5, section 3.2 Competition and Tension between Western Doctors and the Inter-generational Healers.

3.4 Mixing Up of Terms

Part 1 of Chapter 3 pointed out that the Sri Lankan Government generally uses the words 'indigenous medicine'[23] and 'traditional medicine'[24] interchangeably to refer to traditional healing systems. It is argued that these terms should not be used in this way as they do not mean the same thing; nor does the Sri Lankan Government treat them in the same way. In elaborating this argument in Chapter 3, it was argued that one of the issues with the Sri Lankan Government using the terms indigenous medicine and traditional medicine is that, it threatens the concept of authenticity of healing practice. As identified through interviews, the terms indigenous or traditional healing do not necessarily mean a healing system that originated in Sri Lanka. For example, traditional healing systems covered under the scope of the Ministry of Indigenous Medicine are: Ayurveda (healing system adopted from North India),[25] Siddha (healing system adopted from South India), Unani (healing system adopted from Arabs) and Desheeya Chikitsa (indigenous system of medicine in Sri Lanka).[26] Only the last of these is usually claimed to have originated from Sri Lanka. Not properly identifying and classifying the living practices of healing and wellbeing threatens the possibilities of recognising, supporting and regulating the diverse cultural heritage of healing in Sri Lanka.

3.5 Not Having Clarity on Terms

Part 1 of Chapter 3 pointed to the issue of not having clarity of terms used to refer to healing practices in Sri Lanka. To support this argument the chapter provided two examples. The first was in relation to different definitions of 'indigenous health care,' and the second was the lack of a proper definition for what is 'traditional Sinhala medicine.' Part 1 of Chapter 4 also discussed how the diversity and complexity of practices around terms cause difficulties for them in having clarity for different groups and people. The terms Ayurveda and Deshiya Chikitsa are examples

---

[23] Indigenous medicine is used in the context of 'Ministry of Indigenous Medicine', 'Institute of Indigenous Medicine.'

[24] Traditional medicine is used in the context of 'National Institute of Traditional Medicine.'

[25] This is how Ministry of Indigenous Medicine has introduced Ayurveda. (See: http://www.indigenousmedimini.gov.lk/ (last retrieved 20 February 2019)

[26] Ministry of Indigenous Medicine: Herbal Medicines in Sri Lanka. http://www.indigenousmedimini.gov.lk/index.html (last retrieved 20 February 2019).

of this.[27] It was suggested that there are many forms of Ayurveda, for example Keraminiya Ayurveda, Siddha Ayurveda and Hybrid Ayurveda. These differences are not well marked or clearly recognised. The analysis given of Deshiya Chikithsa,[28] by depicting what Deshiya Chikithsa is referred to in different platforms revealed that there is no agreed upon definition for Deshiya Chikitsa. Not having clarity of terms used for traditional healing practices is problematic for government determination of its scope of recognition, support and regulation of healing.

3.6 Issues in the Administration of Traditional Health Care

Part 2 of Chapter 4 has discussed the national level and provincial level structures that are in place to provide traditional health care services. Here it is argued that because the provincial Ayurveda departments are managed by nine different administrative structures it is difficult to administratively coordinate, monitor the services, and maintain standards. Since the delivery of traditional healing is administrated by different administrative structures it has been difficult to maintain the same standards of government support and regulation of traditional health care facilities within different provinces.

3.7 Ayurvedisation of Healing

In all the Government sponsored traditional healing systems emphasis has been placed on the Ayurvedisation of indigenous and traditional healing practices. The Ayurverdisation of healing is evident in government administration, public education,[29] public hospitals and curative services,[30] government sponsored medicines and drugs[31] and public sponsored

[27] Chapter 3, section 1. 6.

[28] Chapter 3, section 1. 6.

[29] Chapter 4, part 3 has portrayed how Ayurveda education has received prominence by establishing the Ayurveda Education and Hospital Board, training inter-generational healers (also known as traditional healers), Ayuveda by National Institute of Traditional Medicine; Offering Ayurveda Degrees and Post-Graduate Qualifications from both Institute of Indigenous Medicine and Gampaha Wickramarchchi Ayurveda Institute; and introducing a Diploma in Ayurveda.

[30] Chapter 4, section 4. 5 has argued how the focus of traditional healing curative services has been mainly on Ayurveda.

[31] Chapter 4, part 5 has argued that Ayurveda medicines and drugs have received attention from the Government of Sri Lanka in terms of standardising, sponsoring the production of and distribution to Government hospitals and dispensaries under the purview of the Ministry of Indigenous Medicine.

research.[32] When the Government gives priority to Ayurveda and when the Government classifies the diverse practices of traditional healing as 'Ayurveda', the diversity of traditional healing practices tends to be overlooked. As a result of Ayurvedisation of traditional healing practices, the diverse forms of traditional healing practices face the threat of existence.

3.8 Westernisation of Healing

The Sri Lankan Government frameworks to support and regulate traditional healing practices are informed and influenced by biomedical frameworks. This is illustrated in: part 2 of Chapter 5 where it is argued that government administration of the traditional health care system has contributed to adopting a biomedical framework for traditional healing; part 3 of Chapter 5 where it is argued that as part of Government efforts of universalising the traditional healing education system adopting English as the medium of instruction;[33] part 4 of Chapter 5 where it is argued that hospitals and curative services for traditional healing that are sponsored by the Government have contributed to the adoption of Western styled places of treatment for traditional healing; and part 6 of Chapter 5 that has argued that government sponsored research has adopted a biomedical research framework to support the Western concepts of universalisation and standardisation of knowledge.

The diverse knowledge systems of healing that are part of the rich cultural heritage of Sri Lanka either originated in Sri Lanka or were adopted from other countries. Each of these healing practices has its own cultural connotations based on values, beliefs, faiths which it was originally based on. The different knowledge frameworks of healing practices were what has contributed towards the richness of cultural heritage in traditional healing. Adopting biomedical frameworks is a means of uniforming all healing practices. Such interventions have counterproductive impact on healing practices as it threatens the cultural attributes and diversities among healing knowledge and practices.

---

[32] Chapter 4, part 6 has argued that the Government has focused on Ayurveda in both research and gardens.

[33] Chapter 4, section 3.3 Institute of Indigenous Medicine, University of Colombo and Chapter 5, section 3.4 Gampaha Wickremarachchi Ayurveda Institute have adopted English as the official language of instructions.

3.9 Socio-economic and cultural challenges that threaten the existence of Inter-generational healers

Part 2 of Chapter 5 has argued that largely due to the diverse, unstructured and informal character of inter-generational healing, inter-generational healers in the present day face many challenges including, lack of employment opportunities,[34] secretive knowledge, [35] and formal induction to Ayurveda education.[36] Section 2.1 of Chapter 5 has argued that the lack of employment opportunities has challenged the survival of inter-generational healing and practice. Section 2.2 of Chapter 5 has analysed how secretive knowledge has made it possible to keep the knowledge system alive for many generations. In this section it was discussed how secret inter-generational knowledge systems worked well when the caste system was alive in Sri Lanka as families followed the family trade for livelihood. In this section[37] it is argued, in an open economic social system, where the caste does not have a significant impact on career, where the knowledge systems are formalised and accessible to all interested persons, and where the price of a good or service is determined by market economies, protecting secretive knowledge is no longer a viable option. In section 2.4 of Chapter 5 it was shown how inter-generational healers tend to obtain formal education in recognised traditional healing practices (mainly Ayurveda and to a lesser extent, Siddha, Unani, Homeopathy and Acupuncture) to gain recognition for their healing practice. Here it is suggested that when an inter–generational healer acquires a formal education in healing, the healer can no longer be called an inter-generational healer. Section 2.4 of Chapter 5 has argued inter-generational healers following formal Ayurveda education for government recognition has challenged the informal, unstructured knowledge base of inter-generational healers by inducting them to a formal knowledge of traditional healing. Healing practices thrive in a country as part of cultural heritage only if it is traditional, contemporary and living, and at the same time, inclusive, representative and community based.[38] Government interventions on inter-generational healing and socio-economic and cultural challenges faced by

---

[34] Chapter 5, section 2.2.1.
[35] Chapter 5, section 2. 2.2.
[36] Chapter 5, section 2. 2.4.
[37] Chapter 5, section 2. 2.2 Secretive Knowledge.
[38] See UNESCO, *What is Intangible Cultural Heritage?* http://www.unesco.org/culture/ich/index.php?pg=00002 (last retrieved 20 February 2019).

inter-generational healers threaten the existence of inter-generational healing practice and the intangible cultural aspects of healing.

Conclusion

Sri Lanka possesses diverse forms of living practices related to healing and wellbeing that contribute to the rich and diverse cultural heritage of the country. As discussed and illustrated in the book, many of these healing and wellbeing practices were adopted from other countries, while others originated in Sri Lanka. Some healing practices are informal and unique while some others are formal. The healing knowledge systems and practices are based on values, beliefs of the healers and the community. The practice of diverse healing systems based on diverse knowledge systems contribute towards the richness of the cultural heritage of the country. Cultural dynamics of the healers and communities has played a prominent role in establishing and maintaining the sacredness, effectiveness and uniqueness of the living healing and wellbeing practices in Sri Lanka.

With trends in globalisation and formalisation of knowledge, countries around the world are losing touch with traditional practices related to healing and wellbeing. Formalisation and standardisation of all healing practices has several impacts. First, only healing practices that are proven effective by Western scientific knowledge have been recognised. Second, in the process of recognising and regulating healing practices the Government tends to follow a biomedical framework that loses the cultural connotations attached to the healing practice, such as ambience of the place of practice and traditions of performing healing. Third, only the knowledge of healing is transmitted by formal government sponsored education, not the cultural aspect of healing. All the above mentioned impacts have caused a loss of traditional cultural aspects of healing.

This book has pointed out the Government of Sri Lanka plays an important role in recognising, supporting and regulating traditional practices related to healing and wellbeing, yet currently the Government does not recognise and positively regulate the traditional cultural aspects of healing. Government's non recognition of cultural heritage aspects of the living healing systems of Sri Lanka, therefore, has threatened the survival of rich and diverse cultural heritage of healing.

REFERENCES

Secondary Sources

Abramson, P. R. (1992) *A Case for Case Studies*, Thousand Islands, CA: Sage Publications.

Aryasinghe, A. (2000) *The Deities and Demons of Sinhala Origin*, Nugegoda: Deepanee Printers and Publishers (Pvt.) Ltd.

Aguirre, A. A., Ostfeld, R. S., Tabor, G.M., House C. and Pearl M. C. (eds.) (2002). *Conservation Medicine: Ecological Health in Practice*, New York: Oxford University Press.

Aguirre, A. A., Ostfeld, R., and Daszak, P. (2012). *New Directions in Conservation Medicine: Applied Cases of Ecological Health,* US: Oxford University Press.

Alatas, S. F. (2006) *Alternative Discourses in Asian Social Science: Responses to Eurocentrism*, New Delhi: Sage Publications.

Alatas, S. H. (1969) 'Academic Imperialism,' Lecture delivered to the History Society, University of Singapore, 26th September 1969.

Alatas, S. H. (1972) 'The Captive Mind in Development Studies' 34(1) *International Social Science Journal,* 9.

Alatas, S. H. (1974) 'The Captive Mind and Creative Development' 36(4) *International Social Science Journal,* 691.

Alatas, S. H. (2000) 'Intellectual Imperialism: Definition, Traits and Problems' 28 *Southeast Asian Journal of Social Science,* 23.

Altbach, P. (1977) 'Servitude of the Mind? Education, Dependency and Neo-colonialism' 79 *Teachers College Record,* 187.

Aluvihare, A. (2012) 'Surgical Instruments at the Alahana Parivena Hospital in Polonnaruwa' paper presented at the SAARC International Conference on Archaeology of Buddhism: Recent Discoveries in South Asia, Colombo: SAARC Cultural Centre, August.

Amaradasa R and De Silva M. (2001) 'Evolution and Structure of Science and Technology in Sri Lanka' 6 (1) *Sage Journals Online.*

Anderson, C. S. (2003) '"For Those Who are Ignorant:" A Study of the Bauddha Adahilla' in J. C. Holt, J. N. Kinnard, and J. S. Walters. (eds.) *Constituting Communities: Theravada Buddhism and the Religious Cultures of South and Southeast Asia*, Albany: State University of New York Sunny Press.

Anderson, C. (2009) 'Critical Indigenous Studies: From Difference to Destiny' in 15 (2) *Cultural Studies Review*.

Anderson, J. (2010) *Indigenous Traditional Knowledge and Intellectual Property*, North Carolina: Centre for the Study of the Public Domain Duke University School of Law. http://web.law.duke.edu/cspd/pdf/ip_indigenous-traditional knowledge.pdf (last retrieved 20 February 2019).

Anderson, J. (2012) 'On Resolution, Intellectual Property and Indigenous Knowledge Disputes Prologue' 2 (1) *Landscapes of Violence*.

Antons, C. (2009) 'Introduction,' in Christoph Antons (ed.) *Traditional Knowledge, Traditional Cultural Expressions and Intellectual Property Law in the Asia-Pacific Region*, Alphen aan den Rijn: Kluwer Law International.

Atkinson, P. Coffey, A. and Delamont S. (2003) *Key Themes in Qualitative Research: Continuities and Dangers*. New York: Rowan and Littlefield.

Atkinson, R. (1998) *Life Story Interview,* Sage.

Axt, J. R. et al. (1993) *Biotechnology, Indigenous Peoples and Intellectual Property Rights*, Congressional Research Service, The Library of Congress, Washington DC.

Babbie, E. (1998) *The Practice of Social Research* (5th ed.) Belmont, CA: Wadsworth.

Ben-Yishai, A. (2013) *Common Precedents: The Presentness of the Past in Victorian Law and Fiction,* USA: OUP.

Biber-Klemm, S. (1998) *Legal Protection of Genetic Information and Related Traditional Knowledge, Synbook* NRP 42, Swiss National Science Foundation, 1.

Bigus, O. E., Hadden, S. G. and Glaser Barney G. (1994) 'The Study of Basic Social Processes' in B. G. Glaser (ed.) *More Grounded Theory Methodology: A Reader,* Mill Valley, CA: Sociology Press, 38.

Bond G. D. (1988) *The Buddhist Revival in Sri Lanka: Religious Tradition, Reinterpretation and Response*, University of South Carolina, Delhi: Shri Jainendra Press.

Booth, W. C., Colomb, G. G. and Williams J. M. (1995, 2003) *The Craft of Research*, Chicago and London: The University of Chicago Press.

Brahmachari, S. K. (2011) *Traditional Knowledge Digital Library (TKDL) An Effective and Novel Tool for Protection of India's Traditional Knowledge Against Bio-Piracy*, Government of India: Press Information Bureau http://www.tkdl.res.in/tkdl/PressCoverage/PIB_120811.pdf (last retrieved 20 February 2019).

Braudel, F. (1982-4) *Civilization and Capitalism: 15th– 18th Centuries* (three volumes). London: William Collins.

Brown, J., Nora M. and Michael B., (eds.) (2005) *The Protected Landscape Approach: Linking Nature, Culture and Community*, IUCN-The World Conservation Union.

Bubela, T. and Gold, E. R. (2012) *Genetic Resources and Traditional Knowledge: Case Studies and Conflicting Interests*, Cheltenham and Massachusetts: Edward Elgar.

Calabresi G. and Melamed A. D. (1972) 'Property Rules, Liability Rules and Inalienability: One View of the Cathedral' 85 (6) *Harvard Law Review*, 1089.

Carbone, J. (2012) 'A Capabilities-based Framework' in Tania Bubela and Richard E. Gold (eds) *Genetic Resources and Traditional Knowledge: Case Studies and Conflicting Interests*, Cheltenham and Massachusetts: Edward Elgar, 339.

Champagne, D. (2007) 'In Search of Theory and Method in American Indian Studies' in 31 (3) *American Indian Quarterly*.

Chandler, A. D. (1990) *Scale and Scope: The Dynamics of Industrial Capitalism*, Cambridge, MA: The Belknap Press of the Harvard University Press.

Charmaz, K. (1983), 'The Grounded Theory Method: An Explication and Interpretation' in R. M. Emerson (ed.), *Contemporary Field Research,* Boston: Little Brown, 109.

Charmaz, K. (1990), 'Discovering Chrome Illness: Using Grounded Theory' 30 *Social Science and Medicine*, London: Sage, 1161.

Charmaz, K. (1995) 'Grounded Theory' in J.A. Smith, R. Harre and L.V. Langenhove (eds.), *Rethinking Methods in Psychology*, London: Sage. 27.

Charmaz, K. (2003) 'Grounded Theory' in J. A. Smith (ed.), *Qualitative Psychology: A Practical Guide to Research Methods*, London: Sage. 81.

Charmaz, K. (2006) *Constructing Grounded Theory: A Practical Guide through Qualitative Analysis*, London, Thousand Oaks, New Delhi: Sage.

Coates, D. (2000) *Models of Capitalism: Growth and Stagnation in the Modern Era*, Polity Press.

Conway, D. (2009) 'Indigenizing Intellectual Property Law: Customary Law, Legal Pluralism and the Protection of Indigenous Peoples' Rights, Identity and Respirces,' in Texas Wesleyan Law Review, pp 301-347

Coomaraswamy, A. K. (1909) *Essays in National Idealism*, Colombo: Colombo Apothecaries Co. Ltd.

Coomaraswamy, A. K. (1946) 'Indian Culture and English Influence,' An Address to Indian Students and Their Friends, Massachusetts Institute of Technology, January 1944

Coomaraswamy, A. K. *East and West*, Colombo: Ola Books Ltd.
Cooray, A. (2015) 'The Reception of Roman-Dutch Law in Sri Lanka in *7 (3), The Comparative and International Law Journal of Southern Africa*, Institute of Foreign and Corporate Law. 295-320.
Cooray, A. (2015) 'The Reception of Islamic Law in Sri Lanka and Its Interplay with Western Legal Traditions' in V. V. Palmer, M. Y, Mattar, and A. Koppel (eds.) *Mixed Legal Systems, East and West,* Burlington: Ashgate Publishing Company, 213.
Coperahewa, S. (2009) 'The Language Planning Situation in Sri Lanka' in 10 (1) *Current Issies in Language Planning.*
Coperahewa, S. (2011) 'The Language Planning Situation in Sri Lanka' in R. B. Kaplan, and R. B. Baldauf (eds.) *Language Planning in the Asia Pacific – Hong Kong, Timor-Leste and Sri Lanka*. Oxon: Routledge.
Corti, L. (2004) 'Secondary Data in Your Research,' in M. Lewis-Beck, A. E. Bryman, and F. Liao (eds.) The SAGE Encyclopaedia of Social Science Research Methods. SAGE, 20.
Correa, C. M. (2000) 'Options for the Implementation of Farmers Rights at the National Level' *Working Paper No. 8*, South Centre, 31.
Cottier, T. (1997) 'The Protection of Genetic Resources and Traditional Knowledge in International Law: Past, Present and Future' Discussion Paper submitted to the International Conference on Creativity and Innovation, Grassroots, Centre for Management in Agriculture, Indian Institute of Management, Ahmedabad, India, 11-14 January 1997.
Cox P.A. (1997) 'Indigenous People and Conservation' in *Biodiversity and Human Health* in F. Grifo and J. Rosenthal (eds.) Covelo, Califiornia: Island Press.
Cutting, J. (2002) *Pragmatics and Discourse,* London: Routledge.
Darian-Smith, E. and Fitzpatrick, P. (eds.) (1999) *Laws of the Postcolonial*, Ann Arbor: The University of Michigan Press.
Das, E. (2005) *History and Status of Homeopathy Around the World*, New Delhi: B. Jain Publishers (Pvt) Ltd.
Dean, B. and Levi, J. M. (2003) *At the Risk of Being Heard*, Ann Arbor: The University of Michigan Press.
de Soto, H. (2000) *The Mystery of Capital*, Great Britain: Bantam Press.
De Silva, N. (2015) 'Sri Lanka's Traditional Knowledge about Health and Wellbeing: History, Present Status and the Need for Safeguarding.' in S. Garg (ed.) *Traditional Knowledge and Traditional Cultural Expression of South Asia*, Colombo: SAARC Cultural Centre. 40.
De Silva, N. (2014) 'Traditional Knowledge as Cultural Heritage in Sri Lanka: Post-Colonial Interpretation' in V *SAARC Culture*, Colombo: SAARC Cultural Centre, 23.

De Silva, K. M. (1998) *Reaping the Whirlwind: Ethnic Conflict, Ethnic Politics in Sri Lanka,* New Delhi: Penguin Books.

De Silva, K.M. (1981) *A History of Sri Lanka*, Colombo: Vijitha Yapa Publishers.

De Silva, P. and Punchihewa, A. G. (2011) *Socio-Anthropological Research Project on Vaddha Community in Sri Lanka*, Colombo: Department of Sociology, University of Colombo and Ministry of Culture and Arts.

Dharmadasa, K. N. O. (2011) 'Creolization as a Mechanism for Language Survival: The Case of the Vedda Language in Sri Lanka' paper presented at the SAARC Conference on Diminishing Cultures of South Asia. Kandy: SAARC Cultural Centre, July.

Dharmadasa, K. N. O. (1991) *Language, Religion and Ethnic Assertiveness: The Growth of Sinhalese Nationalism in Sri Lanka*, Michigan: University of Michigan Press.

Dharmadasa, K. N. O. and Samarasinghe, S. W. R. de A. (eds.) (1990) *The Vanishing Aborigines: Sri Lanka's Veddas in Transition*, Colombo: International Centre for Ethnic Studies (ICES).

Dharmadasa, K.N.O. (1974) 'The Creolization of an Aboriginal Language: The Case of the Vedda in Sri Lanka,' XVI (2) *Anthropological Linguistics*, 96.

Dhammarama, (Ven.) P. A. (2005) *Gods and their Origin in Sri Lanka: The Buddhist and the Concept of Divinity*, Dehiwela: Sri Devi Publishers.

Dias, L. (2002) *Sinhala-Tamil Nationalism and Sri Lanka's East Coast Veddas*, http://vedda.org/east-coast-veddas.htm (Last Retrieved on 20 February 2019).

Dietrich, H. J. (1958) 'Hahnemann's Capacity for Greatness- Samuel Hahnemann and Hahnemann Medical College.' 93(2) *The Hahnemannian*, 35.

Dilmah Conservation (2013) *Traditional Communities in Sri Lanka: The Ahikuntaka*, Peliyagoda: Ceylon Tea Services PLC. http://www.dilmahconservation.org/wp-content/uploads/2015/05/AHIKUNTAKA-BOOK-Without-crop-marks.pdf (Last retrieved 20 February 2019).

Dissanayake, D. (2009) *Health Care in Ancient Sri Lanka*, Address on 31 August 2008 at Royal Asiatic Society, Colombo. https://www.academia.edu/14877493/Healthcare_in_Ancient_Sri_Lanka (Last retrieved 20 February 2019.

Dissanayake, D. (2012) *Health Care in Ancient Sri Lanka* in the Saadhu Blog. http://saadhu.com/blog/2012/08/ancient-healthcare/ (Last retrieved on 20 February 2019).

Dissanayake, W. (2005) *Enabling Traditions- Four Sinhala Cultural Intellectuals*. Boralasgamuwa: Visidunu Prakashakayo (pvt.) Ltd.

Downes, D. R. and Laird, S. A. (1999) 'Sharing the Benefits of Biodiversity: Access Regimes and Intellectual Property Rights' *Science, Technology and Development Discussion Paper N°6*, Center for International Development and Belfer Centre for Science and International Affairs, Cambridge, Massachusets, USA: Harvard University.

Downes, D. R. and Laird, S. A. (1999a) *Registries of Local and Indigenous Knowledge Relating to Biodiversity: Risks and Potential for Managing Access and Benefit Sharing,* Prepared for UNCTAD Biotrade Initiative.

Downes D.R. and Laird S.A. (1999b) with contributions by Dutfield G. and Wynberg R. *Innovative Mechanisms for Sharing Benefits of Biodiversity and Related Knowledge: Case Studies on Geographical Indications and Trademarks*, prepared for UNCTAD Biotrade Initiative.

Downes D.R. and Laird S.A. (1999c) with contributions by Dutfield G, Mays TD and Casey J. *Community Registries of Biodiversity-Related Knowledge: The Role of Intellectual Property in Managing Access and Benefit,* prepared for UNCTAD Biotrade Initiative.

Drahos, P. (2014) *Intellectual Property, Indigenous People and their Knowledge,* Cambridge University Press.

Durkheim, E. (1915) *The Elementary Forms of the Religious Life*, New York; London: George Allen and Unwin: Free Press.

Durning A.T. (1992) *Guardians of the Land: Indigenous Peoples and the Health of the Earth,* Worldwatch Paper no. 112, Washington, DC, Worldwatch Institute.

Dutfield, G. (2006) *Protecting Traditional Knowledge: Pathways to the Future,* Issue Paper No. 26, Geneva: International Centre for Trade and Sustainable Development.

Dutfield, G. (2006) *Protecting Traditional Knowledge: Pathways to the Future,* (Issue Paper No. 16) Geneva: International Centre for Trade and Sustainable Development.
http://www.pmg.org.za/files/docs/100907ictsd.pdf (last retrieved 20 February 2019)

Dutfield, G. (2000) 'Developing and Implementing National Systems for Protecting Traditional Knowledge: A Review of Experiences in Selected Developing Countries.' Geneva: UNCTAD Expert Meeting on Systems and National Experiences of Protecting Traditional Knowledge, Innovation and Practices. (30 October – 1 November 2000)
http://r0.unctad.org/trade_env/docs/dutfield.pdf (last retrieved 20 February 2019)

Dutfield, G. (2000) *Intellectual Property Rights, Trade and Biodiversity: Seeds and Plants Varieties,* Earthscan and IUCN, London.

Dutt, B. B. (1925) *Town Panning in Ancient India,* New Delhi: Gyan Publishing House.

Eschenbruch, N. (2005) 'Rationalist, Magician, Scharlatan? Samuel Hahnemann and Homeopathy from the Viewpoint of Homeopathy' 94 (11) *Schweiz. Rundsch. Med. Prax.* (In German), 443.

Fanon, F. (1963) *The Wretched of the Earth*, New York: Grove Press.

Fecteau, L. (2001) 'The Ayahuasa Patent Revocation: Raising Questions About Current U.S. Patent Policy' 21 BC *Third World Law Journal* 69, 84.

Fernando, D. (1999) 'Healthcare System in Transition III. Sri Lanka, Part I. An Overview of Sri Lanka's Healthcare System' in 22 (1) *Journal of Public Health Medicin*e, 14. http://jpubhealth.oxfordjournals.org/content/22/1/14.full.pdf (last retrieved 20 February 2019)

Fink, A. (2005) *Conducting Research Literature Reviews – From Internet to Paper*, Thousand Oaks, London, New Delhi: Sage Publications.

Firouzeh, N. (2004) 'Globalisation and Homogenisation of Culture: The Role of Mass Medias in Developing Countries' in 12 *Human Ecology Special Issue,* 235.

Forsyth, M. (2013) 'How Can the Theory of Legal Pluralism Assist the Traditional Knowledge Debate?' in 33 *Intersections: Gender and Sexuality in Asia and the Pacific.* http://intersections.anu.edu.au/issue33/forsyth.htm#n7 (last retrieved 20 February 2019)

Four Directions Council (1996). *Forests, Indigenous Peoples and Biodiversity: Contribution of the Four Directions Council to the Secretariat of the Convention on Biological Diversity*, Lethbridge, Four Directions Council.

Fourmile, H. (1995) 'Protecting Indigenous Property Rights in Biodiversity' in Sultan R. (ed) *Eco-Politics IX: Perspectives on Indigenous Peoples Management of Environmental Resources*, Darwin: Northern Land Council.

Frawley, D. (2000) *Ayurvedic Healing.* 2d ed. Wisconsin: Lotus Press.

Fulcher, J. (2004) *Capitalism. A Very Short Introduction*, Oxford: Oxford University Press.

Fylan, F. (2005) 'Semi Structured Interviewing' in Miles, Jeremy and Gilbery, Paul (eds) *A Handbook of Research Methods for Clinical and Health Psychology*, Oxford: Oxford University Press. 65.

Gaillet, L. L. (2012) '(Per)Forming Archival Research Methodologies' in 64 (1) *College Composition and Communication Special Issue: Research Methodologies*, Urbana: National Council of Teachers of English http://search.proquest.com.libraryproxy.griffith.edu.au/docview/1081830956?accountid=14543 (Last Retrieved on 20 February 2019)

Gamage, G. (2007) *Law and the Judicial System of Ancient and Medieval Sri Lanka,* Diulapitiya: Saraswathi Publishers.

Gampaha Wickramarachchi Ayurveda Institute (2011) *Annual Report 2011.* Gampaha: Gampaha Wickramarachchi Ayurveda Institute.

Gandhi, M. (1994) *The Gandhi Reader: A Source Book of His Life and Writings,* Homer A. Jack (ed.) New York: Grove Press. (First published in 1956 by Indiana University Press)

Garreau, F. H. (1985) 'The Multinational Version of Social Science with Emphasis Upon the Discipline of Sociology,' 33(3) *Current Sociology,* 1.

Geiger, W. (trans) (1960) *Mahavamsa or the Great Chronicle of Ceylon*, Colombo: Ceylon Government Information Department.

Glaser, B. G. (ed.) (1994) *More Grounded Theory*, Mill Valley, CA: The Sociology-Press.

Glaser, B. G. (1992) *Basics of Grounded Theory Analysis*, Mill Valley, CA: The Sociology Press.

Glaser, B. G. and Strauss Anslem L. (1965) *Awareness of Dying*, Chicago: Aldine.

Glaser, B. G. and Strauss Anslem L. (1967) *The Discovery of Grounded Theory*, Chicago: Aldine.

Goonetilake, S. (1998) *Towards a Global Science- Mining Civilizational Knowledge*, New Delhi: Vistaar Publications.

Gray, J. (1998) *False Dawn: The Delusions of Global Capitalism*, Granta.

GRAIN and Kalpavriksh (2002) *Traditional knowledge of biodiversity in Asia-Pacific: Problems of piracy and protection* http://www.grain.org/article/entries/81-traditional-knowledge-of-biodiversity-in-asia-pacific-problems-of-piracy-and-protection#_edn1 (last retrieved 20 February 2019)

Gray, A (1999) 'Voices of the Earth: Introduction' in: D.A. Posey (ed.) *Cultural and Spiritual Values of Biodiversity: A Complementary Contribution to the Global Biodiversity Assessment*. London/Nairobi, Intermediate Technology Publications/UNEP.

Graziano, A. M. and Raulin, M. L. (2004) *Research Methods: A Process of Inquiry* (5th ed.) Boston, New York, San Francisco: Pearson Education Group.

Griffiths, J. (1986) 'What is Legal Pluralism' *24 Journal of Legal Pluralism* pp 1-55.

Griffith University (2012) *Griffith University Code for the Responsible Conduct of Research.* http://policies.griffith.edu.au/pdf/Code%20for%20the%20Responsible%20Conduct%20of%20Research.pdf (Last retrieved 20 February 2019)

Gunasekara, S. and Rajapakse R. (2007) '*Law and Policies in Sri Lanka relating to Protection of Plant Generic Resources*' in *Our Common Heritage? Farmers' Rights to Plant Generic Resources in Sri Lanka*, Colombo: Law and Society Trust.

Gunasinghe, A. (2012) *Shanthikarma, Roga Wayapashamana Vidhi ha Budhu Samaya*, (Sinhala). Published by the Author.

Gunatilake G. (1998) *Equity in Health – The Case of Sri Lanka*, Colombo: Marga Institute.

Gunawardena J. (2006) *Chapter III: Traditional Crop Varieties, Intellectual Property Rights and International Conventions in An Uncertain Future: Traditional Plant Varieties and their Crop Wild Relatives in Sri Lanka,* Colombo: Law and Society Trust.

Gunawardena, D. (1994) *Dadabimen Dadabimata* (2nd Print) Colombo: Dayawansha Jayakodi and Company. (Sinhala)

Gunawardena, D. (2003) *Veddas' The Indigenous People of Sri Lanka – 1* (New Revised Edition). A Guide to the Study of Veddas' Language and Culture. Kandy: Simple Wisdom.

Gunawardene, P., *Sri Lanka Parliament Debate Hansard* (14 June 1956)

Gupta, A. (1999), 'Rewarding Creativity for Conserving Diversity in Third World: Can IPR Regime Serve the Needs of Contemporary and Traditional Knowledge Experts and Communities in Third World?' in T. Cottier, P. Widmer and K. Schindler, (eds.), *Strategic Issues of Industrial Property Management in a Globalising Economy*. Oxford, Portland and Oregon: Hart Publishing. 119.

Gupta, V. K. *Traditional Knowledge Digital Library (TKDL)* India: Council of Scientific and Industrial Research. http://www.csir.res.in/# (last retrieved 8 September 2014)

Guruge, A.W. P. (1975) *Buddhism- The Religion and It's Culture*, (2nd Print- 1984), Dehiwala: Sridevi Printing Works.

Guruge, A.W.P. (2007) 'Henry Steel Olcott in Sri Lanka: Death Centennial Tribute' in *Theosophical History, 13 (1)*, 10.

Hamilton, T. (2009) *Immortal Longings: F. W. H. Myers and the Victorian Search for Life After Death,* Imprint Academic.

Hannum, H. (2011) 'New Developments in Indigenous Rights.' 28 (649) *Virginia Journal of International law,* 1988. Available at SSRN:

http://papers.ssrn.com/sol3/papers.cfm?abstract_id=1957812 (last retrieved 20 February 2019)

Harankaha, M. H. A. *A Review on the Proposed Act for the Protection of New Plant Varieties (Breeders Rights) – A Critical Analysis*. University of Colombo. http://www.cmb.ac.lk/wp-content/uploads/2014/02/A-REVIEW-ON-THE-PROPOSED-ACT-FOR-THE-PROTECTION-OF-NEW-PLANT-VARIETIES.pdf (last retrieved 20 February 2019)

Hardt M. and Negri A. (2000) *Empire*, Cambridge: Harvard University Press.

Harris, M. (2013) 'Emergent Indigenous Identities: Rejecting the Need for Purity' in *The Politics of Identity: Emerging Indigeneity*, Sydney: UTSePress. Pp 10-25

Harris, M., Carlson B. and Poata-Smith E. (2013) 'Indigenous Identities and the Politics of Authenticity' in *The Politics of Identity: Emerging Indigeneity*, Sydney: UTSePress. pp1-9.

Haverkort B., and Reijntjes, C. (2010) 'Diversities of Knowledge Communities, their Worldviews and Sciences: On the Challenges of their Co-evolution' in S.M. Subramanian and B. Pisupati, (ed.) *Traditional Knowledge in Policy and Practice: Approaches to Development and Human Well-Being*, Tokyo, New York, Paris: United Nations University. 12.

Hill, R. M. (1993) *Archival Strategies and Techniques*, California and New Delhi: Sage Publications, Inc. http://srmo.sagepub.com.libraryproxy.griffith.edu.au/view/archival-strategies-and-techniques/SAGE.xml (Last Retrieved on 20 February 2019)

Hirimuthugodage, D. (2013) *Biodiversity as a Cornerstone of Sustainable Development: A Sri Lankan Perspective*, The Island Online. http://www.island.lk/index.php?page_cat=article-details&page=article-details&code_title=79554 (last retrieved 20 February 2019).

Holsti, O. R. (1968) *Content Analysis for the Social Sciences and the Humanities*, Reading, MA: Addison-Wesley.

Holt, J. (ed.) (2011) *The Sri Lanka Reader: History, Culture, Politics,* Durham and London: Duke University Press Books.

Homeopathy Medical Council (2010) *Annual Report of the Homeopathic Medical Council 2010*.

Horner, I. B. (trans) (1975) *The Minor Anthologies of the Pali Cannon (Part III): 'Chronicle of Buddhas' (Buddhavamsa) and 'Basket of Conduct' (Cariyapitaka)*, Oxford: Pali Text Society.

Hussein, A. (2009) *Zeylanica: A Study of the Peoples and Languages of Sri Lanka*, Colombo: Neptune Publications (Pvt.) Ltd.

IIM (2012) *Annual Report- 2012*, Institute of Indigenous Medicine, University of Colombo.

International Society for Ethnobiology (ISE), *International Society of Ethnobiology Code of Ethics 2006* (with 2008 additions) available at http://www.ethnobiology.net/what-we-do/core-programs/ise-ethics-program/code-of-ethics/ (last retrieved 10 February 2015)

Jan, S. (1983) 'Patterns of Legislation Concerning Traditional Medicine' in Robert, H. Banner man et. al. (eds:) *Traditional Medicine in Health Care Coverage*. Geneva, WHO, 290.

Jayasekera H. L. S. '*The Sources of Sinhalese Customary Laws*' in 1 (1) *The Journal of Ceylon Laws*.

Jayathilaka, D. B. (1934) *Sri Saranankara- Lankawe Anthima Sangarajayan Wahanse*, Colombo: Lankahinahawa.

Jayawardena, K. (2012) *Nobodies to Somebodies: The Rise of the Colonial Bourgeoisie in Sri Lanka*, Colombo: SSA.

Jaysasekera, M. L. S. (1984) *Customary Laws of Sri Lanka in their Historical and Cultural Background*, Sri Lanka: Ministry of Cultural Affairs.

Johns, T. and Eyzaguirre, P. B. (2006). 'Linking Biodiversity, Diet and Health in Policy and Practice.' *Proceedings of the Nutrition Society*, 65(2), 182.

Jones, M. (2009) *The Hospital System and Health Care, Sri Lanka, 1815 – 1960,* New Delhi: Orient Blackswan.

Jorgensen, D. L. (1989) *Participant Observation: A Methodology for Human Studies*, 15. London: SAGE.

Kamardeen, N. (2013) 'Proposed Plant Variety Legislation in Promoting Economic Growth.' In *Sunday Times, Business Times*. http://www.sundaytimes.lk/131110/business-times/proposed-plant-variety-legislation-in-promoting-economic-growth-68091.html (last retrieved 20 February 2019)

Kandaswamy, P.N. (1979) *History of Siddha Medicine*, Madras.

Kannangara, A. P. (2011) *A Survey of Social Change in an Imperial Regime*, Colombo: Vijitha Yapa Publications.

Karem, J. (2001) 'On the Advantages and Disadvantages of Postcolonial Theory for Pan-American Study' in 1 (3) *CR: The New Centennial Review,* 87. https://muse.jhu.edu/login?auth=0&type=summary&url=/journals/new_centennial_review/v001/1.3karem.html (last retrieved 20 February 2019)

Katiresu, C. S. A (1907, 2010) *Hand Book of The Thesawalamai* (1907), Montana: Kessinger Publishing LLC.

Kayne, S. (2006). 'Samuel Hahnemann (1755–1843): the Founder of Modern Homeopathy' 36 (2) *Pharmaceutical historian*.

Kelly (2005) *Report on Threats to the Practice and Transmission of Traditional Knowledge Regional Report: Asia and Australia*, Australian Institute of Aboriginal and Torres Strait Islander Studies (AIATSIS). http://aiatsis.gov.au/sites/default/files/products/research_outputs_submission/2006-convention-on-biological-diversity.pdf (Last retrieved 20 February 2019)

Kidwell, C.S. (2009) 'American Indian Studies: Intellectual Navel Gazing or Academic Discipline?' in 33 (1) *The American Indian Quarterly,* 1.

Kiene T. (2011) *The Legal Protection of Traditional Knowledge in the Pharmaceutical Field: An Intercultural Problem in the International Agenda*, Münster: WaxmannVerlag GmbH.

Kipuri, N. (2009) 'Chapter II: Culture' in *State of the World Indigenous Peoples*, New York: Department of Economic and Social Affairs, United Nations, 51.

Kotagama, S. (2013) Special Lecture on 'Traditional Knowledge and Biodiversity' delivered at the SAARC Regional Seminar on Traditional Knowledge and Traditional Cultural Expressions of South Asia. (30 April 2013) Sigiriya: SAARC Cultural Centre.

Kumar, V. (2002) *Vastushastra.* New Dawn/ Sterling.

Kumar, V. (2000) *Systems and National Experiences for Protecting Traditional Knowledge, Innovations and Practices –Sri Lanka*. Geneva: UNCTAD Expert Meeting on Systems and National Experiences for Protecting Traditional Knowledge, Innovations and Practices (30 October – 1 November 2000) http://r0.unctad.org/trade_env/docs/srilanka.pdf (last retrieved 20 February 2019)

Kusumaratane, S. (2005) *Indigenous Medicine in Sri Lanka- A Sociological Analysis*, Nugegoda: Sarasavi Publishers.

Latour, B. (2004) 'Why Has Critique Run out of Steam? From Matters of Fact to Matters of Concern' 30(2) *Critical Inquiry.* 225.

Lawrence, W. (2002) 'Indigenous People and the Environment: Convergence from Nordic Perspective (Norway)' in 20 *UCLA Journal of Environmental Law & Policy.*

Le Masurier C. J. R. and Panabokke T. B. (eds.) (1880) *Niti Niganduwa a Code of Law Belonging to the Last Days of the Kandyan Period,* Colombo: Government Press.

Leanne F. (2001) 'The Ayahuasa Patent Revocation: Raising Questions About Current U.S. Patent Policy' 21 *BC Third World Law Journal* 69.

Lee, R. W. (1946) *The Elements of Roman Law: With a Translation of the Institutes of Justinian*, London: Sweet and Maxwell.

Leslie, C. (1992) ‘8 - Interpretation of Illness: Syncretism in Modern Ayurveda’ in Charles M. Leslie and Allan Young (eds) *Paths to Asian Medical Knowledge*. Berkeley: University of California Press Berkeley, 177.

Lenora, R. B. (1954) ‘Progress of Ayurveda’ in *Silver Jubilee Souvenir*. Colombo: Government College of Indigenous Medicine (English language section). 4.

Lindemann, G. (2011) 'On Latour’s Social Theory and Theory of Society, and His Contribution to Saving the World' 34(1) *Human Studies* 93.

Lodha R, Bagga A. (2000) ‘Traditional Indian Systems of Medicine.’ 29(1) *Ann Acad Med* Singapore, 37.

Lofland, J. and Lofland, L. H. (1995) *Analysing Social Settings,* 3rd ed. Belmont, CA: Wordsworth.

Lofland, J. (1974) ‘Styles of Reporting Qualitative Field Research.’ *American Sociologist.* 9: 101-111.

Lofland, J. (1976) *Doing Social Life: The Qualitative Study of the Human Interactions in Natural Settings,* New York: Wiley.

Longhurst, R. (2010) ‘Semi Structured Interviews and Focus Groups’ in, Nicholas Clifford, Shaun French and Gill Valentine, (eds) *Key Methods in Geography*. SAGE, 103.

Lowe W. N. S. (2007) *Evolution of the Compulsory Service System (Rajakariya) in Sri Lanka,* Kelaniya: University of Kelaniya.

MacKay, F., *A Guide to Indigenous Peoples’ Rights in the International Labour Organization*, Forest Peoples Programme. http://www.forestpeoples.org/sites/fpp/files/publication/2010/09/iloguideiprightsjul02eng.pdf (last retrieved 20 February 2019)

Mackenzie, E. R. and Rakel, B. (2006) *Complementary and Alternative Medicine for Older Adults: A Guide to Holistic Approaches to Healthy Aging*, Springer.

Madan, T. N. (1966) ‘For a Sociology of India,’ 9 *Contributions to Indian Sociology*, 9.

Malinowski, B. K. (1935) *Coral Gardens and their Magic*, New York: Dover.

Malinowski, B. K. (1948) *Magic, Science and Religion and Other Essays,* Glencoe, Illinois: The Free Press.

Matthews, J. (2000) ‘Religion in the Social Sciences: A Socio-epistemological Critique,’ 56 *Akademika*, 85.

Meegaskumbura, P.B. (1990) 'Religious Beliefs of the Veddas in Relation to their Word view' in K.N.O. Dharmadasa Samarasinghe, S. W. R. de A. (eds.) *Vanishing Aborigines*, 99.

Meissner, M. (1992) 'Samuel Hahnemann—the Originator of Homeopathic Medicine.' 30 (7–8) *Krankenpflege Journal*, 364.

Moreton- Robinson, A. (ed.) (2004) 'Whiteness, Epistemology and Indigenous Representation' in *Whitening Race: Essays in Social and Cultural Criticism*, Canberra: Aboriginal Studies Press.

Morris, B. (1988) *Anthropological Studies of Religion*, Cambridge: Cambridge University Press.

Motwani, K. (1955) *Colonel H. S. Olcott, a Forgotten Page in American History*, Madras: Ganesh.

Mugabe, J. (1999) *Intellectual Property Protection and Traditional Knowledge: An Exploration in International Policy Discourse*, Nairobi: ACTS Press.

Munzer, S. and Rustiala, K. (2009) 'The Uneasy Case for Intellectual Property Rights in Traditional Knowledge' 27 *Cardozo Arts & Entertainment Law Journal* 37, 38.

Murphet, H. (1972) *Hammer on the Mountain, Life of Henry Steel Olcott (1832-1907)*, Wheaton: Theosophical Publishing House.

Nagel, J. (1993), 'Constructing ethnicity: creating and recreating ethnic identity and culture', in Yetman, N. (ed.), *Majority and Minority: The Dynamics of Race and Ethnicity in American Life*, 6th ed., Boston, MA: Allyn and Bacon.

Narayanaswamy V. (1975) *Introduction to the Siddha System of Medicine*, T. Nagar, Madras (Chennai): Research Institute of Siddha Medicine.

Neuman W. L. (2000) *Social Research Methods – Qualitative and Quantitative Approaches* (4th ed.) MA: Allyn and Bacon.

Neuman W. L. (1994) *Social Research Methods – Qualitative and Quantitative Approaches* (2nd ed.) MA: Allyn and Bacon.

Nijar, G. S. (1996) *In Defense of Indigenous Knowledge and Biodiversity: a Conceptual Framework and Essential Elements of a Right Regime*, Third World Network Briefing Paper N° 1. Penang, Malaysia.

Nordstrom, C. R. (1988) 'Exploring Pluralism – The Many Faces of Ayurveda' in 27 (5) *Social Science and Medicine,* 479.

Nordstrom, C. R. (1989) 'Ayurveda: A Multilectic Interpretation' in 28 (9) *Social Science and Medicine,* 963.

Obeyesekere, G. (1970) 'Religious Symbolism and Political Change in Ceylon' in 1 *Modern Ceylon Studies*, 43.

Obeyesekere, G. (1970) 'The Idiom of Demonic Possession: A Case Study.'4 *SSMed,* 97.

Obeyesekere, G. (1977) 'Psycho-cultural Exegesis of a Case of Spirit Possession in Sri Lanka' in Vincent Crapanzaro and Vivian Garrison (eds) *Case Studies in Spirit Possession,* New York: John Wiley and Sons.

Obeyesekere, G. (1977) 'Theory and Practice of Psychological Medicine in the Ayurvedic Tradition' in 1 (2) *Culture, Medicine and Psychiatry,* 155.

Obeyesekere, G. (1978) 'The Firewalkers of Kataragama: the Rise of *Bhakti* Religiosity in Buddhist Sri Lanka' in 37 (3) *Journal of Asian Studies*, 457.

Obeysekere, G. (2002) 'Where Have All the Väddas Gone? Buddhism and Aboriginality in Sri Lanka' in Neluka Silva (ed.) *The Hybrid Island: Culture Crossing and the Invention of Identity in Sri Lanka*, Colombo: Social Scientists'' Association, 1.

Pahuja, S. (2011) *Decolonising International Law: Development, Economic Growth and the Politics of Universality*, Cambridge: Cambridge University Press.

Pal, Madhabendranath (1991) 'The Tridosha Theory.' In 10 (3) *Ancient Science of Life,* 144-155. http://www.ncbi.nlm.nih.gov/pmc/articles/PMC3331283/pdf/ASL-10-144.pdf (Last retrieved 20 February 2019)

Pathmeswaran, A., Nugegoda, D. B., Post, E. (2008) *Report of the Independent Evaluation: The Anti Leprosy Campaign Sri Lanka 2008.* Colombo.

Patton, M. Q. (2002) *Qualitative Research and Evaluation Methods*. Sage Publications, Inc.

Patwardhan, B.; Warude, D.; Pushpangadan, P. and Bhatt, N. (2005) 'Ayurveda and Traditional Chinese Medicine: A Comparative Overview' in 2 (4) *Evidence-Based Complementary and Alternative Medicine*, 465.

Perera M. A, L. R. (1996) 'Health Care Services in Sri Lanka, the Success Story of the Century' in *Health for all – today?* Colombo: SIRHA, Faculty of Medicine.

Perera, A. (2011) 'Plant Variety Protection in Sri Lanka and its Impact on Sri Lanka's Agricultural Economy: A Critical Analysis' in 14 (3-4) *The Journal of World Intellectual Property*, 301-333. http://onlinelibrary.wiley.com/doi/10.1111/j.1747-1796.2011.00420.x/abstract (last retrieved 20 February 2019)

Perera, D. (2013) 'Ayurvedization of Indigenous Medical Knowledge' Lecture delivered on 30 December 2013 at the Royal Asiatic Society, Colombo 7.

Parry, J. (1986) The Gift, the Indian Gift and the 'Indian Gift' in *Man, New Series, Vol. 21, No. 3,* pp. 453-473 https://www2.warwick.ac.uk/fac/arts/history/ecc/events/writingrights/workshopprogramme/readingmaterials/parry_-_gift_indian_gift.pdf (last retrieved 21 April 2016)

Pesek, T. J., Helton, L. R., and Nair, M. (2006) 'Healing across cultures: Learning from traditions' in 3 (2) *EcoHealth,* 114.

Pieris, R. (1964) 'Vedda and Sinhalese Kinship,' in 64 (139) *Man*, 118.

Pongsiri, M. J., Roman J., Ezenwa, V.O., Goldberg, T.L., Koren, H. S., Newbold, S. C., Ostfeld, R. S., Pattanayak, S. K. and Daniel J. Salkeld, D. J. (2009) 'Biodiversity loss affects global disease ecology' in 59, (11) *Bioscience*, 945.

Posey D.A. (1999) 'Introduction: Culture and Nature – The Inextricable Link' in *Cultural and Spiritual Values of Biodiversity – A Complementary Contribution to the Global Biodiversity Assessment.* London and Nairobi: Intermediate Technology Publications/UNEP.

Posey D.A., (ed.) (1996). *Traditional Resource Rights: International Instruments for Protection and Compensation for Indigenous Peoples and Local Communities*, Gland, Switzerland, IUCN.

Prematilleke, L. and Aluvihare, A. (2012) 'The Archaeology of Buddhist Monastic Hospitals in Ancient Lanka' paper presented at the SAARC International Conference on Archaeology of Buddhism: Recent Discoveries in South Asia, Colombo: SAARC Cultural Centre. August.

Prothero, S. R. (1996) *The White Buddhist, the Asian Odyssey of Henry Steel Olcott*, Bloomington: Indiana University Press.

Raj, S. J. and Harman, W. P. (2006) *Dealing with Deities – The Ritual Vow in South Asia*, New York: State University of New York Press.

Ramanna, A. and Udgaonkar, S. (2005) 'Intellectual Property Rights in South Asia: Opportunities and Constraints for Technology Transfer' in S. C. Babu and A. Gulati (eds.) *Economic Reforms and Food Security: The Impact of Trade and Technology in South Asia*, New York: Food Products Press and International Business Press.

Reyes-García, V., et al. (2013), 'Evidence of Traditional Knowledge Loss Among a Contemporary Indigenous Society,' 34 (4) *Evolution and Human Behavior,* 249. http://dx.doi.org/10.1016/j.evolhumbehav.2013.03.002 (last retrieved 20 February 2019)

Rizza, E. (1994). 'Samuel Hahnemann: A Mystical Empiricist. A Study of the Origin and Development of the Homeopathic Medical System' in 6 (3) *Medicina nei secoli*, 515.

Robinson, D. (2010) *Confronting Biopiracy: Challenges, Cases and International Debates*, London: Earthscan.

Rodrigues, E. B. (2012) 'Property Rights, Biocultural Resources and Two Tragedies: Some Lessons from Brazil' in T. Bubela, and E. R. Gold (eds.) *Genetic Resources and Traditional Knowledge. Case Studies and Conflicting Interests*, Northampton: Edward Elgar, 113.

Rodriguez-Navarro, G. E. (2000) 'Indigenous Knowledge as an Innovative Contribution to the Sustainable Development of the Sierra Nevada of Santa Marta, Colombia: The Elder Brothers, Guardians of the "Heart of the World"' in 29 (7) *AMBIO: A Journal of the Human Environment.*

Rural Advancement Foundation International. (1994) *Conserving Indigenous Knowledge: Integrating Two Systems of Innovation*, An Independent Study by the Rural Advancement Foundation International, New York: United Nations Development Programme.

Saberwal, S. (1968) 'The Problem' in 112 *Seminar,* Special Issue on Academic Colonialism, New Delhi, 10-13.

Said, E. (1993) *Culture and Imperialism,* London: Chatto and Windus.

Saks, M. (2008) 'Plural Medicine and East-West Dialogue' in Dagmar Wujastyk, and Frederick M. Smith (eds.) *Modern and Global Ayurveda: Pluralism and Paradigms*. Albany, NY, USA: State University of New York Press, 2008, 29.

Samaraweera, V. (1997) 'The Muslim Revivalist Movement: 1880-1915' in *Sri Lanka: Collective Identities Revisited*, M. Roberts (ed), Colombo: Marga Institute.

Saunders, M., Lewis, P. and Thornhill A. (1997, 2009) *Research Methods for Business Students*, Essex: Pearson Education Limited.

Scott, J. and Marshall, G. (2005) *A Dictionary of Sociology*, Oxford University Press.

Seligmann, C. G. and Seligmann, B. Z. (1911) *The Veddas*. Cambridge: Cambridge University Press.

Sayer, D. (1991) *Capitalism and Modernity*, Routledge.

Silva, K. T. (1991) 'Ayurveda, Malaria and the Indigenous Herbal Tradition in Sri Lanka' in 33 (2) *Social Science and Medicine*, 153.

Simpson, B. (1997) 'Possession, Dispossession and the Social Distribution of Knowledge Among Sri Lankan Ritual Specialists.' *The Journal of the Royal Anthropological Institute, Vol 3, No 1*, pp 43-59 http://www.jstor.org.libraryproxy.griffith.edu.au/stable/3034364?pq-origsite=summon&seq=1#page_scan_tab_contents (last retrieved 20 February 2019)

Singh, A. and Schmidt, P. (2000) *Postcolonial Theory and the United States Race, Ethnicity and Literature,* Mississippi: University Press of Mississippi.

Sinha, V. (1997) 'Reconceptualizing the Social Sciences in Non-Western Settings: Challenges and Dilemmas,' 25 (1) *Southeast Asian Journal of Social Science, 167.*

Siriweera, W. I. *Ayurveda Hospitals in Ancient Sri Lanka* (Summary of a guest lecture delivered at the sixth International Medical Congress organised by the Peradeniya Medical School Alumni Association and the Faculty of Medicine) http://sinhalanet.com/ayurveda.html (last retrieved on 19 February 2013)

Shiva, V. (2000) 'The World on the Edge' in W. Hutton and A. Giddens (eds) *On the Edge: Living with Global Capitalism*, London: Jonathan Cape.

Smith, L. W. (1978) 'An Evolving Logic of Participant Observation, Educational Ethnography and Other Case Studies' in L. Shulman (ed.) *Review of Research in Education*. Itasca, IL: Peacock

Snyder, W. M. (1997) 'Communities of Practice: Combining Organizational Learning and Strategy – Insights to Create a Bridge to the 21st Century. Academy pf Management Conference – 1997.

Social Policy Analysis Research Centre (2009) *PADHI (Psychosocial Assessment of Development and Humanitarian Interventions) Conceptual Framework to Understand the Determinants of Wellbeing in Sri Lanka*. Colombo: Social Policy Analysis Research Centre (SPARC)

Soni, R. L. and Kantipalo, (Bhikkhu) (2006) *Life's Highest Blessings – The Maha Mangala Sutta*. http://www.accesstoinsight.org/lib/authors/soni/wheel254.html (Last retrieved 20 February 2019).

Spencer, J. (ed) (1990) *Sri Lanka: History and the Roots of Conflict,* Routledge.

Sri Lanka Resource Centre for Indigenous Knowledge (SLRCIK) (1996) Proceedings of the First National Symposium on Indigenous Knowledge and Sustainable Development, 19-20 March, Colombo: SLRCIK.

Stake, R. E. (1994) 'Case Studies' in N. K. Denzin and Y. S. Lincoln (eds*)* *Handbook of Qualitative Research*, Thousand Oaks, CA: Sage Publications.

St. Claire, D. (1978) *David St. Clair's Lessons in Instant ESP,* Prentice-Hall.

Stern, P. N. (1994) 'The Grounded Theory Method: Its Uses and Processes' in B. G. Glaser (ed.), *More Grounded Theory: A reader,* Mill Valley, CA: The Sociology Press, 116.

Steven M. and Kal R. (2009) 'The Uneasy Case for Intellectual Property Rights in Traditional Knowledge' 27 *Cardozo Arts and Entertainment Law Journal* 37, 38.

Stiglitz J.E. (1999) 'Knowledge as a Global Public Good' in I. Kaul, et al. (eds.) *Global Public Goods: International Cooperation in the 21st Century*, Oxford, OUP, 320.

Stone, P. et al (1966) *The General Inquirer: A Computer Approach to Content Analysis in the Behavioral Sciences*, Cambridge, MA: MIT Press.

Strauss, A. L. and Corbin, J. M. (1990) *Basics of Qualitative Research: Grounded Theory Procedures and Techniques*, Newbury Park, CA: Sage.

Strauss, A. L. and Corbin, J. M. (1994) 'Grounded Theory Methodology: An Overview' in N. K. Denzin and Y. S. Lmcoln (eds.), *Handbook of Qualitative Research*, Thousand Oaks, CA: Sage, 273.

Strauss, A. L. (1987) *Qualitative Analysis for Social Scientists*, New York: Cambridge University Press.

Subasinghe, W. (2005) 'Gypsy Culture and Society in the Changing World: A Sociological Analysis' presented at the 10th International Conference on Sri Lankan Studies. 16-18 December 2005, University of Kelaniya.

Subramanian S.M. and Pisupati, B. (eds.) (2010) *Traditional Knowledge in Policy and Practice: Approaches to Development and Human Well-Being*, Tokyo, New York, Paris: United Nations University.

Swaminathan, J. M. *Need of IP Policies for R and D Institutes and Industries*, http://www.juliusandcreasy.com/inpages/publications/pdf/need_of_ip_policies_for_r.pdf (last retrieved 20 February 2019)

Talaat, W, Asma, W. I, Mohd N. and Lokman, H.M. (2012) 'Traditional Knowledge on Genetic Resources: Safeguarding the Cultural Sustenance of Indigenous Communities,' in 8 (7) *Asian Social Science.*

Talagala, C. (2012) *Enforcement of Intellectual Property Rights in Sri Lanka: Some Issues*, Social Science Research Network. http://papers.ssrn.com/sol3/papers.cfm?abstract_id=2136251 (last retrieved 20 February 2019)

Parsons, Talcott. (1970). *The System of Modern Societies*, New York

Parsons, Talcott. (1977). *Social Systems and the Evolution of Action Theory*, New York

Parsons, Talcott. (1978). *Action Theory and the Human Condition*, New York

Tobin, B. M. (2013) 'Bridging the Nagoya Compiance Gap: The Fundamental Role of Customary Law in Protection of Indigenous Peoples' Resource and Knowledge Rights.' *9/2 Law Environment and Development Journal*, iv. Pp 142-162.

Tobin, B. (1997), 'Know-how Licenses Recognising Indigenous Rights Over Collective Knowledge,' 4 *Bulletin of the Working Group on Traditional Resource Rights*, 17.

Turner, V. (1977) 'Symbols in African Ritual' in J. L. Dolgin, D. S. Kemnitzer and D. M. Schneider (eds) *Symbolic Anthropology: A Reader in the Study of Symbols and Meanings*, New York: Columbia University Press, 183.

Twarog S. and Kapoor P. (ed.) (2004) *Protecting and Promoting Traditional Knolwdge: Systems, National Experiences and International Dimensions*, Geneva: United Nations Conference on Trade and Development document (UNCTD/DITC/TED/10) http://unctad.org/en/docs/ditcted10_en.pdf (last retrieved 20 February 2019)

Twarog, S. and Kapoor, P. (ed.) (2004) *Protecting and Promoting Traditional Knowledge: Systems, National Experiences and International Dimensions*, Geneva: UNCTD (UNCTAD/DITC/TED/10)

Twarog, S. (2003) '*Preserving, Protecting and Promoting Traditional Knowledge: National Actions and International Dimensions*' in *Progressing Towards the Doha Development Agenda: Selected Papers on Trade and Development Research Issues for Asian Countries*, Inamoand Xuto, ITD and ADB

Ullman, D. (2007) *The Homeopathic Revolution – Why Famous People and Cultural Heroes Choose Homeopathy*, Berkely, CA: North Atlantic Books.

Uragoda, C. G. (1987) *A History of Medicine in Sri Lanka*, Colombo: Sri Lanka Medical Association.

Uragoda, C. G. (1995) 'Health Principles Reflected in Ancient Ruins' in, 36 *Science Education Series (Ancient Artefacts and Monumental Structures)*, 48. http://thakshana.nsf.ac.lk/slstic/NA-129/NA_129.pdf (last retrieved on 20 February 2019)

Uragoda, C. G. (2000) *Traditions of Sri Lanka: A Selection with a Scientific Background*, Rathmalana: Vishva Lekha Printers (2nd ed. 2008).

Uyangoda J. (1998) *Caste and Sinhalese Society, Culture and Politics*, Colombo: Social Scientists Association.

Walpola, R. (1956) *History of Buddhism in Ceylon*, Dehiwela: The Buddhist Cultural Centre (3rd ed. 1993).
Walsh, C. (2009) 'The Plurinational and Intercultural State: Decolonization and State Re-founding in Ecuador', *Kult 6 - Special Issue, Epistemologies of Transformation: The Latin American Decolonial Option and its Ramifications* 65.
Wanninayaka, P. B. (1982) *Ayurveda in Sri Lanka*, Colombo: Ministry of Health of Sri Lanka.
Warnapala, Y. and Silva. K. *Z-Score Demystified: A Critical Analysis of the Sri Lankan University Admission Policy,* Journal of Case Studies in Education. http://www.aabri.com/manuscripts/10741.pdf (last retrieved on 20 February 2019)
Warusawitharane, C. (2012) *Kem: Curious Beliefs* exploresrilanka.lk/2012/07/kem-curious-beliefs/ (Last Retrieved on 20 February 2019)
Wax, R. H. (1971) *Doing Field Work: Warnings and Advice,* Chicago: University of Chicago Press.
Waxler-Morrison, E. N. (1988) 'Plural Medicine in Sri Lanka: Do Ayurvedic and Western Medical Practices Differ?' in 27 (5) *Social Science and Medicine*, 531.
Wickremasinge, D.M.de Z. (1900) *Catalogue of the Sinhalese Manuscripts in the British Museum*, London: The British Museum.
Wickramasinghe, N. (2006) *Sri Lanka in the Modern Age: a History of Contested Identities*, Honolulu: University of Hawaii Press.
Wickremasinghe, N. (2014) *Sri Lanka in Modern Age- A History*, Oxford University Press
Wickramasinghe S. (2006) 'Development of the National Agricultural Research System in Sri Lanka with Special Reference to Food Crops Sub-Sector: Issues Related to Science Policy' in *Journal of the National Science Foundation of Sri Lanka 34(2),* National Science Foundation, Colombo, 69.
Wickremasinghe S. (2008) 'Science and Technology Structure, Statistical System and the Current Scenario in Sri Lanka' in Seetha I. Wickremasinghe and V.K. Gupta (eds.) *Science and Technology Policy and Indicators for Development: Perspective from Developing Countries*, Tri Nagar: Daya Publishing House, 57.
Wiessner, S. (2011) 'The Cultural Rights of Indigenous Peoples: Achievements and Continuing Challenges' in 22 (1) *The European Journal of International Law,* 121.

Wiessner, S. (2008) 'Indigenous Sovereignty: A Reassessment in Light of the UN Declaration on the Rights of Indigenous Peoples,' 41 *Vanderbilt Journal of Transitional Law,* 1141.

Wijesekera, N. D. (1964) *Veddas in Transition*. Colombo: M.D. Gunasena and Co. Ltd.

WIPO (2001). *Intellectual Property Needs and Expectations of Traditional Knowledge Holders*, Geneva: WIPO.

Wijesekera, N. (1987) *Deities and Demons Magic and Masks (Part 1),* Colombo: M. D. Gunasena and Co. Ltd.

WIPO, *Intellectual Property and Traditional Knowledge*, (Booklet no 2) http://www.wipo.int/edocs/pubdocs/en/tk/920/wipo_pub_920.pdf (last retrieved 20 February 2019)

Witharana D. (2006). 'Flying Without Wings: Good Governance and Development in a Shrinking Local Policy Space – GATS and Reforms,' paper presented at International Conference on Governance and Development, Kandy.

Witharana D., Amarasuriya H., Geeganage J., Gunaratne R., Hemaratne T., Seneviratne W. (2009) *Intellectual Property Rights and Access to Knowledge Initiatives in Sri Lanka*. Nawala: OUSL.

Wolffers, I. (1985) *Factors that Influence Patients in Sri Lanka in their Choice between Ayurvedic and Western Medicine,* 291 British Medical Journal, 970.

Wolffers, I. (1987) *Changing Traditions in Health Care, Sri Lanka*. Leiden: Ph.D. Dissertation.

Wolffers, I. (1989) 'Traditional Practitioners and Western Pharmaceuticals in Sri Lanka' in Geest (ed.) *The Context of Medicines in Developing Countries: Studies in Pharmaceutical Anthropology*, 47.

Wood, E. M. (1999) *The Origin of Capitalism*, Monthly Review Press.

Wujastyk, D. and Smith, F. M. (eds.) (2008) *Modern and Global Ayurveda: Pluralism and Paradigms*, Albany, NY, USA: State University of New York Press.

Yogasundaram, N. (2010) *A Comprehensive History of Sri Lanka from Prehistoric Times to the Present*, Colombo: Vijitha Yapa Publishers.

Young, R. J. C. (2003) *Postcolonialism- A Very Short Introduction*, Oxford: Oxford University Press.

Government Material

Ayurveda Medical Council www.ayurvedicmedicoun.gov.lk/ (last retrieved 20 February 2019)

Department of Ayurveda (2013) *New Year Handbook- 2012- 2013.* Navinna: Department of Ayurveda

Department of Ayurveda (2014) *New Year Handbook- 2013- 2014.* Navinna: Department of Ayurveda

Department of Ayurveda http://www.ayurveda.gov.lk/ (last retrieved 20 February 2019)

Department of Ayurveda, Central Province - http://www.ayurvedacpc.org/ (last retrieved 20 February 2019)

Department of Ayurveda, Western Province – http://www.itrdi.wpc.gov.lk/?dt_portfolio=department-of-ayurveda-western-province (last retrieved 20 February 2019)

Department of Census and Statistics of Sri Lanka http://www.statistics.gov.lk/ (last retrieved 20 February 2019)

Department of Medical and Sanitary Services (1949) *Administrative Report of the Director of Medical and Sanitary Services for 1948.* Colombo: Department of Medical and Sanitary Services.

Department of National Planning (2006). *Mahinda Chinthana: Vision for a New Sri Lanka: A Ten Year Horizon Development Framework 2006-2016 – Discussion Paper.* Department of National Planning, Ministry of Finance and Planning.

Gampaha Wickramarachchi Ayurveda Institute, University of Kelaniya. www.kln.ac.lk/institutes/wickramarachchi/ (last retrieved 20 February 2019)

Gampaha Wickramarachchi Siddha Ayurveda Teaching Hospital www.kln.ac.lk/institutes/wickramarachchi/index.php/gampaha-wickramarachchi-ayurveda-teaching-hospital.html (last retrieved 4 September 2015)

GOSL (2005) *Mahinda Chinthanaya - Towards a New Sri Lanka* (Policy Statement for Government of Sri Lanka for Presidential Elections 2005). Government Publication.

Institute of Indigenous Medicine, University of Colombo www.iim.cmb.ac.lk/ (last retrieved 20 February 2019)

Ministry of Education. *Education for All: National Action Plan* – Sri Lanka.

Ministry of Forestry and Environment (1999) Biodiversity Conservation in Sri Lanka: A Framework for Action. http://www.cbd.int/doc/world/lk/lk-nbsap-01-en.pdf. (last retrieved 26 November 2014)

Ministry of Health (1955) *Proposals for the Revival and Development of Indigenous Medicine in Ceylon*, Ceylon: Government Press.

Ministry of Health and Indigenous Medicine, Northern Province http://www.np.gov.lk/index.php?option=com_content&view=article&id=179&Itemid=16 (last retrieved 20 February 2019)

Ministry of Indigenous Medicine www.indigenousmedimini.gov.lk/ (last retrieved 20 February 2019)

NASTEC (2008) *National Science and Technology Policy*, Colombo: National Science and Technology Commission, Ministry of Science and Technology.

National Intellectual Property Office of Sri Lanka http://www.nipo.gov.lk (last retrieved 20 February 2019)

Sri Lanka Ayurvedic Drugs Corporation www.ayurvediccorp.gov.lk/web/ (last retrieved 20 February 2019)

Sessional Papers

Report of the Committee on Indigenous System of Medicine, Sessional Paper 1 of 1927.

Report of a Subcommittee of the Executive Committee of Health on the Board of Indigenous Medicine and the Decisions on the Report by the Executive Committee Sessional Paper 94 of 1935.

The Report on the Commission on Indigenous Medicine. Sessional Paper 24 of 1947 (Acc. No 117, Class No. GP (24))

The Report on Medical and Public Health Organizations of Ceylon. (1950 pt 1- Acc No. 120, Class No. GP (3))

The Report of the Committee on Indigenous Medicine (Sinhalese), 1950 pt 1- Acc No. 120, Class No. GP (17)

The Report on the committee of inquiry on Homeopathy, Vol 1, no 1 of 1956.

The Report on the Organization of Health Services of Ceylon. Volume 1, no 16 of 1956.

The Report of the Committee of Enquiry into Matters relating to the Abolition of Private Practice of Government Medical Officers. Volume 1, no. 22 of 1956.

The Report of the inter departmental committee appointed by the Hon. The minister of health on the grading of specialists in the department of health, the unification of the categories of medical officers and the determination of their seniority on a common service. 1 (9) of 1960.

The Report of the Committee of Inquiry on Mental Health Service in Ceylon, 4 of 1967.

The Report of the Committee of Inquiry into Salaries and other Conditions of Service of Ayurveda Physicians and other Ayurvedic Personnel in Government and Local Government Service, no 8 of 1967.

International Material

ESC, Sub-Commission on the Promotion and Protection of Human Rights (19 June 2000) Human Rights of Indigenous Peoples. Report of the Seminar on the Draft Principles and Guidelines for the Protection of the Heritage of Indigenous Peoples. http://www.ilo.org/dyn/normlex/en/f?p=NORMLEXPUB:11210:0::NO ::P11210_COUNTRY_ID:103172 (last retrieved 20 February 2019)

WIPO-IGC (2001) *Traditional Knowledge and Folklore, Report: First Session*, WIPO/GRTKF/IC/13/11, Geneva: WIPO.

ILO (2009) 'Indigenous and Tribal Peoples' in *Rights in Practice – A Guide to ILO Convention No. 169*, 9.

OAU. African Model Legislation for the Protection of the Rights of Local Communities, Farmers and Breeders, and for the Regulation of Access to Biological Resources. http://www.wipo.int/edocs/lexdocs/laws/en/oau/oau001en.pdf (last retrieved 20 February 2019)

OHCHR Role in Protecting the Rights of the Indigenous Peoples. http://www.ohchr.org/EN/Issues/IPeoples/Pages/IndigenousPeoplesInd ex.aspx (last retrieved 20 February 2019)

Secretariat of the CBD (2002) *Bonn Guidelines on Access to Genetic Resources and Fair and Equitable Sharing of the Benefits Arising out of their Utilization*- http://www.cbd.int/abs/bonn/ (last retrieved 20 February 2019)

CBD and Related Documents. http://www.cbd.int/ (last retrieved 20 February 2019)

UN Declaration on the Rights of Indigenous Peoples: Frequently Asked Questions. http://www.un.org/esa/socdev/unpfii/documents/FAQsindigenousdecla ration.pdf (last retrieved 20 February 2019)

UN General Assembly (2007) United Nations Declaration of the Rights of the Indigenous Peoples. Resolution adopted by the General Assembly, 2 October 2007, A/RES/61/295. http://www.refworld.org/docid/471355a82.html (last retrieved 20 February 2019)

UN. Frequently Asked Questions – Declaration on the Rights of Indigenous Peoples. On Indigenous Peoples: Indigenous Voices.

http://www.un.org/esa/socdev/unpfii/documents/FAQsindigenousdeclaration.pdf (last retrieved 20 February 2019)

UNEP (2000) 'Legal and Other Appropriate Forms of Protection for the Knowledge, Innovations and Practices of Indigenous and Local Communities Embodying Traditional Lifestyles Relevant for the Conservation and Sustainable Use of Biological Diversity.' Ad Hoc Open-Ended Inter-Sessional Working Group on Article 8(j) and Related Provisions of the Convention on Biological Diversity, First Meeting. UNEP/CBD/WG8J/1/2, Seville, Spain, 27-31 March 2000.

UNEP/WIPO (2000) *The Role of Intellectual Property Rights in the Sharing of Benefits Arising from the Use of Biological Resources and Associated Traditional Knowledge: Selected Case Studies*, Conference of the Parties to the CBD at its 5th Meeting, Nairobi. (UNEP/CBD/COP/5/INF26)

UNESCO – Local and Indigenous Knowledge Systems (LINKS) http://www.unesco.org/new/en/natural-sciences/priority-areas/links/ (last retrieved 20 February 2019)

UNESCO – Sri Lanka – (Official information, News and Events, National Cultural Heritage Laws, Video) http://www.unesco.org/new/en/unesco/worldwide/Asia%20and%20the%20Pacific/sri%20lanka (last retrieved 20 February 2019)

UNESCO Recommendation on the Safeguarding of Traditional Culture and Folklore (1989). http://portal.unesco.org/en/ev.php-URL_ID=13141&URL_DO=DO_TOPIC&URL_SECTION=201.html (last retrieved 20 February 2019).

UNESCO- WIPO. Model Provisions for National Laws on the Protection of Expressions of Folklore against Illicit Exploitation and Other Prejudicial Actions. http://www.wipo.int/export/sites/www/tk/en/folklore/1982-folklore-model-provisions.pdf (last retrieved 20 February 2019)

UNPFII http://undesadspd.org/indigenouspeoples/declarationontherightsofindigenouspeoples.aspx (last retrieved 20 February 2019)

WHO (2001) Legal Status of Traditional Medicine and Complementary/Alternative Medicine: A Worldwide Review. http://apps.who.int/medicinedocs/pdf/h2943e/h2943e.pdf (last retrieved 20 February 2019)

WHO (2002) *WHO Traditional Medicine Strategy 2002-2005*. Geneva. http://www.wpro.who.int/health_technology/book_who_traditional_medicine_strategy_2002_2005.pdf (last retrieved 20 February 2019)

WHO (2002) *WHO Traditional Medicine Strategy 2014-2023*. Geneva.

http://www.who.int/medicines/publications/traditional/trm_strategy14_23/en/ (last retrieved 20 February 2019)

WHO, Collaborating Centres for Traditional Medicine – http://www.who.int/medicines/areas/traditional/collabcentres/en/ (last retrieved 20 February 2019)

WHO, South-East Asia Region (SEARO) - http://www.searo.who.int/en/ (last retrieved 20 February 2019)

WHO, Governing Body Documentation – Resolutions, decisions and annexes; Summary and verbatim records. http://apps.who.int/gb/or/ (last retrieved 20 February 2019)

WHO/ IUCN/ WWF (1993) *Guidelines for the Conservation of Medical Plants*, Gland, Switzerland.

WIPO (2001) Intellectual Property Needs and Expectations of Traditional Knowledge Holders. WIPO Report on the Fact-Finding Missions on Intellectual Property and Traditional Knowledge (1998-1999) http://www.wipo.int/edocs/pubdocs/en/tk/768/wipo_pub_768.pdf (last retrieved 20 February 2019).

WIPO (2009) A Legal Framework for the Protection of Traditional Knowledge in Sri Lanka. Working document, version 1 (January 2009) http://www.wipo.int/wipolex/en/text.jsp?file_id=191824 (last retrieved 20 February 2019)

WIPO-IGC, http://www.wipo.int/tk/en/igc/ (last retrieved 20 February 2019)

WIPO- IGC, *List and Brief Technical Explanation of Various Forms in Which Traditional Knowledge may be Found*, Seventeenth Session (WIPO/GRTKF/IC/17/INF/9) http://www.wipo.int/edocs/mdocs/sct/en/wipo_grtkf_ic_17/wipo_grtkf_ic_17_inf_9.pdf (last retrieved 20 February 2019).

WIPO, Laws and Legislative Measures. http://www.wipo.int/tk/en/legal_texts/ (last retrieved on 20 February 2019)

WIPO, Sri Lanka (Laws, Implementing Rules/ Regulations/ IP Legal Literature/ Treaty Memberships) http://www.wipo.int/wipolex/en/profile.jsp?code=LK (last retrieved 20 February 2019)

WIPO. Sri Lanka Profile http://www.wipo.int/wipolex/en/profile.jsp?code=LK (last retrieved 20 February 2019)

WIPO General Assembly (2000) *Twenty-Sixth WIPO General Assembly: Report*, WO/GA/26/10, Geneva: WIPO.

WIPO, Intergovernmental Committee on Intellectual Property and Genetic Resources, Traditional Knowledge and Folklore. (January 23, 2014) *The*

Protection of Traditional Knowledge: Draft Articles. (WIPO/GRTKF/IC/27/4)
http://www.wipo.int/edocs/mdocs/tk/en/wipo_grtkf_ic_27/wipo_grtkf_ic_27_4.pdf (last retrieved 20 February 2019)

WIPO, Intergovernmental Committee on Intellectual Property and Genetic Resources, Traditional Knowledge and Folklore. (December 2007) *The Protection of Traditional Knowledge: Revised Objectives and Principles* WIPO/GRTKF/IC/12/5(c)
http://www.wipo.int/meetings/en/doc_details.jsp?doc_id=89835 (last retrieved 20 February 2019)

WTO Agreement on Trade Related Aspects of Intellectual Property Rights (TRIPS). See:
http://www.wto.org/english/tratop_e/trips_e/t_agm0_e.htm (last retrieved 20 February 2019)

International Law

Agreement on Trade-Related Aspects of Intellectual Property Rights opened for signature 15 April 1994, 1869 UNTS 299 (entered into force 1 January 1995).

Berne Convention for the Protection of Literary and Artistic Works opened for signature 9 September 1986, 828 UNTS 221 (entered into force 5 December 1887).

Cartagena Protocol on Biosafety to the Convention on Biological Diversity opened for signature 29 January 2000, 2226 UNTS 208 (entered into force 11 September 2003).

Convention Establishing the World Intellectual Property Organization, opened for signature 14 July 1967, 848 UNTS 3(entered into force 26 April 1970).

Convention on Biological Diversity opened for signature 5 June 1992, 1760 UNTS 79 (entered into force 29 December 1993).

ILO Convention on Indigenous and Tribal Peoples (No. 169) opened for signature 27 June 1989, 28 ILM 1382 (entered into force 5 September 1991).

International Treaty on Plant Genetic Resources for Food and Agriculture opened for signature 4 November 2002, 2400 UNTS 303 (entered into force 29 June 2004).

Mardid Agreement for the Repression of False or Deceptive Indications of Source on Goods opened for signature 14 April 1891, 828 UNTS 168 (entered into force 1 June 1963).

Nairobi Treaty on the Protection of the Olympic Symbol opened for signature 26 September 1981, 1863 NUTS 367 (entered into force 25 September 1982).

Paris Convention for the Protection of Industrial Property opened for signature 20 March 1883, 161 CTS 409 (entered into force 7 July 1884).

Patent Cooperation Treaty opened for signature 19 June 1970, 1160 UNTS 231 (entered into force 24 January 1978).

The International Union for the Protection of New Varieties of Plants Convention (UPOV) opened for signature 20 December 1996, 2186 UNTS 203 (entered into force 6 March 2002).

Trademark Law Treaty opened for signature 27 October 1994, 2037 UNTS 35 (entered into force 1 August 1996).

UN Declaration on the Rights of Indigenous Peoples adopted by the General Assembly 13 September 20007, UNGA res 61/295.

UNESCO Convention for Safeguarding of the Intangible Cultural Heritage opened for signature 17 October 2003, 2368 UNTS 35 (entered into force April 2006).

UNESCO Convention on the Protection and Promotion of the Diversity of Cultural Expressions opened for signature 20 October 2005, 2440 UNTS 311 (entered into force 18 March 2007).

Universal Copyright Convention, opened for signature 6 September 1952, and revised 24 July 1971, 216 UNTS 132 (entered into force 16 September 1955).

Legislation – Sri Lanka

An Act to amend the Antiquities Ordinance 9 of 1940 (SL)

Ayurveda (Amendment) Act 9 of 1969 (SL)

Ayurveda (Amendment) Law 7 of 1977 (SL)

*Ayurveda Act 31 of 196*1 (SL)

Ayurveda Medical Council Ordinance 46 of 1935 (SL)

Ayurveda Pharmacies Regulation section 21(1) (SL)

Ceylon Ayurveda Medical Council Ordinance 46 of 1935 (SL)

Code of Intellectual Property Act 52 of 1979 (SL)

Gampaha Wickramarachchi Ayurveda Institute Act 30 of 1982 (SL)

Homeopathy Act 7 of 1970 (SL)

Indigenous Medical Ordinance 17 of 1941 (SL)

Institute of Ayurveda Statute No. 1 of 1977 (SL)

Intellectual Property Act 36 of 2003 (SL)

Intellectual Property Regulation 1 of 2006 (SL)

Lepers Ordinance 4 of 1901 (SL)

National Museums Ordinance 1956 (SL)
Palaka Sabhawa of Samastha Lanka Paramparika Ayurveda Vaidya Vidyalaya of Keraminiya Mawanella (Incorporation) Act 1 of 1986 (SL)
Palaka Sabhawa of Samastha Lanka Paranparika Ayurveda Vaidya Vidyalaya of Keraminiya, Mawanella (Incorporation) Act no 1 of 1986 (SL)
Patent Ordinance 1907 (SL)
Plant Variety Bill 2001 (SL)
Regulations on the Antiquities Ordinance 9 of 1940 (SL)
State *Industrial Corporation Act no. 49 of 1957(SL)*
The Constitution of the Democratic Socialist Republic of Sri Lanka 1978 (SL)
University Act No. 1 of 1972 (SL)
University Act No. 16 of 1978 (SL)

Foreign Legislations

Biodiversity Law No. 7788 (Costa Rica)
The Industrial Property Act, 2001 (Kenya)
The Indigenous Peoples Rights Act, 1997 (No. 8371) (Philippines)
Law on Introducing a Protection Regime for the Collective Knowledge of Indigenous Peoples derived from Biological Resources, 2002 (No 27811) (Peru)

Cases

Foster v. Mountford (1976) 29 FLR 233
Tilousi v. Arizona State University, Case No. CV2004-0115 (Ariz Sup Ct, 2004)

Websites

Ayurveda Expo http://ayurveda-expo.lk (last retrieved 20 February 2019)
Charak Samhita- Most complete and authentic Ayurveda book- www.charakasamhita.com/ (last retrieved 20 February 2019)
China Traditional Chinese Medicine Patent Database – http://221.122.40.157/tcm_patent1/englishversion/help/help.html (last retrieved 20 February 2019)
Encyclopaedia of natural cure and remedies www.treatmentguru.com/ (last retrieved 20 February 2019)
Gene Campaign http://genecampaign.org/ (last retrieved 20 February 2019)

Genesys- Gateway to Genetic Resources – https://www.genesys-pgr.org/welcome (last retrieved 20 February 2019)

Griffith University Human Research Ethics – http://www.griffith.edu.au/research/research-services/research-ethics-integrity/human (last retrieved 20 February 2019)

Herbal Net – A Digital Repository in Herbal Medicine http://herbalnet.healthrepository.org/ (last retrieved 20 February 2019) http://www.healthmin.wpc.gov.lk/en/?page_id=215 (last retrieved 20 February 2019)

Information and Communication Technology Agency of Sri Lanka (2014) *Pansiya Panas Jatakaya* http://jathakakatha.lk/english/ (last retrieved 20 February 2019)

Institute of Ayurveda and Alternative Medicine http://www.instituteofayurveda.org/english/history.htm (last retrieved 20 February 2019)

Intellectual Property Protection, China – http://www.chinaipr.gov.cn/guidespatentarticle/guides/agparent/agpguidance/200701/247873_1.html (last retrieved 20 February 2019)

Kenya Industrial Property Institute http://www.kipi.go.ke/index.php/about (last retrieved 20 February 2019)

Korean Traditional Knowledge Portal – http://www.koreantk.com/en/JZ0100.jsp (last retrieved - 20 February 2019)

The Mahavamsa: The Great Chronical of Sri Lanka http://mahavamsa.org/ (last retrieved 20 February 2019)

The Free Dictionary by Farflex www.thefreedictionary.com/mantra (last retrieved 20 February 2019)

Traditional Knowledge Digital Library- http://www.tkdl.res.in/tkdl/langdefault/common/Home.asp?GL=Eng (last retrieved 20 February 2019)

Traditional Knowledge Digital Library of India http://www.tkdl.res.in/ (last retrieved 20 February 2019)

Sri Lanka Legal Material http://www.commonlii.org/lk/ (last retrieved 20 February 2019)

ANNEX - LIST OF INTERVIEWS COMPLETED

1. Mr. Lalith Kannangara The Secretary, Ministry of Indigenous Medicine, Colombo 8.

2. Mr. A. M. P. Abeysinghe, Director (Planning), Ministry of Indigenous Medicine, Colombo 8.

3. Mr. Palitha Weerakoon, Commissioner of Ayurveda, Department of Ayurveda, Navinna, Maharagama

4. Mr. L. H. Thilakaratne, General Manager, Sri Lanka Ayurvedic Drug Corporation, Navinna, Maharagama.

5. Dr. M. U. N. Z. Farzana Senior Lecturer- Unani, IIM, University of Colombo, Colombo 8.

6. Mr. D. W. Gunawardana, Former General Manager, Siddhayurveda Drug Corporation Ltd., Yakkala.

7. Dr. E. A. S. C.S. Edirisuriya, Residential Medical Officer, Wickramarachchi Ayurveda Teaching Hospital, Yakkala.

8. Dr. M. Chithra Nalini, Senior Medical Officer, Wickramarachchi Ayurveda Teaching Hospital, Yakkala.

9. Dr. Saranadasa Devaraja, Siddhaurveda Medical Institute, Siri Vajira, Ghanodaya Pirivena, Mahavita, Yakkala and Senior Medical Advisor, Siddhayurveda Drug Corporation Ltd., Yakkala.

10. Mr. Prabath Gunasekara, Management Assistant, Ayurvedic Medical Council, Navinna, Maharagama.

11. Dr. M. W. S. J. Kumari, Sectional Head (Ayurveda), Institute of Indigenous Medicine, University of Colombo, Colombo 8.

12. Mr. Sunimal Senaratna, Director, Institute of Indigenous Medicine, University of Colombo, Colombo 8.

13. Mr. R. M. P. Rathnayake, Traditional Keraminiya Healer, Kithulgala.

14. Mr. B. A. M. N. D. S. Thejasuya, Diploma in Ayurveda Student and a Keraminiya Practitioner, Kitulgala.

15. Dr. Parakrama, Bandaranaike Ayurveda Research Institute, Navinna, Maharagama.

16. Mr. Gunapala Wanniya Attho, Community Member, Indigenous People's Heritage Centre, Kota Bakina, Dambana.

17. Mr. Dambane Gunawardena, First Vaddha Graduate and the Principal of Dambana Kanishta Vidyalaya, Dambana.

18. VishwakeerthiVanaspathi UruWalige Wanniya Attho, Chief of Sri Lanka Vaddha Community, Kota Bakina, Dambana.

19. Mr. R. M. C. D. S. B. Rajapakse (Chandima), Inter-generational healer (Diploma in Ayurveda Qualified), Bandarawela.

20. Dr. Sr. K. A. S. Sharma Shmi, Astrologer, Hindu Ritual Performer, Sri Badrakaliamman Temple, Bandarawela.

21. Dr. P. G. Punchihewa, Retired Government Servant, Historian and Folklore Writer, Colombo.

22. Mr. Saviman Urugodawatta, Retired Government Servant and a Writer on History and Culture, Nugegoda.

23. Ms. Bindu Urugodawatta, Archaeologist, Nugegoda.

24. Mr. M. C. K. Perera, Owner of the Acupuncture Centre at Rafter's Retreat, Kithulgala.

25. Mr. Sunil Shantha, *Kadum Bidum* Practitioner, Ayurveda Healer, Ratnapura.

26. Mr. H. G. Piyawantha, Secretary General, Samastalanka Deva Bala Saha JothiVidya, Gupta Vidya Sanscruthika Paryekshana Padanama.

27. Mr. S. K. Liyanarachchige, Inter-generational healer, Special Healer - Eyes attached to District Ayurveda Hospital, Matara.

28. Mr. R. P. Udayapala Kapu Mahaththaya, Sri Maha Bodhiya, Anuradhapura.

29. Ms. Rathnawathie, Inter-generational Healer (*Visha Vaidya*), District Hospital, Trincomalee.

30. Dr. Nageshwari, Medical Superintendent, District Ayurveda Hospital, Trincomalee.

31. Dr. Chinthana Nadugala, Ayurveda Doctor, District Ayurveda Hospital, Matara.

32. Ms. W. A. Kusuma Wijesekera, Inter-Generational healer in Serpent Poisoning, District Ayurveda Hospital, Matara.

33. Dr. G. K. Jayasinghe, Drug Standardization Unit, Wayamba Provincial Ayurveda Commissioners Office, Kurunegala.

34. Dr. L. A. J. Siriwardena, Ayurveda Doctor, D. B. Welagedara Ayurveda Hospital, Kurunegala.

35. Dr. A. S. K. N. Senehelatha, Ayurveda Doctor, D. B. Welagedara Ayurveda Hospital, Kurunegala.

36. Dr. Shirani Wimalasekera, Director, D. B. Welagedara Ayurveda Hospital, Kurunegala.

37. Dr. B. M. Chandraweera, Ayurveda Doctor, D. B. Welagedara Ayurveda Hospital, Kurunegala.

38. Dr. Hameed A. Azeez, Visiting Lecturer, Institute of Indigenous Medicine, University of Colombo and Azeez Medical Centre, Kandy Road, Mawanella.

39. Dr. B. Kotawalagedera, Ayurveda Doctor, Ayurveda Hospital, Pallakelle.

40. Dr. T. Weeraratne, Ayurveda Doctor, Ayurveda Hospital, Pallakelle and Secretary, Government Ayurveda Post-Graduate Medical Officers Association.

41. Prof. Piyal A. Marasinghe, Scientific Officer in Charge, Medical Plants Garden, Haldumulla.

42. Ms. B. V. Punchimenike, Cancer Healer, Weda Gedera, Heladiriya, Mawanella, Balangoda.

43. Mr. Jayathissa Herath, Architect, Nugegoda.

44. Prof. Rohan Gunaratna, S. Rajaratnam School of International Relations, Nanyang Technological University, Singapore.

45. Dr. Sanjay Garg, Deputy Director (Research), South Asian Association for Regional Cooperation Cultural Centre, Colombo 7.

46. Mr. W. A. D. Chithrananda, Deputy Registrar, Gampapha Wickramarachchi Ayurveda Institute, Yakkala.

47. Prof. Jayadeva Uyangoda, Department of Political Science and Public Policy, University of Colombo, Colombo.

48. Mr. Sudesh Mantillake, Lecturer, Department of Fine Arts, University of Peradeniya, Peradeniya.

49. Dr. Parakum Ekkanayake, Medical Officer, Sri Lanka Ayurvedic Drug Corporation, Navinna, Maharagama.

50. Mr. A. D. H. Sudesh, Technical Officer II (Lab), Gampaha Wickramarachchi Ayurveda Institute, University of Kelaniya, Kelaniya.

51. Mr. S. D. M. Mahipala, Inter-generational healer – *Jalabithika* and *Sarpavisha,* Yakkala.

52. Mr. P. Weerasinghe, Inter-generational Eye healer, Basawakkulama, Anuradhapura.

53. Mrs. H. D. Karunawathie, Indigenous Healer – *Sarvanga,* Paradikulama Tradition, Anuradhapura.

54. Ven. Kapugama Somalankara, *Visa Vedakama*, Matara.

55. Ven. Kubulgama Piyakeerthi, Sri Mahinda Pirivena, Ayurveda Medical Institute, Gattuwana Road, Kurunegala.

56. Mrs. W. M. Anulawathie, Inter-generational healer - *Kadum Bidum* and *Iru Rudhawa,* Mahiyanganaya.

57. Mr. R. V. Piyadasa, Inter-generational Healer- *Kadum Bidum,* Badulla.

58. Mr. R. M. D. J. Gunasekera, Inter-generational healing practice of- *Sarvanga*. Specialist in Diabetics, Cholesterol and Pressure, Badulla.

59. Mr. Wansinghe Mudiyanselage Sudu Banda, Inter-generational Healer- *Sarvanga* – specialised in stroke and paralysis, Siri Siddhartha Oushadalaya Maligathanna, Pattiyegedera.

60. Ghana Manio, Spirit Healer, Airport Road, Anuradhapura.

61. Mr. W.S Pushpakumara, Spirit Healer, Thissawewa, Anuradhapura.

62. Ms. B.A Anoma Damayanthi, Spirit Healer, Bassawakkulama, Anuradhapura.

63. Mr. R.M Gunathilake, Spirt Healer, 29, Perniyankulama, Anuradhapura.

64. Mr. P. D. Premachandra, Astrologer, 'Shanthi Sevana,' Mahialla, Kurunegala.

65. Mr. Gamini Priyantha, Meditation Master, Theravada Buddhist Meditation, Dhamrivi Foundation, Colombo.

66. Ven. Wellawatte Seelagawesi Thero, Sri Sumedha Meditation Centre, Gomaraya Road, Thawalanthanna.

67. Mr. P. M. Punchibanda, *Manthra Gurukam* Performer, Kurubure Meegahapitiya, Mahiyanganaya.

68. Mr. H. M. Nandasena Herath, Astrologer, Jothirvedi Manikyarahna, Taaraka Ayurvedic Astrology Centre, Badulla.

69. Mr. M. H. Sanjeewa Perera, Coordinating Officer – Religious Affairs, Taaraka Ayurvedic Astrology Centre, Badulla.

70. Mr. P. H. Sumandasa, Astrologer, Seth Kavi Writer, Ella.

71. Ms. Kumari (Psudo name), Spirit Healer, Anuradhapura.

72. Ven. Mihindupura Mahindawansa Nayaka Thero, Spirit Healer, Trincomalee.

73. Mr. Gallage Niroshan Dilantha Kumara, Spirit Healer, Sri Paththini Devalaya, Matara.

74. Mr. K. N. Arnis, Ritual Dancer, Kakanadura.

75. Ms. Leelawathie, Thelagu Palm Reader, Sri Maha Bodhiya, Anuradhapura.

76. Mr. Ishikawa Naohito, Advisor, Thusare: healing through fingers, A Shiatsu Centre. Motivations in establishing the Centre, supporting system, Colombo.

77. Mr. Thusare, Practitioner, Thusare House and Spa, Colombo.

78. Dr. Sunethra Aluthge, Ayurveda Doctor, Siddha Rural Hospital, Trincomalee.

79. Dr. Mrs. M. S. D. Alfreda, Siddha Doctor, District Ayurveda Hospital, Kappalthurai, Trincomalee.

80. Dr. Mrs. T. Nirojini, Siddha Doctor, Panchakarma Medical Officer in Charge, District Ayurveda Hospital, Trincomalee.

81. Dr. Sarojini Wasana Wijesinghe, Ayurveda Doctor, Trincomalee.

82. Dr. Priyani Renuka Weerasooriya, Ayurveda Doctor, Drug Manufacturing Centre, Trincomalee.

83. Ven. Dr. Kehalpannala Chandaloka Thero, Chief Monk and Principal, Medical College of State Corporate Keraminiya, Mawanella.

84. Mr. Ariya (Vedamahathaya), Kadum Bidum, Near Pidurangala Temple, Sigiriya.

85. Mr. H. A. Menaka, Faculty of Law, University of Colombo, Colombo.

86. Mr. Asitha Punchihewa, Researcher, Social Policy Analysis Research Centre, University of Colombo (Co-Authour of the Recent Vaddha Study conducted by Ministry of Culture), Panadura.

87. Mr. Daya Dissanayake, Author of 'The Healer and the Drug Pusher,' Colombo.

88. Prof. Chandrasiri Palliyaguru, Retired Sinhala Professor, University of Kelaniya, Kelaniya.

89. Kalu Mama, Indigenous Healer, Jungle Dweller, Guide to Sinharaja Forest Reserve, Neluwa.

90. Corporal Kumarsinghe V., Army Training School, Maduru Oya.

91. Corporal Sugathadasa, H. M. R. S., Army Training School, Maduru Oya.

92. Maj. Lushantha Warnasiri, Army Training School, Maduru Oya.

93. Mr. S. M. K. Nimal Karunarathne, Horiwila Kadum Bidum Medical Centre, Horiwila, Paalugaswewa.

94. Mr. R. A. Sudath Priyantha, Horiwila Kadum Bidum Medical Centre, Horiwila, Paalugaswewa.

95. Mr. S. M. H. Seneviratne, Horiwila Paramparika Hela Weda Gedera (Horiwila Traditional Sri Lankan Healing House), Horiwila.

96. Mr. Ajith Liyanage, Indigenous Healing Practitioner and Elephant Keeper, Kataragama Devalaya, Kataragama.

97. Mr. K. Premarathne Mendis, (Ambalangoda Kapu Mahathaya) Sri Murthi Devalaya, Devalaya Gedera, Theriyagama, Kataragama.

98. Dr. Sarojini (Psudo name) Kaithady.

99. Dr. S. Sivashanmugarajah, Head, Department of Siddha Medicine, University of Jaffna, Jaffna.

100. Mr. Je Jeyalan, Ayurveda and Siddha Traditional Healer, Sujjeevaah Clinic, Kaiaddyyamman Road, Jaffna.

101. Mr. K. O. Rajarathna, Inter-generational Mental Healer, Sujjeevaah Clinic, Vavuniya.

102. Mr. S. Paranasivamullai, Inter-generational Siddha Healer, Siva Siddha Medical Centre, Jaffna.

103. Dr. S. Srijeevahan, Siddha Doctor, Sivalingam Dispensary, 9/8, Cross Street, Jaffna.

104. Mr. S. Sivalingam, Registrar, Lanka Siddha Ayurveda Medical College, Jaffna.

105. Dr. Kandeepan, Planning Officer, Provincial Department of Indigenous Medicine, Northern Province, Thirunelveli.

106. Mr. Sandan, *Kadum Bidum* Healer, Trincomalee.

107. Mr. G. Punchibanda, Kapumahathaya, Pidurangala Vishnu Devalaya, Sigiriya.

108. Mr. T. Herath Banda, Inter-generational Healer for *Sarpa Visha*, (Snake poisoning), Innamaduwa.

109. Mr. Tennisson Perera, Astrologer, Station Road, Agulana.

110. Mr. R. L. Kularathne, Rasa Medical Practitioner, Sri Mankgala Rasa Osu Hala (Pvt) Ltd, Moratuwa.

111. Mrs. C. Kularatne, Rasa Medical Practitioner, Sri Mankgala Rasa Osu Hala (Pvt) Ltd, Moratuwa.

112. Dr. (Mrs.) Sivayokamalar Harigaran, Vice Principal, Lanka Siddha Ayurvedic Medical College, Power House Road, Chunnakam.

113. Mr. R. M. Premachandra, Inter-generational Nila Healing, Colombo.

114. Ven. Kekirawe Ananda, Kebithigollawa Siri Gauthama Viharaya, Yoda Gas Wewa, Ataweera Gollawa.

115. Ms. K. N. Suneetha, Ritual Dancing Teacher, Sarasavi Kalayathanaya.

116. Dr. R. Maheswaran, "Dwaakai," Thirunnelvely East, Jaffna.

117. Mr. K. Balakrishnan, Astrologer, *Mantra*, K. K. S. Road, Jaffna.